Everything You Need to Know About Old Age Psychiatry...

Everything You Need to Know About
Old Age Psychiatry…

Edited by

ROBERT HOWARD

Senior Lecturer and Consultant in Old Age Psychiatry,
Institute of Psychiatry and Maudsley Hospital, London, UK

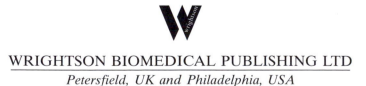

WRIGHTSON BIOMEDICAL PUBLISHING LTD
Petersfield, UK and Philadelphia, USA

Editorial Office:

Wrightson Biomedical Publishing Ltd
Ash Barn House, Winchester Road, Stroud,
Petersfield, Hampshire GU32 3PN, UK
Telephone: 01730 265647
Fax: 01730 260368

British Library Cataloguing in Publication Data
A catalogue record for this book is available from the British Library.

Library of Congress Cataloging in Publication Data
Everything you need to know about old age psychiatry-- / edited by
    Robert Howard.
        p.   cm.
    Includes bibliographical references and index.
    ISBN 1-871816-38-6 (hard cover). -- ISBN 1-871816-38-6
    1. Geriatric psychiatry.   2. Aged--Mental health.   I. Howard,
    Robert, 1961-   .
    [DNLM: 1. Geriatric Psychiatry--methods.   2. Alzheimer Disease.
    3. Dementia--therapy.   4. Dementia--Aged.   5. Mental Disorders-
    -therapy.   6. Mental Disorders--Aged.   WT 150 E93 1999]
    RC451.4.A5E826   1999
    618.97'689--dc21
    DNLM/DLC   99-14082
    for Library of Congress   CIP

ISBN 1 871816 38 6

Composition by Scribe Design, Gillingham, Kent
Printed in Great Britain by Biddles Ltd, Guildford.

Contents

Contributors

Brian H. Anderton, *Professor, Department of Neuroscience, Institute of Psychiatry, De Crespigny Park, London SE5 8AF, UK*

Mark Ardern, *Department of Psychiatry of Old Age, St Charles' Hospital, Ladbroke Grove, London W10 6DZ, UK*

Robert C. Baldwin, *Department of Psychiatry for the Elderly, Psychiatry Directorate, Central Manchester Healthcare Trust, Oxford Road, Manchester M13 9BX, UK*

E. Jane Byrne, *Department of Old Age Psychiatry, Withington Hospital, West Didsbury, Manchester M20 8LR, UK*

Robert Howard, *Section of Old Age Psychiatry, Institute of Psychiatry, De Crespigny Park, London SE5 8AF, UK*

Robin Jacoby, *Professor of Old Age Psychiatry, University of Oxford, The Warneford Hospital, Oxford OX3 7JX, UK*

David Jolley, *Professor of Old Age Psychiatry, Penn Hospital, Wolverhampton WV4 5HN, UK*

Sir Ludovic Kennedy, *President of the Voluntary Euthanasia Society, 13 Prince of Wales Terrace, London W8, UK*

Christopher G. Krasucki, *Section of Old Age Psychiatry, Institute of Psychiatry, De Crespigny Park, London SE5 8AF, UK*

Simon Lovestone, *Section of Old Age Psychiatry, Institute of Psychiatry, De Crespigny Park, London SE5 8AF, UK*

Ian G. McKeith, *Professor of Old Age Psychiatry, Institute for the Health of the Elderly, Newcastle General Hospital, Westgate Road, Newcastle upon Tyne NE4 6BE, UK*

Anthony H. Mann, *Professor of Epidemiological Psychiatry, Institute of Psychiatry, De Crespigny Park, London SE5 8AF, UK*

Vassilis M. Mouratoglou, *Old Age Directorate, The Bethlem and Maudsley NHS Trust, The Maudsley Hospital, Denmark Hill, London SE5 8AZ, UK*

John T. O'Brien, *Department of Psychiatry and Institute for the Health of the Elderly, University of Newcastle upon Tyne, Castleside Unit, Newcastle General Hospital, Newcastle upon Tyne NE4 6BE, UK*

Michael Philpot, *Old Age Psychiatry Directorate, Maudsley Hospital, Denmark Hill, London SE5 8AZ, UK*

Justine Schneider, *Centre for Applied Social Studies, University of Durham, 15 Old Elvet, Durham DH1 3HL, UK*

Robert Stewart, *Section of Old Age Psychiatry, Institute of Psychiatry, De Crespigny Park, London SE5 8AF, UK*

Glenn C. Telling, *MRC Prion Diseases Unit, Imperial College School of Medicine at St Mary's, Norfolk Place, London W2 1PG, UK*

John Wattis, *Medical Director, Leeds Community & Mental Health Services, Meanwood Park Hospital, Tongue Lane, Leeds LS6 4QB, UK*

Preface

This book and the biannual Short Course in Old Age Psychiatry at the Institute of Psychiatry from which it arose have a simple aim: to provide a current and comprehensive digest of the areas whose rapid development will most affect our work as old age psychiatrists. An irony of old age psychiatry has long been that while the clinical work we do is generally perceived as unglamorous and even stigmatizing, those areas of neuroscience and clinical research and ethical and philosophical issues that involve our patients have the highest profiles imaginable. Keeping abreast of advances and developments is now a real challenge and the approach we have followed with our Short Course and the Wrightson books has been to invite acknowledged experts who are also skilled communicators to tackle an area to which they are close in a way that has relevance in the clinic. Updates on progress in the laboratory, controversial or emerging areas of diagnosis and treatment and the ethical debate surrounding physician-assisted suicide are the themes of this book. The book is loosely divided into three unequal parts examining basic research and treatment of dementia and management of functional disorders. The title of both Short Course and book was chosen while I was in a particularly cheerful and expansive state of mind and should be taken as no more than a highly personal view of what an old age psychiatrist needs to know and not as a challenge to the reader to discover essential material that has not been included. With this caveat, I am happy to take full responsibility for any omissions if I can take credit for choosing those authors who to me represent the old age psychiatry equivalent of a fantasy football or cricket team. This is a good place to express my heartfelt gratitude to all the authors for their cheerfully delivered contributions, to Judy Wrightson and her staff for as usual making book production run smoothly and to Margaret Derrick and Lee Wilding for long-suffering and uncomplaining support of Short Course organization.

ROBERT HOWARD
Institute of Psychiatry, January 1999

I

The Dementias:
Laboratory to Clinic

1

Molecular Biology of Alzheimer's Disease

BRIAN H. ANDERTON

Professor, Department of Neuroscience, Institute of Psychiatry, London, UK

Molecular studies of Alzheimer's disease have stemmed initially from investigations of the two principal pathological lesions, neurofibrillary tangles and neuritic plaques. Subsequently the identification of genetic risk factors has influenced molecular approaches, in particular autosomal-dominant mutations in the genes for the amyloid precursor protein (APP) and presenilins 1 and 2 (PS1 and PS2), and the demonstration that possession of one or two copies of the apolipoprotein E ϵ4 allele confers increased risk of development of Alzheimer's disease. The majority of experimental studies into molecular mechanisms of neurodegeneration have been with model systems but, nevertheless, have resulted in considerable advances in understanding and insight into the possible events proceeding in the brain. This chapter will briefly review current knowledge in this regard.

THE PROTEINS OF NEURITIC PLAQUES AND TANGLES

The classical neuritic or senile plaque has a central extracellular deposit or core composed primarily of amyloid β-protein (Aβ) surrounded by dystrophic neurites that are filled with paired helical filaments (PHF). The core has a number of other proteins apparently associated with Aβ; these include apolipoprotein E, and non-amyloid component (NAC) which is a fragment of α-synuclein, another protein of primary neurodegenerative significance since the discovery of mutations in the α-synuclein gene in pedigrees with familial Parkinson's disease (Polymeropoulos *et al.*, 1997; Krüger *et al.*, 1998). Aβ is also found in diffuse deposits without the neuritic involvement and in cerebral blood vessels (Selkoe, 1994a). There is reason

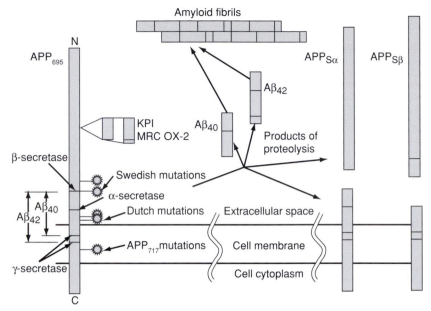

Figure 1. Amyloid precursor protein (APP) exists as several alternatively spliced isoforms, with and without the additional KPI and MRC OX-2 domains. The positions of the Aβ segment and the known mutations are indicated as well as the α-, β- and γ-secretase cleavage sites for generation of $A\beta_{40}$ and $A\beta_{42}$ and subfragments of Aβ. APP_S exists as two slightly different sizes according to whether the intact APP molecule is cleaved at the α- or β-secretase sites. $A\beta_{40}$ and $A\beta_{42}$ both aggregate into neurotoxic fibrils, $A\beta_{40}$ and $A\beta_{42}$ having the greater tendency to aggregate. Although all of these products are diagrammatically shown to occur at the cell surface, many occur intracellularly.

to believe that the earliest signs of Alzheimer changes in the brain may be the appearance of these diffuse Aβ deposits.

Aβ is a short polypeptide of 39–43 amino acids derived by proteolysis from a longer membrane-spanning amyloid precursor protein (APP) (Selkoe, 1994b). The predominant Aβ species appear to be 40 and 42 residues long ($A\beta_{40}$ and $A\beta_{42}$), and depending upon how individual molecules are proteolytically processed, a variety of additional fragments are produced (Figure 1). $A\beta_{42}$ has a greater tendency to aggregate than $A\beta_{40}$, which is significant because it is aggregated Aβ in the form of amyloid fibrils that is neurotoxic, at least to neurons in culture (Iversen *et al.*, 1995). Thus, the proteolytic processing of APP and the effects of mutations in APP and PS1 and PS2 on this process have been subject to intense investigation and will be discussed further below.

Neurofibrillary tangles are intracellular accumulations in neuronal perikarya of paired helical filaments. PHF are also present in more distal regions of neurons where they are observed as neuropil threads as well as being present in the dystrophic neurites of neuritic plaques (Braak et al., 1994). PHF are composed of the microtubule-associated protein, tau, in a hyperphosphorylated state compared with tau isolated from control post-mortem brain (Smith and Anderton, 1994). Studies of biopsy samples have shown that in affected neurons PHF replace the normal cytoskeleton of microtubules and neurofilaments (Flament-Durand and Couck, 1979; Gray et al., 1987). Since a neuron could not survive long without an intact cytoskeleton, studies of tau have focused on understanding how it becomes hyperphosphorylated and the consequences of hyperphosphorylation on microtubule function, as well as factors that promote tau aggregation into PHF.

APP PROCESSING AND Aβ PRODUCTION

The identification of mutations in the APP gene are essentially proof that APP function must be disturbed in Alzheimer's disease. Most attention has focused on production and deposition of Aβ; however, since abundant diffuse deposits of Aβ in the post-mortem brain are not correlated with dementia, it is quite possible that it is not Aβ deposition that is the crucial event but rather some, as yet unknown, function of APP that is disrupted which triggers Alzheimer's disease.

It has, nevertheless, been shown that mutations in APP that cause Alzheimer's disease result in either an increase in the total amount of Aβ production or an increase in the ratio of $A\beta_{42}:A\beta_{40}$ produced (Suzuki et al., 1994; Citron et al., 1994). Both are predicted to result in increased aggregation and deposition of Aβ in the brain. Mutations in PS1 and PS2 have also been demonstrated to increase the ratio of $A\beta_{42}:A\beta_{40}$ produced (Duff et al., 1996; Xia et al., 1997; Citron et al., 1997) and so these mutations are also consistent with Aβ production and aggregation being an important pathogenic event. The site(s) of APP processing are not fully determined since there is evidence for cell surface proteolysis as well as intracellular processing (Checler, 1995; Chyung et al., 1997; Ikezu et al., 1998; Haass et al., 1998). However, the current consensus is that cleavage at the C-terminus of Aβ, the so-called γ-secretase site, takes place in the endoplasmic reticulum and Golgi apparatus. Cleavage of γ-secretase to produce $A\beta_{42}$ seems likely to be in the endoplasmic reticulum whereas alternative γ-secretase cleavage to produce $A\beta_{40}$ may predominantly take place in the Golgi apparatus (Figure 2). Thus, the trafficking of APP and the residence time in these intra-cellular compartments en route to the cell surface may be the determining

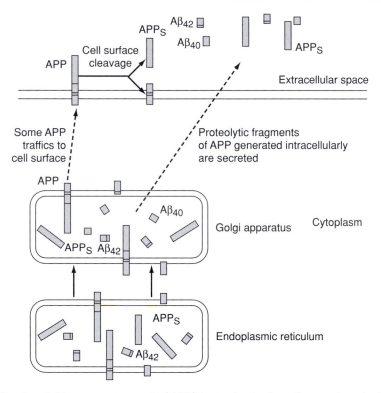

Figure 2. Amyloid precursor protein (APP) is synthesized on the rough endoplasmic reticulum and some traffics to the cell surface where it may be processed. Other molecules are apparently proteolytically processed whilst APP is still in the endoplasmic reticulum, with γ-secretase activity that generates preferentially $A\beta_{42}$ predominating over γ-secretase that generates $A\beta_{40}$. $A\beta_{40}$ is probably generated in the Golgi apparatus or other endosomal compartment. Thus, the residence time for APP in different intracellular compartments may be the critical factor in determining the ratio of $A\beta_{40}:A\beta_{42}$ secreted by cells.

factor that regulates the production of $A\beta_{40}$ and $A\beta_{42}$. This would be consistent with knowledge of PS subcellular location since PS1 and PS2 are multiple-pass membrane proteins (Figure 3), predominantly restricted to the endoplasmic reticulum (Kovacs *et al.*, 1996; Mattson *et al.*, 1998) and mutations in PS1 and PS2 may therefore influence trafficking of APP. However, it is not known whether this is the mechanism rather than PS1 and PS2 exerting a regulatory influence on one or more γ-secretase activities, nor whether mutations in APP affect susceptibility to proteolysis at different amino acid residues or if they too can affect APP processing.

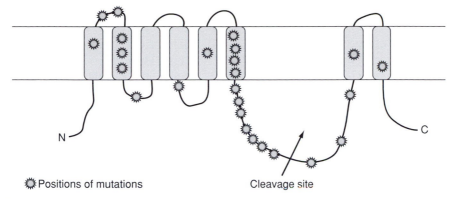

Figure 3. A diagram of presenilins 1 and 2 showing that the polypeptide chain traverses the endoplasmic reticulum membrane multiple times with a large loop domain now known to be located on the cytoplasmic side. The approximate positions of many of the known mutations in PS1 are shown.

TAU AND PHF

Studies both *in vitro* and in transfected cells have shown that tau promotes microtubule assembly and bundling (Kanai *et al.*, 1992). Phosphorylation of tau, particularly by members of the proline-directed protein kinase family at up to 17 serine or threonine residues that are immediately followed in the amino acid sequence by a proline (SP and TP motifs), impairs these assembly and bundling properties of tau (Trinczek *et al.*, 1995; Lovestone *et al.*, 1996b; Utton *et al.*, 1997). Tau in PHF (PHF-tau) has been shown by sequencing to be phosphorylated at 25 sites so far and more may yet be discovered (Morishima-Kawashima *et al.*, 1995; Hanger *et al.*, 1998). Of these 25 sites many are SP or TP motifs. Thus, proline-directed protein kinases may be particularly important in tau pathology, and probably the strongest *in vivo* candidate kinase, is glycogen synthase kinase-3β (GSK-3β) (Muñoz-Montaño *et al.*, 1997; Hong *et al.*, 1997; Lovestone *et al.*, 1999).

Phosphorylation of tau by GSK-3β could contribute to the observed loss of microtubules because the phosphorylated tau is less potent as a promoter of microtubule assembly and bundling. However, there is as yet no evidence that hyperphosphorylation of tau promotes its aggregation into PHF. In fact, it has been shown that fragments of tau can be induced to form PHF *in vitro*, as can intact but unphosphorylated tau by the addition of certain proteoglycans or even RNA (ribonucleic acid) (Wille *et al.*, 1992; Crowther *et al.*, 1992; Kampers *et al.*, 1996; Goedert *et al.*, 1996).

APOLIPOPROTEIN E

Possession of one or two copies of the ε4 allele of apolipoprotein E is the genetic factor that influences the development of Alzheimer's disease in the greatest number of individuals. However, we still have little idea as to the mechanism. *In vitro* studies have shown that apolipoprotein ε4 apparently promotes aggregation of Aβ more potently than apolipoprotein ε3, although there are other studies that support an opposite effect (Strittmatter *et al.*, 1993; LaDu *et al.*, 1994). In tissue culture, apolipoprotein ε3 promotes more extensive neurite outgrowth and branching of neurites and this may be mediated by an interaction with intracellular tau (Nathan *et al.*, 1994, 1995; Puttfarcken *et al.*, 1997; DeMattos *et al.*, 1998). This would be an unexpected mechanism because apolipoproteins are not regarded as being capable of gaining access to the cytoplasm. However, it has been shown that this does occur in the case of apolipoprotein E and there is experimental evidence that the expression of tau may influence the greater retention in the cytoplasm of apolipoprotein ε3 over apolipoprotein ε4 (Lovestone *et al.*, 1996a). Clearly, more studies are required before a consistent and convincing proposed mechanism for the observed genetic influence of apolipoprotein E allotypes emerges.

THE OVERALL PATHOGENIC PROCESS

The apparent early deposition of Aβ and the identification of mutations in the APP gene led to the proposal that abnormal APP processing was the initial pathogenic event and that other pathological features followed in the so-called 'amyloid cascade hypothesis' (Hardy and Higgins, 1992). However, it was not clear whether production of neurofibrillary tangles was part of this sequence of events or if they are produced independently. This is still the case, but recent discoveries of mutations in tau in familial cases of frontotemporal dementia with parkinsonism linked to chromosome 17 (FTDP-17) have demonstrated the pathogenic importance of tangles (Spillantini *et al.*, 1998; Poorkaj *et al.*, 1998; Hutton *et al.*, 1998).

The brains of cases of FTDP-17 often show the presence of neurofibrillary tangles composed of hyperphosphorylated tau aggregated into either PHF or straight filaments. There are no deposits of Aβ. Thus, the neurodegeneration in these individuals is the direct result of tau mutations and tangle formation. In human brain tau exists as six alternately spliced isoforms (Figure 4). The mutations so far identified are coding mutations which may either affect binding of tau to microtubules or affect alternative splicing such that more tau is expressed with 4-repeat motifs of the tubulin-binding domain instead of the alternative 3-repeat tau. The number of repeats also affects

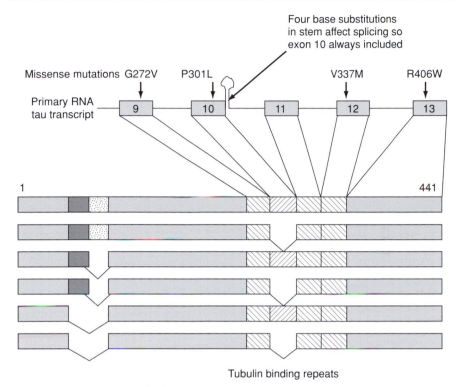

Figure 4. The six brain isoforms of tau are generated by alternative splicing of a primary RNA transcript and the relationship between the encoded exons and the domains of tau are shown. In FTDP-17 four point mutations have been found that give rise to amino acid changes and four that affect the stem loop structure which results only in tau being synthesized with four tubulin binding domains.

the binding of tau to microtubules (Preuss *et al.*, 1997). Thus, although the mechanism by which these tau mutations result in neurodegeneration is not known, the presently favoured view is that microtubule stability/bundling is affected and an excess of tau not bound to microtubules then aggregates to form PHF or straight filaments (Figure 5).

Thus, together, the FTDP-17 cases with tangles but without Aβ pathology and Alzheimer's disease caused by APP mutations having both Aβ plaques and neurofibrillary tangles are the strongest evidence for the amyloid cascade hypothesis, with tau genetically placed downstream of APP (Figure 6). The tau mutations in FTDP-17 demonstrate the primary pathogenic importance of tau/tangles and argue against tangle formation being an unimportant epiphenomenon in Alzheimer's disease. We are therefore thrown back into finding the biochemical link between APP/Aβ and tau/PHF.

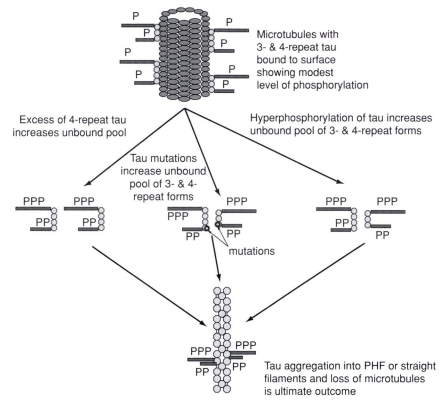

Figure 5. Possible mechanisms whereby microtubule disassembly may occur as a result of tau abnormalities.

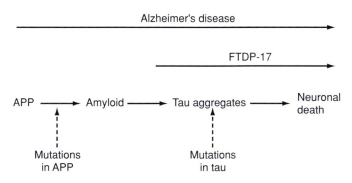

Figure 6. A scheme depicting the amyloid cascade hypothesis.

NOTCH/WINGLESS SIGNALLING

Presenilins have been shown genetically in *Caenorhabditis elegans* to play a role in Notch signalling. The Notch pathway is important in determining cell fate in development but Notch is still expressed in the adult nervous system, and mutations in Notch 3 have been shown to be the genetic lesion in a rare stroke condition, cerebral autosomal-dominant arteriopathy with subcortical infarcts and leucoencephalopathy syndrome (CADASIL) (Joutel *et al.*, 1996). Notch signalling can also be influenced by another developmental signalling pathway in *Drosophila*: the wingless pathway; its mammalian

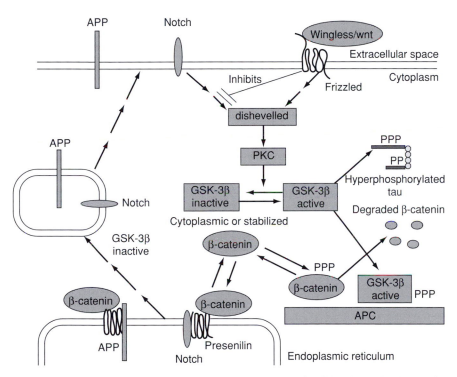

Figure 7. The hypothetical relationships between the Notch and wingless/wnt pathways and tau hyperphosphorylation and trafficking of APP. Presenilins may affect Notch signalling by regulating the trafficking of active Notch to the cell surface where it acts as a receptor. The wingless/wnt pathway inhibits Notch signalling at the level of dishevelled but downstream in both pathways is GSK-3β. GSK-3β phosphorylates adenomatous polyposis coli protein (APC) and possibly β-catenin as the mechanism for regulating the cytoplasmic concentration of β-catenin, known as 'stabilization'. β-catenin has been found to bind presenilins but it remains to be demonstrated that this affects the regulation of APP processing. However, a possible link between APP processing and tau phosphorylation is apparent.

homologue is the wnt pathway. The wingless/wnt pathway includes GSK-3β and one of its substrates, β-catenin (Dale, 1998). It has now been shown that β-catenin forms a complex with PS1 (Zhou *et al.*, 1997; Yu *et al.*, 1998) and, since GSK-3β is a strong candidate as a tau kinase, these may therefore be intriguing pieces in the jigsaw that may reveal the biochemical links between APP and tau (Figure 7). However, for the present they are only isolated pieces and more work will be required to determine whether they are important in demonstrating that the amyloid cascade is a reality and no longer a hypothesis.

ACKNOWLEDGEMENT

Some of the work referred to in this chapter was supported by the Medical Research Council, Wellcome Trust, Research into Ageing, Alzheimer's Disease Society, Parkinson's Disease Society and Glaxo Wellcome Research and Development.

REFERENCES

Braak, E., Braak, H. and Mandelkow, E.-M. (1994). A sequence of cytoskeleton changes related to the formation of neurofibrillary tangles and neuropil threads. *Acta Neuropathol (Berl)* **87**, 554–567.

Checler F. (1995). Processing of the β-amyloid precursor protein and its regulation in Alzheimer's disease. *J Neurochem* **65**, 1431–1444.

Chyung, A.S.C., Greenberg, B.D., Cook, D.G., Doms, R.W. and Lee, V.M.Y. (1997). Novel β-secretase cleavage of β-amyloid precursor protein in the endoplasmic reticulum intermediate compartment of NT2N cells. *J Cell Biol* **138**, 671–680.

Citron, M., Vigo-Pelfrey, C., Teplow, D.B. *et al.* (1994). Excessive production of amyloid β-protein by peripheral cells of symptomatic and presymptomatic patients carrying the Swedish familial Alzheimer disease mutation. *Proc Natl Acad Sci USA* **91**, 11993–11997.

Citron, M., Westaway, D., Xia, W.M. *et al.* (1997). Mutant presenilins of Alzheimer's disease increase production of 42-residue amyloid β-protein in both transfected cells and transgenic mice. *Nat Med* **3**, 67–72.

Crowther, R.A., Olesen, O.F., Jakes, R. and Goedert, M. (1992). The microtubule binding repeats of tau protein assemble into filaments like those found in Alzheimer's disease. *FEBS Lett* **309**, 199–202.

Dale, T.C. (1998). Signal transduction by the Wnt family of ligands. *Biochem J* **329**, 209–223.

DeMattos, R.B., Curtiss, L.K. and Williams, D.L. (1998). A minimally lipidated form of cell-derived apolipoprotein E exhibits isoform-specific stimulation of neurite outgrowth in the absence of exogenous lipids or lipoproteins. *J Biol Chem* **273**, 4206–4212.

Duff, K., Eckman, C., Zehr, C. *et al.* (1996). Increased amyloid-β42(43) in brains of mice expressing mutant presenilin 1. *Nature* **383**, 710–713.

Flament-Durand, J. and Couck, A. (1979). Spongiform alterations in brain biopsies of presenile dementia. *Acta Neuropathol (Berl)* **46**, 159–162.

Goedert, M., Jakes, R., Spillantini, M.G., Hasegawa, M., Smith, M.J. and Crowther, R.A. (1996). Assembly of microtubule-associated protein tau into Alzheimer-like filaments induced by sulphated glycosaminoglycans. *Nature* **383**, 550–553.

Gray, E.G., Paula Barbosa, M. and Roher, A. (1987). Alzheimer's disease: paired helical filaments and cytomembranes. *Neuropathol Appl Neurobiol* **13**, 91–110.

Haass, C., Grünberg, J., Capell, A. *et al.* (1998). Proteolytic processing of Alzheimer's disease associated proteins. *J Neural Transm* **105**, 159–167.

Hanger, D.P., Betts, J.C., Loviny, T.L.F., Blackstock, W.P. and Anderton, B.H. (1998). New phosphorylation sites identified in hyperphosphorylated tau (PHF-tau) from Alzheimer's disease brain using nanoelectrospray mass spectrometry. *J Neurochem* **71**, 2465–2476.

Hardy, J.A. and Higgins, G.A. (1992). Alzheimer's disease: the amyloid cascade hypothesis. *Science* **256**, 184–185.

Hong, M., Chen, D.C.R., Klein, P.S. and Lee, V.M.Y. (1997). Lithium reduces tau phosphorylation by inhibition of glycogen synthase kinase-3. *J Biol Chem* **272**, 25326–25332.

Hutton, M., Lendon, C.L., Rizzu, P. *et al.* (1998). Association of missense and 5'-splice-site mutations in *tau* with the inherited dementia FTDP-17. *Nature* **393**, 702–705.

Ikezu, T., Trapp, B.D., Song, K.S., Schlegel, A., Lisanti, M.P. and Okamoto, T. (1998). Caveolae, plasma membrane microdomains for α-secretase-mediated processing of the amyloid precursor protein. *J Biol Chem* **273**, 10485–10495.

Iversen, L.L., Mortishire-Smith, R.J., Pollack, S.J. and Shearman, M.S. (1995). The toxicity *in vitro* of β-amyloid protein. *Biochem J* **311**, 1–16.

Joutel, A., Corpechot, C., Ducros, A. *et al.* (1996). *Notch3* mutations in CADASIL, a hereditary adult-onset condition causing stroke and dementia. *Nature* **383**, 707–710.

Kampers, T., Friedhoff, P., Biernat, J. and Mandelkow, E.M. (1996). RNA stimulates aggregation of microtubule-associated protein tau into Alzheimer-like paired helical filaments. *FEBS Lett* **399**, 344–349.

Kanai, Y., Chen, J. and Hirokawa, N. (1992). Microtubule bundling by tau proteins *in vivo*: analysis of functional domains. *EMBO J* **11**, 3953–3961.

Kovacs, D.M., Fausett, H.J., Page, K.J. *et al.* (1996). Alzheimer-associated presenilins 1 and 2: neuronal expression in brain and localization to intracellular membranes in mammalian cells. *Nat Med* **2**, 224–229.

Krüger, R., Kuhn, W., Müller, T. *et al.* (1998). Ala30Pro mutation in the gene encoding α-synuclein in Parkinson's disease. *Nat Genet* **18**, 106–108.

LaDu, M.J., Falduto, M.T., Manelli, A.M., Reardon, C.A., Getz, G.S. and Frail, D.E. (1994). Isoform-specific binding of apolipoprotein E to β-amyloid. *J Biol Chem* **269**, 23403–23406.

Lovestone, S., Anderton, B.H., Hartley, C., Jensen, T.G. and Jorgensen, A.L. (1996a). The intracellular fate of apolipoprotein E is tau dependent and apoe allele-specific. *NeuroReport* **7**, 1005–1008.

Lovestone, S., Hartley, C.L., Pearce, J. and Anderton, B.H. (1996b). Phosphorylation of tau by glycogen synthase kinase-3beta in intact mammalian cells: the effects on the organization and stability of microtubules. *Neuroscience* **73**, 1145–1157.

Lovestone, S., Davis, D.R., Webster, M.-T. *et al.* (1999). Lithium reduces glycogen synthase kinase-3 induced tau phosphorylation – effects in living cells and in neurons at therapeutic concentrations. *Biol Psychiatry* in press,

Mattson, M.P., Guo, Q., Furukawa, K. and Pedersen, W.A. (1998). Presenilins, the endoplasmic reticulum, and neuronal apoptosis in Alzheimer's disease. *J Neurochem* **70**, 1–14.

Morishima-Kawashima, M., Hasegawa, M., Takio, K. *et al.* (1995). Proline-directed and non-proline-directed phosphorylation of PHF-tau. *J Biol Chem* **270**, 823–829.

Muñoz-Montaño, J.R., Moreno, F.J., Avila, J. and Díaz-Nido, J. (1997). Lithium inhibits Alzheimer's disease-like tau protein phosphorylation in neurons. *FEBS Lett* **411**, 183–188.

Nathan, B.P., Bellosta, S., Sanan, D.A., Weisgraber, K.H., Mahley, R.W. and Pitas, R.E. (1994). Differential effects of apolipoproteins ϵ3 and ϵ4 on neuronal growth *in vitro*. *Science* **264**, 850–852.

Nathan, B.P., Chang, K.C., Bellosta, S. *et al.* (1995). The inhibitory effect of apolipoprotein E4 on neurite outgrowth is associated with microtubule depolymerization. *J Biol Chem* **270**, 19791–19799.

Polymeropoulos, M.H., Lavedan, C., Leroy, E. *et al.* (1997). Mutation in the α-synuclein gene identified in families with Parkinson's disease. *Science* **276**, 2045–2047.

Poorkaj, P., Bird, T.D., Wijsman E. *et al.* (1998). Tau is a candidate gene for chromosome 17 frontotemporal dementia. *Ann Neurol* **43**, 815–825.

Preuss, U., Biernat, J., Mandelkow, E.M. and Mandelkow, E. (1997). The 'jaws' model of tau-microtubule interaction examined in CHO cells. *J Cell Sci* **110**, 789–800.

Puttfarcken, P.S., Manelli, A.M., Falduto, M.T., Getz, G.S. and LaDu, M.J. (1997). Effect of apolipoprotein E on neurite outgrowth and β-amyloid-induced toxicity in developing rat primary hippocampal cultures. *J Neurochem* **68**, 760–769.

Selkoe, D.J. (1994a). Alzheimer's disease: a central role for amyloid. *J Neuropathol Exp Neurol* **53**, 438–447.

Selkoe, D.J. (1994b). Normal and abnormal biology of the β-amyloid precursor protein. *Annu Rev Neurosci* **17**, 489–517.

Smith, C. and Anderton, B.H. (1994). Dorothy Russell Memorial Lecture. The molecular pathology of Alzheimer's disease: are we any closer to understanding the neurodegenerative process? *Neuropathol Appl Neurobiol* **20**, 322–338.

Spillantini, M.G., Murrell, J.R., Goedert, M., Farlow, M.R., Klug, A. and Ghetti, B. (1998). Mutation in the tau gene in familial multiple system tauopathy with presenile dementia. *Proc Natl Acad Sci USA* **95**, 7737–7741.

Strittmatter, W.J., Weisgraber, K.H., Huang, D.Y. *et al.* (1993). Binding of human apolipoprotein E to synthetic amyloid β peptide: isoform-specific effects and implications for late-onset Alzheimer disease. *Proc Natl Acad Sci USA* **90**, 8098–8102.

Suzuki, N., Cheung, T.T., Cai, X.-D. *et al.* (1994). An increased percentage of long amyloid β protein secreted by familial amyloid β protein precursor (βAPP_{717}) mutants. *Science* **264**, 1336–1340.

Trinczek, B., Biernat, J., Baumann, K., Mandelkow, E.M. and Mandelkow, E. (1995). Domains of tau protein, differential phosphorylation, and dynamic instability of microtubules. *Mol Biol Cell* **6**, 1887–1902.

Utton, M.A., Vandecandelaere, A., Wagner, U. *et al.* (1997). Phosphorylation of tau by glycogen synthase kinase 3β affects the ability of tau to promote microtubule self-assembly. *Biochem J* **323**, 741–747.

Wille, H., Drewes, G., Biernat, J., Mandelkow, E.M. and Mandelkow, E. (1992). Alzheimer-like paired helical filaments and antiparallel dimers formed from microtubule-associated protein tau *in vitro*. *J Cell Biol* **118**, 573–584.

Xia, W.M., Zhang, J.M., Kholodenko, D. *et al.* (1997). Enhanced production and oligomerization of the 42-residue amyloid β-protein by Chinese hamster ovary cells stably expressing mutant presenilins. *J Biol Chem* **272**, 7977–7982.

Yu, G., Chen, F.S., Levesque, G. *et al.* (1998). The presenilin 1 protein is a component of a high molecular weight intracellular complex that contains β-catenin. *J Biol Chem* **273**, 16470–16475.

Zhou, J.H., Liyanage, U., Medina, M. *et al.* (1997). Presenilin 1 interaction in the brain with a novel member of the Armadillo family. *NeuroReport* **8**, 2085–2090.

Everything You Need to Know About Old Age Psychiatry . . .
Edited by Robert Howard
©1999 Wrightson Biomedical Publishing Ltd

2

Risk Factors for Alzheimer's Disease

ANTHONY H. MANN

Professor of Epidemiological Psychiatry, Institute of Psychiatry, London, UK

INTRODUCTION: CHANGING CONCEPTS

The epidemiologist and the biological researcher are beginning to come together. Until now, although both have seen themselves as searching for the cause of disease, their activities have seemed incompatible. The former studied community populations, trying to discover how the disease is distributed and, more specifically, who is at risk and why; the latter tracked the processes whereby the disease developed and affected individuals to produce the clinical state. Laboratory research focused on small, selected (in the epidemiologist's mind) samples attending specialist clinics, while the epidemiologist was searching for external exposures or environmental factors in large community samples. The specific focus of much laboratory research has been the identification of a gene or genes that would explain the familial nature of many cases.

This dichotomy has reflected the traditional view of disease onset: independent roles for genes and environment. The goal has been to discover how much each contributed. However, the discovery that the genotype can influence the environment to which the individual is exposed through life has changed this perspective. For example: life-events – quintessential external exposures – have been shown to have a heritability of around 40% (Plomin *et al.*, 1990). The genotype can also act to modify the impact of an exposure by affecting, for example, coping mechanisms (the capacity to solve problems and seek support). Heritability here is claimed to be around 30% (Kendler *et al.*, 1991). In epidemiological language, therefore, the genotype can act as a confounder or effect modifier, distorting or masking associations between an external exposure and disease onset by affecting both or the relationship between them. Thus, the epidemiologist has to consider the genotype as an important variable in research, its effect being best controlled by the use of genetically sensitive designs involving families, siblings or twins. At the same time, gene research has not found a particular variation that explains the onset of Alzheimer's disease, except in rare familial cases with early onset. The major results have been a susceptibility gene, ApoE ∈4, that does not entirely explain disease onset and whose impact may vary between cultures (Osuntokun *et al.*, 1995). Thus, environmental exposures must still be important. The coming together of epidemiological and biological research means that gene studies can move from small case–control studies, in which clearly defined cases (often selected for this purpose) are compared for the proportion carrying a particular gene, to controls from the normal elderly population (see review by Holmes, 1997). Case–control studies of this type will provide evidence of a gene's importance, but may well overestimate its predictive power in representative community samples, where the prevalence of dementia is actually low, because of large numbers of false positives (Ben Schlomo *et al.*, 1993). Studies of the genotype in community populations are necessary to quantify individual- and population-attributable risks. Fortunately, DNA extraction from cheek scrapes has made collection of biological materials possible on a large scale, outside hospitals and specialist centres.

A second shift, relevant to researching Alzheimer's disease risk, is the re-evaluation of the strict categorical approach to the diagnosis of dementia, Alzheimer's disease, vascular dementia and Lewy body dementia being the three major subtypes. The publication of international consensus criteria for Alzheimer's disease (McKhann *et al.*, 1984) was a crucial step in furthering research. These criteria, which could be readily applied, were based upon an assumption, however, that there was a pure pathology for Alzheimer's disease, so that all those with dementia who could have other possible causes of brain pathology could only be classified as 'possible' Alzheimer's disease. Not surprisingly, these criteria were shown to have diagnostic accuracy among specific, clinic samples of patients with likely Alzheimer's dementia in predicting the post-mortem appearance of Alzheimer's pathology. Their use, too, has allowed research to be comparable between centres and between countries. Similar criteria for the diagnosis of vascular dementia and Lewy body dementia have followed (Roman *et al.*, 1993; McKeith *et al.*, 1996). Paradoxically, however, the results of some of this research, particularly the study of risk from cardiovascular disease, have begun to challenge the boundaries created by these criteria. Further, post-mortem studies of brain material from representative community samples of subjects with dementia indicate more mixed pathologies than the clinical *in vivo* diagnosis would suggest (Holmes *et al.*, 1999). Under these circumstances, the clinical criteria are not so accurate. The concept of vascular dementia is particularly challenged (Rao and Howard, 1998).

The ground, therefore, is shifting. Givens of Alzheimer's disease research a few years ago are no longer so. Thus any review of risk factors now will be inconclusive and a repeat in a few years' time may well look different. The state of play in 1991, at the time of the publication of the EURODEM meta-analysis, then a major step forward in epidemiological research, will be the starting-point of this chapter and developments since that date will then be reviewed.

THE TRADITIONAL RISK FACTORS

Age

Increasing age remains a robust risk factor for the prevalence of dementia in the population, the rate doubling every 5.1 years of age (Jorm et al., 1987). The EURODEM meta-analysis of pooled cross-sectional data from 11 European centres provided a weighted average prevalence rate of 1.4% for dementia for those between 65 and 69, rising to 21.5% for those between 85 and 89 (Hofman et al., 1991). It has still not been established whether the risk continues to rise at the same rate beyond the age of 90. Incidence studies are still few, but there seems to be an age-related rise from approximately 1.5% to 2% per annum for those between 70 and 79 to 3–5% per annum for those between 80 and 89 (Copeland et al., 1992; Boothby et al., 1993). Of course, age is a number that reflects the passage of time during which various events possibly relevant to the onset of Alzheimer's disease can occur. For example, there is more time for genes to be expressed, more time for the impaired cell maintenance of older age to become manifest, and more time for an individual to meet a significant external exposure or for the number of exposures to accumulate.

Individual risk factors

Table 1 shows the results of the EURODEM meta-analysis (Jorm et al., 1991) which summarized the state of knowledge so far as risk factors were concerned. The importance of family history of dementia and Down's syndrome, of head trauma and depression, were a significant confirmation of results from case–control studies conducted earlier in the USA (Kokmen et al., 1991; French et al., 1985) and Australia (Broe et al., 1990). Since 1991, more research has been published on depression, head injury and smoking as risk factors, but the discovery of the role of ApoE ε4 genotype has radically altered the landscape. In addition, attention has been focused on previous intellectual attainment and particularly on the role of cardiovascular risk factors.

Table 1. Risk factors for AD (modified from EURODEM studies, 1991).

Risk factor	Relative risk (95% CI)
Family history of dementia	3.5 (2.6–4.6)
Family history of Down's syndrome	2.7 (1.2–5.7)
Family history of Parkinson's disease	2.4 (1.0–5.8)
Hypothyroidism	2.3 (1.0–5.4)
Head trauma	1.8 (1.3–2.7)
	F = 0.9 (0.4–1.7)
	M = 2.7 (1.6–4.4)
Depression	1.9 (1.1–3.3)
Maternal age	(15–19 years) = 1.5 (0.8–3)
	(40+) = 1.7 (1.0–2.9)
Epilepsy	1.6[a]
Herpes zoster/simplex	1.15[a]
Alcohol	1[a]
Smoking (ever smoked)	0.8[a]

[a]Ninety-five per cent confidence intervals for relative risk value include 1, i.e. the association may be due to chance.

Environmental exposures

The presence of aluminium in plaques in the brain of those with Alzheimer's disease has led to considerable interest in aluminium consumption during life and the chances of developing dementia. A positive association between rate of onset of dementia in the UK and aluminium in water levels was reported by Martyn *et al.* (1989). There were difficulties in being sure of the level of exposure without accurately defining the water supply to a particular area. A review of the evidence on this topic was noncommittal, as the possibility of confounding had not been eliminated (Doll, 1993). The EURODEM analyses provided no evidence for links between Alzheimer's disease and occupational exposure to solvents or lead. In contrast, a population case–control study in Canada did report that occupational exposure to glue, pesticides and fertilizers elevated risk (Canadian Study of Health and Aging, 1994) and a study of the treated incidence of early-onset dementias in Scotland showed considerable clustering in certain industrialized areas (Whalley *et al.*, 1995). There was a fivefold increase in the prevalence rate of Alzheimer's disease when African-Americans in Indianapolis were compared with Africans in Ibadan. In the latter group, amyloid plaques and neurofibrillary tangles were reported as rare among random autopsy samples (Hendrie *et al*, 1995). All these findings suggest that exposure during life to some environmental toxin cannot yet be excluded as a possible risk factor.

THE ApoE GENOTYPE

At the time of the EURODEM studies, the importance of the ApoE genotype for the development of Alzheimer's disease was not yet known. Its three variants (ϵ2, ϵ3 and ϵ4) were studied for their effect on lipoprotein levels, those homologous for the ϵ4 variant being at risk for hypercholesterolaemia. The first papers linking ApoE ϵ4 to an increased risk of Alzheimer's disease were published in 1993 (Strittmatter *et al.*, 1993; Poirier *et al.*, 1993), its importance being raising the risk for late-onset Alzheimer's disease in particular. These and much subsequent research on this topic were case–control studies, in which dementia subjects were referred to and assessed in specialist centres and became the cases; normal elderly people became the controls. The results of these studies were summarized by Holmes (1997). It seems that the possession of ApoE ϵ4 at least doubles the chance of Alzheimer's disease, whether familial or sporadic in type. However, as indicated above, studies of this type will establish the importance of an exposure, but may well overemphasize its powerfulness; thus there is a need for a population approach.

An important study in this respect, was that by Kuusisto *et al.* (1994) in Finland. Nine hundred and eighty people, aged between 69 and 79 years, were studied. Six hundred and fifty-two had no ϵ4 alleles, of whom 19 (2.9%) developed Alzheimer's disease. Two hundred and seventy-seven (28.2%) had one allele, of whom 21 (7.6%) developed the disease and only 28 (2.9%) were homologous for ϵ4 allele, of whom six (21.4%) developed Alzheimer's disease. In terms of the numbers of cases that arose in this population, more cases arose from those who had one allele than those who had two, although the possession of the latter significantly elevated risk in a small number of people. There have been no other comparable population studies of this type. However, two special populations have been reported: those aged 85 in Stockholm (Skoog *et al.*, 1997) and a cohort of elderly subjects recruited to a hypertension trial (Prince *et al.*, 1999). In the former, the ϵ4/ϵ4 combination was was present in 4.6% of the population and one or more ϵ4 allele in 43%. In the latter, ϵ4/ϵ4 allele was present in 0.5% and at least one ϵ4 allele in 14.6%. In both there was a significant association between ϵ4 allele and the presence of Alzheimer's disease, but the double combination only contributed a small number of cases to the total. It should be emphasized that many people with that high-risk combination, however, do not develop any dementia (13 out of 32 in the 85-year-old Stockholm cohort). Further, only five were diagnosed as probable Alzheimer's disease. Tang *et al.* (1996) have shown that the ϵ4 allele is not universally powerful. In a mixed ethnic study in New York, only the white elderly subjects with dementia were shown to be at increased risk with the possession of the ϵ4 allele. The Afro-American and Hispanic elders in the same community did not show this association. A lack of association between ApoE ε4 and Alzheimer's disease has been reported in Nigeria (Osuntokun *et al.*, 1995). It may also have a different effect at different ages (Breitner *et al.*, 1998).

Cross-sectional studies will be bedevilled by survivor bias: a possible difference in longevity for those with and without ApoE ε4 genotype with dementia. Furthermore, some subjects at a cross-section may yet develop dementia. Longitudinal studies would be a way to get around these difficulties, and some are beginning to appear. Tilvis *et al.* (1998) followed three birth cohorts aged 75, 80 and 85 for five years. Twenty-seven per cent of the population had an ApoE ε4 allele. Those with this allele performed worse at baseline upon cognitive testing and at the five-year follow-up. Forty-eight per cent of those with ApoE ε4 allele had died within the five years, compared with 37% of those without – a hazard ratio of 1.61 for all causes of death. Death associated with a dementia was more likely, with an elevated risk of 3.24. There is, therefore, some suggestion here of a differential survival rate.

It seems certain that the possession of ApoE ε4 makes some individuals susceptible to Alzheimer's disease, presumably more vulnerable to the action of other factors. The epidemiological evidence does not suggest it to be causative of Alzheimer's disease in itself; the mechanism remains to be elucidated.

CARDIOVASCULAR RISK FACTORS

The consensus criteria for Alzheimer's disease (McKhann *et al.*, 1984) exclude from the diagnosis of probable Alzheimer's disease those with overt evidence of cardiovascular disease. These criteria imply that atherosclerosis can be researched only in association with cognitive impairment or dementia in general, but not, by definition, with probable Alzheimer's disease. Vascular disease and hypertension can be associated with impaired cognitive performance. However, a case–control study, based upon the Medical Research Council's Elderly Hypertension Trial, provided a different perspective (Prince *et al.*, 1994). There were good baseline vascular risk factors measures for those people without dementia recruited from general practices into a treatment trial of hypertension. Follow-up over the following 10 years showed that 50 subjects had developed dementia, with 31 having dementia of Alzheimer type. There were associations of borderline significance between the onset of Alzheimer's disease and a range of vascular risk factors (smoking, hypertension, evidence of ischaemia on the electrocardiogram (ECG)) in those without a family history of dementia. Subsequently, in a community population study in Rotterdam, current vascular status was assessed extramurally using ultrasonography to measure the thickness of the walls of the common carotid artery and the presence of carotid plaques

(Hofman *et al.*, 1997). Peripheral vascular disease was assessed using the ratio of ankle to brachial systolic blood pressure. An atherosclerosis score computed from these three measures was significantly associated with the presence of all dementias *and* for those meeting criteria for Alzheimer's disease. This study provided important evidence, therefore, for an association between atherosclerosis and dementia of all clinical types.

Risk factors for vascular disease, in particular hypertension and diabetes, rather than overt manifestations of cardiovascular disease, have also been examined in relationship to Alzheimer's disease. There may be an elevated risk in diabetes (Leibson *et al.*, 1997). One longitudinal study of blood pressure levels and dementia indicated that systolic and diastolic pressures were raised 10 years before the onset of both Alzheimer's disease and vascular disease (Skoog *et al.*, 1996). In the years immediately preceding dementia onset, however, the blood pressure level fell. The role of smoking has been controversial. The EURODEM meta-analysis and a subsequent report from the Rotterdam survey suggested a protective effect, particularly in the latter study, for those with a family history, when the odds ratio for dementia was reduced to 0.2 (Brenner *et al.*, 1993). These findings contrasted with those from the Medical Research Council cohort and the Canadian Study of Aging which suggested an elevated risk from smoking for Alzheimer's disease in those without a family history and a suggestion of a dose–response effect (Prince *et al.*, 1994). In a follow-up over two years of the Rotterdam cohort, 146 incident cases of dementia were detected, 105 with Alzheimer's disease (Ott *et al.*, 1998). Smokers had an increased risk of all dementias, including Alzheimer's disease, of 2.2, but the risk was greater for those smokers without the ApoE ϵ4 gene (4.6). Smoking would, therefore, seem to be an important risk factor for the development of dementia and probably of Alzheimer's disease, but its impact is modified by the genotype.

Given the known effects of ApoE ϵ4 status on lipid level, the interactions between cardiovascular status and risk, genotype and dementia become of considerable interest. Hofman *et al.* (1997) showed a marked effect in their Rotterdam sample. There were 246 dementia cases and 928 nondemented controls whose ApoE ϵ4 status was known. The age-adjusted odds ratio for all dementias was 4.5 for those with severe atherosclerosis and ApoE ϵ4, but if only ApoE ϵ4 or atherosclerosis were present then the risk of dementia was not increased. The same interaction applied for the Alzheimer's disease cases, with an odds ratio of 3.9 for those with ApoE ϵ4 and atherosclerosis. So far as risk is concerned, the association between smoking and Alzheimer's disease is affected by ApoE ϵ4 status, as shown above. Jarvik *et al.* (1995) suggested that total cholesterol may also be higher in those with ApoE ϵ4 and Alzheimer's disease compared with those without the genotype, and speculated on the role of cholesterol as a mechanism for the genes effect. However, this hypothesis was not supported in a recent follow-up study of the Medical Research Council's elderly hypertensive cohort. ApoE ε4 and dementia status were established in 370 survivors of the cohort, 12 years after recruitment to the hypertension trial. As reported earlier, ApoE ε4 status was strongly associated with dementia, but the association became stronger (rather than weaker) if cardiovascular risk factors, including total cholesterol, were controlled in the analysis (Prince *et al.*, 1999). The relationship between cardiovascular status and its risk factors, clinical Alzheimer's disease and genotype, remains of considerable research interest. No conclusions can be drawn at the moment.

HEAD INJURY

Head trauma has been reported as a risk factor for Alzheimer's disease (Mortimer *et al.*, 1985), its importance being confirmed in the EURODEM analysis (odds ratio 1.8). Mayeux *et al.* (1993) compared patients with Alzheimer's disease and controls in a New York community survey. The odds ratio for a history of head injury in those with Alzheimer's disease was 3.7 (1.4–9.7) compared with controls, the rates being highest for those who had their head injury late in life. First-degree relatives of patients with onset before 70 also had a raised risk of Alzheimer's disease (odds ratio 2.5 (1.1-5.6)). The relatives who had experienced a head injury had a greatly increased chance of dementia (5.9 (2.3–4.58)), but the head injuries of relatives of controls also had an elevated risk (6.9 (2.5–18.9)). The authors concluded that both head injury and family history contributed to the onset of Alzheimer's disease.

DEPRESSION

The influence of depression in early life on the later onset of Alzheimer's disease was suggested in the EURODEM analysis. Henderson *et al.* (1992) suggested a broader definition of 'nervous breakdown' as also a risk factor and Agbayewa (1986) reported all forms of psychiatric disorder to be more common in patients with Alzheimer's disease. In his study, hospitalized Alzheimer patients were compared with medical and surgical inpatients. Methodological problems in researching this risk factor need to be overcome. The psychiatric disorder must be established as being distinct from a prodrome of Alzheimer's disease and its diagnosis should have some independent confirmation from case-notes. Cooper and Holmes (1998) recently addressed these issues in the Camberwell Dementia Register of 559 subjects, in which all dementia subtypes were represented. Twelve and a half per cent had a history of psychiatric problems, clearly distinct from the onset of dementia, schizophrenia and unipolar affective disorders being the commonest diagnoses. No distinguishing features of the current clinical dementia were found when those with and without a previous psychiatric history were compared. However, comparison with a control group of elderly Camberwell residents showed that only 3.4% of these had a psychiatric history, an estimated odds ratio of 3.6 for previous psychiatric history being associated with dementia. Psychiatric illness, rather than just depression, therefore, may be a risk factor, but the mechanism has yet to be established.

PREVIOUS EDUCATIONAL ATTAINMENT

Those with lower educational levels seem to be at greater risk of dementia as exemplified in the Canadian Study of Health and Aging (1994). The odds ratio for those with less than six years of education developing dementia was four and a half times greater than for those with more than 10 years' education. A similar disparity was reported in China – in a completely different culture (Zhang *et al.*, 1990). Ascertainment bias, poorly educated people performing less well on tests that require literacy, has been discounted for such findings. A brain 'reserve' theory is now postulated (Satz, 1993). This suggests that a certain amount of brain cell loss produces a greater effect in poorly endowed individuals than in those with greater intellectual powers; otherwise better educated individuals would show a greater amount of pathology at the same severity of dementia. Schmand *et al.* (1997) speculated that education level, as it depends on opportunities as much as intelligence, may be an invalid measure of brain reserve. From an Amsterdam study of 2063 elders who were followed up for four years, IQ (intelligence quotient) was assessed using the DART, a Dutch version of the National Adult Reading Test. Education, gender and occupational level were also recorded. There was a correlation of 0.51 between the DART score and educational level. While age remained the strongest predictor of the 152 incident cases, IQ was nearly as powerful, a high IQ having a strongly protective effect. The level of education did not appear in their regression model.

Premorbid ability has been taken a step further with the publication of the 'nun' study. Snowden *et al.* (1996) followed a cohort of 93 nuns who received cognitive testing in late life and post-mortem examination of the brains was carried out. Essays written at around the age of 22, at the time of admission to the convent, were examined for grammatical complexity and ideas density and the measures in these two areas quantified. It turned out, in this unique cohort – in which the environment was largely controlled through life in an enclosed order – that low ideas density predicted poor cognitive function and clinical Alzheimer's disease at the end of life. The diagnosis was confirmed by the high density of neurofibrillary tangles at post-mortem in those who died. This cohort was subsequently used to illustrate the brain 'reserve' theory by describing a subject without evident dementia who, at post-mortem, showed an abundance of neurofibrillary tangles (Snowden, 1997).

The brain 'reserve' theory, as measured by tests of intelligence or linguistic ability, may be useful to formulate the reason why some individuals seem to be at risk. The relationship between the genotype and these variables reflecting 'brain reserve' will be of considerable interest.

ANTI-INFLAMMATORY DRUGS

Case–control studies have suggested lower rates of Alzheimer's disease in those with arthritic conditions (Broe *et al.*, 1990). The explanation seemed to lie in the use of nonsteroidal anti-inflammatory drugs (NSAIDs) (Breitner, 1996). Two control studies suggested an inverse relationship between NSAID consumption and Alzheimer's disease. In a larger study, Stewart *et al.* (1997) obtained prescription data on community residents between 1980 and 1995 who were also screened for the onset of dementia and Alzheimer's disease. They reported an inverse association between the use of NSAIDs (but not paracetamol or aspirin) and the onset of dementia. There was a dose–response effect, use for more than two years having a greater effect. While this was an exciting report, there are methodological limitations. It was a *post hoc* analysis, and it is not clear how 'blindness' to the classification of medication occurred. Most importantly, the prescriptions were non-random.

It is not yet clear whether the effect of NSAIDs is specifically on dementia, or whether they may be active through their effect on cognitive function. In an analysis of the data for the Medical Research Council's hypertension trial, changes in measures of cognitive function using the Paired Associate Learning Test (PALT) and Trail-Making Test (TMT) over four years and the consumption of NSAIDs were compared. NSAIDs were used by approximately 15% of this sample. An effect of NSAID use in preventing PALT score decline was found, particularly when controlling for the effect of age and gender and the use of benzodiazepines (Prince *et al.*, 1998). Younger subjects seemed to benefit more. No effect, however, was found on changes in the TMT. The authors made some observations concerning further research on this topic, particularly on the need to control for polypharmacy, as NSAID users were also likely to be taking many other drugs. A large prospective cohort study with careful measurement of all other forms of medication consumption is now needed. Confounding, by indication or contraindication of use of these drugs which may also be a cause of other risk factors for Alzheimer's disease (e.g. cardiovascular), can only be avoided by random allocation of NSAIDs. This would be hard to achieve over a long period.

The importance of such findings has led to the consideration of treatments. Rogers *et al.* (1993) reported some improvement in Alzheimer's disease with indomethacin. Richards *et al.* (1997) examined the cognitive function of older men at high risk of coronary heart disease (as judged by a risk factor score) who had been recruited five years earlier as participants in a random controlled trial to investigate the benefit of anticoagulation by warfarin or aspirin in preventing stroke or coronary heart disease. Those taking aspirin had significantly better performance (particularly on frontal lobe tests) after five years' use of this drug. This study, too, was *post hoc* and the conclusions were dependent on an assumption of the initial randomization into treatment groups being free of bias in terms of cognitive ability. Again, the role of NSAIDs is intriguing, with considerable potential for further research.

CONCLUSIONS

It is probably no longer tenable to see Alzheimer dementia as a typical disease with a discrete pathology and a unique cause. Clinical dementia often occurs in the presence of mixed pathology, with both Alzheimer's pathology and cardiovascular changes present to some extent, but the proportions varying. Application of strict diagnostic criteria will force clinicians into too stark a categorical position. If vascular disease is important, does it act as a second brain insult, bringing forward clinical dementia, as suggested by Snowden and Riley (1997)? A follow-up study from Dublin of Alzheimer patients with and without magnetic resonance imaging (MRI) evidence of vascular disease did not support this view (Swanwick *et al.*, 1996). No change in the rate of decline in the two groups was evident. The damage from cardio-vascular disease could be occurring at a level at which overt disease cannot be detected by MRI. If the importance of vascular disease and its risk factors continues to be confirmed, there are exciting possibilities for prevention.

A 'susceptibility' gene has been established. Its mode of action is, as yet, unclear, as the evidence that it acts through promoting cardiovascular disease is not at all certain. More studies, in which the interplay of the genotype and risk factor are evaluated, will be important (as in the Rotterdam study). Variation in brain 'reserve' does seem to be important in understanding why some risk factors may be important for some people and may be a phenotypic representation of an underlying genotype. More, too, is yet to be discovered about the relationship and action of a previous psychiatric illness in promoting Alzheimer's disease. Finally, NSAIDs do seem to offer some chance of amelioration, although there will need to be much better research, other than the evidence of the *post hoc* reanalyses currently available.

REFERENCES

Agbayewa, M.O. (1986). Earlier psychiatric morbidity in patients with Alzheimer's disease. *J Am Geriatr Soc* **34**, 561–564.

Ben Schlomo, Y., Lewis, G. and McKeigue, P. (1993). ApoE4 and Alzheimer's disease [Letter]. *Lancet* **34**, 310.

Boothby, H., Blizard, R., Livingston, G. and Mann, A.H. (1993). The Gospel Oak Study stage III: the incidence of dementia. *Psychol Med* **24**, 89–95.

Breitner, J.C. (1996). Inflammatory processes and antiinflammatory drugs in Alzheimer's disease: a current appraisal. *Neurobiol Aging* **17**, 789–794.

Breitner, J.C., Jarvik, G.P., Plassman, B.L., Saunders, A.M. and Welsh, K.A. (1998). Risk of Alzheimer's disease with the epsilon4 allele for apolipoprotein E in a population-based study of men aged 62–73 years. *Alzheimer Dis Assoc Disord* **12**, 40–44.

Brenner, D.E., Kikull, W.A., van Belle, G. *et al.* (1993). Relationship between cigarette smoking and Alzheimer's disease in a population-based case–control study. *Neurology* **43**, 293–300.

Broe, G.A., Henderson, A.S., Creasey, H. *et al.* (1990). A case–control study of Alzheimer's disease in Australia. *Neurology* **40**, 1698–1707.

Canadian Study of Health and Aging (1994). Risk factors for Alzheimer's disease in Canada. *Neurology* **44**, 2073–2080.

Cooper, B. and Holmes, C. (1998). Previous psychiatric history as a risk factor for late-life dementia: a population-based case–control study. *Age Ageing* **27**, 181–188.

Copeland, J.M.R., Davidson, I.A., Dewey, M.E. *et al.* (1992). Alzheimer's disease, other dementias, depression and pseudodementia: prevalence, incidence and three-year outcome in Liverpool. *Br J Psychiatry* **161**, 230–239.

Doll, R. (1993). Review: Alzheimer's disease and environmental aluminium. *Age Ageing* **22**, 138–153.

French, L.R., Schuman, L.M., Mortimer, J.A. *et al.* (1985). A case–control study of dementia of the Alzheimer type. *Am J Epidemiol* **121**, 414–421.

Henderson, A.S., Jorm, A.F., Korten, A.E. *et al.* (1992). Environmental risk factors for Alzheimer's disease: their relationship to age of onset and to familial or sporadic types. *Psychol Med* **22**, 429–436.

Hendrie, H.C., Osuntokun, B.O., Hall, K.S. *et al.* (1995). Prevalence of Alzheimer's disease and dementia in two communities: Nigerian Africans and African Americans. *Am J Psychiatry* **152**, 1485–1492.

Hofman, A., Rocca, W.A., Brayne, C. *et al.* (1991). The prevalence of dementia in Europe: a collaborative study of 1980–1990 findings. *Int J Epidemiol* **20**, 736–748.

Hofman, A., Ott, A., Breteler, M.M.B. *et al.* (1997). Atherosclerosis, apolipoprotein E and prevalence of dementia and Alzheimer's disease in the Rotterdam Study. *Lancet* **349**, 151–154.

Holmes, C. (1997). Apolipoprotein E: implications and applications. In: Holmes, C. and Howard, R. (Eds), *Advances in Old Age Psychiatry*. Wrightson Biomedical, Petersfield, pp. 33–40.

Holmes, C., Cairns, N., Lantos, P.L. and Mann, A. (1999). The validity of current clinical criteria for Alzheimer's disease, vascular dementia and dementia with Lewy bodies. *Br J Psychiatry* in press.

Jarvik, G.P., Wijsman, E.M., Kukull, W.A., Schellenberg, G.D., Yu, C. and Larson, E.B. (1995). Interactions of apolipoprotein E genotype, total cholesterol level, age and sex in prediction of Alzheimer's disease. *Neurology* **45**, 1092–1096.

Jorm, A.F., Korten, A.E. and Henderson, A.S. (1987). The prevalence of dementia: a quantitative integration of the literature. *Acta Psychiatr Scand* **76**, 465–479.

Jorm, A.F., van Duijn, C.M., Chandra, V. *et al.* (1991). Psychiatric history and related exposures as risk factors for Alzheimer's disease: a collaborative re-analysis of case–control studies. EURODEM Risk Factors Research Group. *Int J Epidemiol* **20** (suppl 2), S43–S47.

Kendler, K.S., Kessler, R.C., Heath, A.C. *et al.* (1991). Coping: a genetic epidemiological investigation. *Psychol Med* **21**, 337–346.

Kokmen, E., Beard, R.N., Chandra, V. *et al.* (1991). Clinical risk factors for Alzheimer's disease: a population-based case-control study. *Neurology* **41**, 1393–1397.

Kuusisto, J., Koivisto, K., Kervinen, K. *et al.* (1994). Association of apolipoprotein E phenotypes with late-onset Alzheimer's disease; population-based study. *BMJ* **309**, 636–638.

Leibson, C.L., Rocca, W.A., Hanson, V.A. *et al.* (1997). Risk of dementia among persons with diabetes mellitus: a population-based cohort study. *Am J Epidemiol* **145**, 301–308.

Martyn, C.N., Barker, D.J.P., Osmond, C. *et al.* (1989). Geographical relation between Alzheimer's disease and aluminium in drinking water. *Lancet*, **i**, 58–65.

Mayeux, R., Ottman, R., Tang, M.-X. *et al.* (1993). Genetic susceptibility and head injury as risk factors for Alzheimer's disease among community-dwelling elderly persons and their first-degree relatives. *Ann Neurol* **33**, 494–501.

McKeith, I.G., Galasko, D., Kosaka, K. *et al.* (1996). Consensus guidelines for the clinical and pathologic diagnosis of dementia with Lewy bodies (DLB): report of the consortium on DLB International Workshop. *Neurology* **47**, 1113–1124.

McKhann, G., Drachman, D., Folstein, M., Katzman, R., Price, D. and Stadlan, E.M. (1984). Clinical diagnosis of Alzheimer's disease. Report of the NINCDS-ADRDA work group under the auspices of the Department of Health and Human Services Task Force on Alzheimer's Disease. *Neurology* **34**, 939–944.

Mortimer, J.A., French, R.L., Hutton, J.T. and Schuman, L.M. (1985). Head injury as a risk factor for Alzheimer's disease. *Neurology* **35**, 264–267.

Osuntokun, B.O., Sahota, A., Ogunniyi, A.O. *et al.* (1995). Lack of association between apolipoprotein E episilon 4 and Alzheimer's disease in elderly Nigerians. *Ann Neurol* **38**, 463–465.

Ott, A., Slooter, A.J.C., Hofman, A. *et al.* (1998). Smoking and risk of dementia and Alzheimer's disease in a population-based cohort study: the Rotterdam Study. *Lancet* **351**, 1840–1843.

Plomin, R., Lichtenstein, P., Pedersen, N.L. *et al.* (1990). Genetic influence on life events during the last half of the life span. *Psychol Aging* **5**, 25–30.

Poirier, J., Davignon, J., Bouthillier, D., Kogan, S., Bertrand, P. and Gauthier, S. (1993). Apolipoprotein E polymorphism and Alzheimer's disease. *Lancet* **342**, 697–699.

Prince, M., Cullen, M. and Mann, A. (1994). Risk factors for Alzheimer's disease and dementia: a case–control study based on the MRC elderly hypertension trial. *Neurology* **44**, 97–104.

Prince, M., Rabe-Hesketh, S. and Brennan, P. (1998). Do antiarthritic drugs decrease the risk for cognitive decline? *Neurology* **50**, 374–379.

Prince, M., Lovestone, S., Cervilla, J. *et al.* (1999). The association between ApoE and dementia is mediated neither by vascular disease nor its risk factors in an aged cohort of survivors with hypertension (submitted).

Rao, R. and Howard, R. (1998). Vascular dementia: dead or alive. *Int J Geriatr Psychiatry* **13**, 277–284.

Richards, M., Meade, T.W., Peart, S., Brennan, P.J. and Mann, A.H. (1997). Is there any evidence for a protective effect of antithrombotic medication on cognitive function in men at risk of cardiovascular disease? Some preliminary findings. *J Neurol Neurosurg Psychiatry* **62**, 269–272.

Rogers, J., Kirby, L.C., Hempelman, S.R. *et al.* (1993). Clinical trial of indomethacin in Alzheimer's disease. *Neurology* **43**, 1609–1611.

Roman, G.C., Tatemichi, T.K., Erkinjuntti, T. *et al.* (1993). Vascular dementia: diagnostic criteria for research studies: report of the NINDS-AIREN International Workshop. *Neurology* **43**, 250–260.

Satz, P. (1993). Brain reserve capacity on symptom onset after brain injury: a formulation and review of evidence for threshold theory. *Neuropsychology* **7**, 273–295.

Schmand, B., Smit, J.H., Geerlings, M.I. and Lindeboom, J. (1997). The effects of intelligence and education on the development of dementia. A test of the brain reserve hypothesis. *Psychol Med* **27**, 1337–1344.

Skoog, I., Lernfeldt, B., Landahl, S. *et al.* (1996). 15-year longitudinal study of blood pressure and dementia. *Lancet* **347**, 1141–1145.

Skoog, I., Hesse, C., Aevarsson, O. *et al.* (1997). A population study of apoE genotype at the age of 85: relation to dementia, cerebrovascular disease and mortality. *J Neurol Neurosurg Psychiatry* **64**, 37–43.

Snowden, D.A. and Riley, K.P. (1997). Aging and Alzheimer's disease: lessons from the nun study. *Gerontologist* **37**, 150–156.

Snowden, D.A., Kemper, S.J., Mortimer, J.A., Greiner, L.H., Wekstein, D.R. and Markesbery, W.R. (1996). Linguistic ability in early life and cognitive function and Alzheimer's disease in late life. Findings from the nun study. *JAMA* **275**, 528–532.

Snowden, D.A., Greiner, L.H., Mortimer, J.A. *et al.* (1997). Brain infarction and the clinical expression of Alzheimer's disease. The nun study. *JAMA* **277**, 813–817.

Stewart, W.F., Kawas, C., Corrada, M. and Metter, E.J. (1997). Risk of Alzheimer's disease and duration of NSAID use. *Neurology* **48**, 626–632.

Strittmatter, W.J., Saunders, A.M., Schmechel, D. *et al.* (1993). Apolipoprotein E: high avidity in binding to amyloid and increased frequency of type 4 allele in late onset Alzheimer's disease. *Proc Natl Acad Sci U S A* **90**, 1977–1981.

Swanwick, G.R.J., Kirby, M., Coen, R.F. *et al.* (1996). Effects of co-existent cerebrovascular disease on rate of progression in Alzheimer's disease. *Ir J Psychol Med* **13**, 91–93.

Tang, M.-X., Maestre, G., Tsai, W.Y. *et al.* (1996). Relative risk of Alzheimer's disease and age-at-onset distribution based on ApoE genotypes among elderly African-Americans, Caucasians and Hispanics in New York City. *Am J Hum Genet* **58**, 574–584.

Tilvis, R.S., Strandberg, T.E. and Juvak, K. (1998). Apolipoprotein E, phenotypes, dementia, and mortality in a prospective population sample. *J Am Geriatr Soc* **46**, 712–715.

Whalley, L.J., Thomas, B.M., McGonigal, G. *et al.* (1995). Epidemiology of presenile Alzheimer's disease in Scotland (1974–88) I. Non-random geographical variation. *Br J Psychiatry* **167**, 728–731.

Zhang, M., Katzman, R., Salmon, D. *et al.* (1990). The prevalence of dementia and Alzheimer's disease in Shanghai, China: impact of age, gender and education. *Ann Neurol* **27**, 428–437.

Everything You Need to Know About Old Age Psychiatry . . .
Edited by Robert Howard
©1999 Wrightson Biomedical Publishing Ltd

3

Clinical Genetics of Alzheimer's Disease

SIMON LOVESTONE

Section of Old Age Psychiatry, Institute of Psychiatry, London, UK

Progress on understanding the genetic aetiology of Alzheimer's disease has been extremely rapid. Over the past few years we have come to understand that Alzheimer's disease (AD) is properly thought of as a collection of disorders with a common end-point but with differing genetic aetiologies, and increasingly other disorders resulting in a dementia have been defined molecularly (Blacker and Tanzi, 1998; Roses, 1996). This progress demands a clinical response; the questions are, who is to respond, why, and in what way? This chapter will attempt to address these questions, drawing upon experience gained in other conditions such as Huntington's disease and on the experience of talking to families either at risk of AD or, as will be shown to be equally likely, subject to unwarranted concerns about risk of AD.

MOLECULAR GENETICS AND NEURODEGENERATIVE DISEASES

The inheritable dementias include Alzheimer's disease (Roses, 1997) and frontotemporal degeneration. Some forms of the latter have a mutation in the tau gene (Spillantini *et al.*, 1998a; Spillantini *et al.*, 1998b); others have been linked to chromosome 3 and yet other forms are part of the frontotemporal motor neurone disease complex (Neary *et al.*, 1990), some of which seem to be inherited in an autosomal-dominant manner. Other inheritable dementias include the prion disorders and secondary dementias such as Huntington's disease. Other neurodegenerative diseases with a clearly autosomal-dominant inheritance include CADASIL (Ruchoux and Maurage, 1997) which can be associated with AD (Gray *et al.*, 1994) and some cases of Parkinson's disease (Polymeropoulos *et al.*, 1997). In addition to autosomal-dominant inherited neurodegenerative disorders, there appears to be some genetic risk involved in progressive supranuclear palsy, possibly mediated through polymorphisms in the tau gene (Higgins *et al.*, 1998) and also a clear genetic risk for AD where family history is the largest single risk factor (Slooter and van Duijn, 1997; van Duijn *et al.*, 1994). This molecular complexity only adds to the difficulty in determining the appropriate clinical response – many genes cause disorders that either share symptoms or, although with a different genetic aetiology, have an identical clinical and neuropathological outcome.

The clinical response to genetic discoveries in AD is quite different for early-onset familial and for late-onset AD. Early-onset familial AD is rare. When there is an informative pedigree it is often autosomal-dominant and the genetics are manifest both to clinicians and to families. Late-onset AD, on the other hand, is extremely common and the genetics less obvious. For many years the understanding of the inheritance of AD escaped clinicians and others involved in research. Although a family history is one of the strongest risk factors for AD (Slooter and van Duijn, 1997) many individuals with AD have no family history – so-called sporadic cases. However, careful pedigree studies have consistently demonstrated a high cumulative incidence in first-degree relatives rising to 50% or more by the age of 90 years (Korten *et al.*, 1993; Huff *et al.*, 1988; Martin *et al.*, 1988; Farrer *et al.*, 1989; Sadovnick *et al.*, 1989). It does seem as though the major explanation of sporadic cases of AD is simply absence of family living to the age of onset of the disorder. Although the importance of genetic factors in the aetiology of late-onset AD has not been appreciated until relatively recently it is possible that some relatives of patients have been more concerned about inheriting Alzheimer's disease than is generally realized. There is some evidence suggestive of this in a telephone helpline for those concerned about dementia: the most frequently raised subject was that of genetics (Harvey *et al.*, 1998).

Three genes have been associated with early-onset familial AD: the amyloid precursor protein (APP) gene and the presenilin (PS1 and PS2) genes on chromosomes 21, 14 and 1 respectively (reviewed in Hardy, 1996). Mutations in PS1 are the most frequently found and mutations in PS2 the least common. Even so, all are rare (Schellenberg *et al.*, 1991; Cruts *et al.*, 1998). It is almost certain that at least one other autosomal-dominant AD gene remains to be discovered. For early-onset familial AD the identification of mutations in the APP gene or the presenilin genes raises the possibility both of predictive and diagnostic testing. Diagnostic testing is the less problematical in many ways, although important questions remain as to how many families carry an identified mutation. Initial screens of known autosomal-dominant families suggested that more than 70% of such families would carry a mutation in one of the APP or presenilin genes. More recent population-based studies suggest that the frequency of mutations in the PS genes in early-onset familial and nonfamilial AD might be considerably lower than this (Cruts *et al.*, 1998). However, finding a mutation in a patient with AD determines the molecular diagnosis in that individual and, despite some concerns about penetrance (Rossor *et al.*, 1996), raises the possibility of predictive testing for all at-risk relatives.

PREDICTIVE TESTING IN AUTOSOMAL-DOMINANT CONDITIONS

Predictive testing should follow Huntington's disease (HD) guidelines in which affected individuals would be tested first and unaffected relatives would be offered appropriate counselling, a process that takes a minimum of four months (Simpson and Harding, 1993). Psychiatrists have played an important part in developing the protocols used in HD and psychiatric issues certainly present themselves during the extended counselling programme (Scourfield *et al.*, 1997). Undergoing this counselling and learning one's status as a carrier or not of an HD mutation would be expected to be a daunting prospect and an important question remains as to how many individuals would want to avail themselves of such a process. When asked, a majority of those at risk of HD indicated that they would want to receive this information although the results of testing programmes thus far suggest that actually a minority proceed to full testing (Adam *et al.*, 1993); almost certainly a self-selection process is at work in those presenting themselves for testing (Decruyenaere *et al.*, 1995). Only one case has been reported of predictive testing for AD and importantly, it was found that an individual carrying the mutation subsequently became depressed on being given this information (Lannfelt *et al.*, 1995). Perhaps more surprising is the finding consistent across a number of studies that even receiving good news, at least for HD, can increase psychological distress at follow-up (Bloch *et al.*, 1992; Wiggins *et al.*, 1992). The reason for this is almost certainly twofold. First, those receiving good news will, of course, have relatives, often many relatives, who either carry the disease gene or are already affected by the disease. Those not carrying the gene might be expected to suffer from survivor guilt. Secondly, individuals at risk of HD often comment that their life has been put on hold. Relationships may have been ended, the decision not to have children may have been taken and careers may not have been pursued as actively as they otherwise would have been. The impact of living with the risk of Huntington's disease has been graphically described. When told that they do not in fact carry the gene, this results in a considerable change in circumstances and a re-evaluation which can lead in some individuals to increased stress (Wahlin *et al.*, 1997; Hayden *et al.*, 1995). Some studies do suggest that the adverse events occurring in those with increased risk tend to occur immediately after receiving bad news, whereas those receiving good news tend to have adverse events later, suggesting perhaps such a re-evaluation process (Lawson et al., 1996). However, at one-year follow-up, those receiving both good and bad news were found to have less depression and increased well-being (Bloch et al., 1992; Wiggins et al., 1992). Longer-term follow-up does show some differences between those at high and low risk although after longer follow-up those in the high-risk group are nearing the age at which they might expect to experience symptoms (Taylor and Myers, 1997)

GENETIC TESTING AND LATE-ONSET ALZHEIMER'S DISEASE

For late-onset AD the situation is entirely different. One gene only has been identified that increases risk, the apolipoprotein E gene (ApoE) (reviewed in Growdon, 1998; Strittmatter and Roses, 1996). The relationship of ApoE to AD is complex. Many studies have suggested that one variant, ApoE ϵ2, is protective, while the ApoE ϵ4 allele increases risk. More recently, evidence has been provided suggesting that apoE modulates when and not if an individual will suffer from AD (Meyer et al., 1998). This emphasizes the point that many individuals carrying two copies of the risky allele, apoE ϵ4, do not suffer from AD and equally a large number of individuals who do suffer from the condition do not carry a single ϵ4 allele. ApoE, and almost certainly other genes yet to be identified or confirmed, increase risk but are not determinative. The clinical consequences for such nondeterminative risk genes include diagnostic testing, susceptibility testing and testing for clinical management.

Some evidence has suggested that ApoE genetic testing might increase diagnostic certainty in AD (Alzheimer's Association and National Institute for Aging, 1998; Mayeux et al., 1998; Farlow, 1997; Post et al., 1997). Prospective studies to post-mortem have only been performed on a research-based population but nonetheless demonstrate some value in diagnostic ApoE testing; one study suggested 100% positive predictive value and another huge collaborative study of more than 2000 patients suggested a very significant increase in diagnostic specificity in combining clinical diagnosis with ApoE testing (Mayeux et al., 1998; Relkin et al., 1996). However, research populations are unlikely to be typical for AD and in studies to date subjects have received an intensive clinical investigation and diagnosis and have already received a firm NINCDS-ADRDA-based diagnosis (National Institute for Neurological, Communicable Diseases and Stroke/Alzheimer's Disease and Related Disorders Association). For diagnostic testing to be useful, it is likely that it would have to be proven to have a benefit in those clinical subjects where diagnosis is difficult – atypical dementias or early in the course of the dementia. For this, community-based prospective studies to post-mortem are needed although they may be difficult to perform. It is possible that combining ApoE genotyping with neuroimaging or some other investigation would aid early detection of AD (Small *et al.*, 1996). However, most consensus groups that have considered the adjunctive use of ApoE genotyping in diagnosis agree that while this may become a useful tool, at present the data are insufficient to recommend it (Lovestone, 1998).

The second potential use of ApoE genotyping is in susceptibility testing. While prediction will never be possible for a nondeterminative risk gene, it is clear that ApoE and almost certainly other genes, increase risk, and that if this could be quantified reliably, then this information might be of some interest. Seshadri *et al.* (1995), in a meta-analysis of studies of individuals over the age of 65, demonstrated that lifetime risk at retirement was 0.15 for AD increasing to 0.29 for those with at least one ApoE ε4 allele. They concluded that as this was not determinative, predictive testing was not possible. However, whether individuals would be interested to learn of a doubling of risk at this critical time has not been empirically determined.

Finally, it has been suggested that ApoE testing might be of some use in clinical management. Some evidence suggests that response to acetylcholinesterase inhibitors is moderated by ApoE response (Poirier *et al.*, 1995; Farlow *et al.*, 1998; Richard *et al.*, 1997). This is very much in line with the considerable attention given to the burgeoning field of pharmacogenomics in general, and for AD this will become important if in the future compounds can be directed to those most likely to respond based upon genotypic analysis. However, for each individual to whom a compound is directed, another has been denied treatment and there are ethical consequences arising from this use of genetics.

THE UK ALZHEIMER'S DISEASE GENETICS CONSORTIUM

Because of the ethical and clinical issues arising from this rapid growth in understanding of the genetic basis of the neurodegenerative disorders, the UK Alzheimer's Disease Genetics Consortium was founded (Lovestone and Harper, 1994; Lovestone *et al.*, 1996). This is a collection of clinicians in the fields of genetics, neurology, old age psychiatry, general practice and others, together with the lay societies (Alzheimer's Disease Society, Alzheimer's Disease International, Genetics Interest Group) and representatives from research and clinical genetics laboratories. Together, the Consortium meets to discuss research findings and to consider the consequences of this for patients and their families. In brief, the Consortium has agreed to date that predictive testing for AD should follow Huntington's disease guidelines for early-onset familial AD, but is not recommended for late-onset AD. With regard to diagnostic testing and testing for clinical management, more data are needed and there are important issues that remain to be resolved. For both of these forms of genetic testing and for research, consent is an important issue and the Consortium, in evidence presented in response to the Lord Chancellor's 'Who Decides?' paper, agrees that consent should be obtained from patients where they are capable, and where they are not capable to give informed consent, agreement should be sought from relatives. In all cases agreement or consent should be explicitly for nondisclosure. That is, it should be agreed in advance whether results should be made available to patients and their families and where a test is performed in a research context, then the results of the tests should never be relayed back to families. In all cases individual patients with dementia should give assent at least.

A GENETICS CLINIC FOR LATE-ONSET ALZHEIMER'S DISEASE FAMILIES

The author and colleagues have become increasingly concerned that relatives of patients with AD have concerns about inheriting dementia and are often not able to access reliable and up-to-date information. A Dementia Genetics Clinic was established at the Maudsley Hospital to meet some of these concerns. The aims of the clinic were to offer information to relatives and to provide a preliminary assessment prior to genetic counselling for those for whom it was appropriate. The clinic is run in conjunction with the Regional Genetics Service based at Guy's Hospital and for the past two years on average approximately one patient has been seen each month. The clinic has deliberately kept a low profile and has not been advertised widely but is open referral and patients are accepted from general practitioners, specialists and self-referral, without geographical constraints.

Table 1 gives the details of the first 20 patients seen in the clinic. It is notable that the majority are women, a finding that reflects similar results for HD. It is also notable that those seen in the clinic do not come from unusually multiply affected families – those seen are not particularly familial. The number of relatives of those seen affected by AD is actually rather small. Equally surprising was the finding that the time of onset of the affected member of the family was not predominantly early and that in nearly half of the families seen, autosomal-dominant AD could be excluded from a pedigree analysis alone. One concern prior to starting the clinic was that it would be providing a service to two groups of patients – the unnecessarily and mildly worried, referred by themselves, and the highly familial and appropriately worried, referred by specialist care. Neither prediction has yet been borne out. Many more patients than expected were referred from

Table 1. Characteristics of first 20 patients seen in the Dementia Genetics Clinic at the Maudsley Hospital, London.

Characteristics of those referred	Mean age (range) years	Female gender	Referral source	Referral area
	46 (23–75)	75%	1 self 10 primary care 7 specialist care	3 local 10 regional 7 national

Characteristics of family pedigree	First-degree relatives affected	Second-degree relatives affected	Youngest age of onset in family	Autosomal-dominant excluded
	1.6 range 1–4	2.6 range 1–5	50–80 years	In 45% by pedigree analysis

Psychiatric morbidity	Previous assessment in secondary care	Concerned	Anxious	Depressed
	6 (30%)	2 (10%)	8 (40%)	8 (40%)

primary care. At present what happens to those patients referred to a regional genetics clinic in the absence of a specialist AD clinic is not known. Very few highly familial, early-onset, autosomal-dominant families were referred.

However, those seen are moderately distressed individuals. Many have sought help in other contexts, having had multiple referrals to neurologists or psychologists, some having had extensive investigations including magnetic resonance imaging and others having received repeated psychometry. All individuals seen were clearly not suffering from dementia and in most cases were two or more decades younger than the age of onset in their relatives. Their anxieties regarding memory were not assuaged by investigations but were readily addressed by placing in an accurate context their concerns regarding inheriting AD. Eight out of the 20 individuals were very anxious and a further eight were clinically depressed, either receiving treatment from a specialist or were referred after having been seen in a clinic.

In summary, the expectations of the clinic were that a majority of individuals would be from early-onset familial autosomal-dominant families although it was expected a number of individuals from less clearly genetic AD families would be seen. In fact, the vast majority of patients seen have very few affected family members; despite this, the level of psychiatric morbidity was very considerable and these individuals often spend considerable time, and indeed NHS resources, in attempting to get further information. In their search for further information they often receive intensive

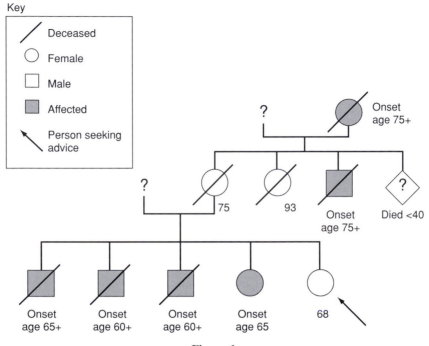

Figure 1.

investigations themselves, not something that they had expected or found helpful in many cases. The four family trees illustrate some of the individuals seen. In Figure 1, a 68-year-old lady presented having witnessed late-onset dementia in all four of her siblings. A maternal uncle and maternal grandfather were also affected by late-onset dementia. At presentation she was very concerned about her own memory and risk of suffering from AD which she estimated at far greater than 50%. She had taken a number of actions based upon this risk estimate including making a will and establishing enduring power of attorney. Pedigree analysis demonstrated that the link individual between herself and her second-degree-affected family members was entirely clear of dementia at the age of 75. Nothing was known about her other parent. Autosomal-dominant AD cannot be excluded formally but is extremely unlikely given such a pedigree although she is, simply by virtue of having affected first-degree family members, at somewhat increased risk. Genetic testing would not be appropriate in this family.

In contrast, the 55-year-old man presenting with two older brothers affected at the age of 60 or 62 (Figure 2) clearly did not have an autosomal-dominant family tree. On presentation, he believed that he was at 50% risk

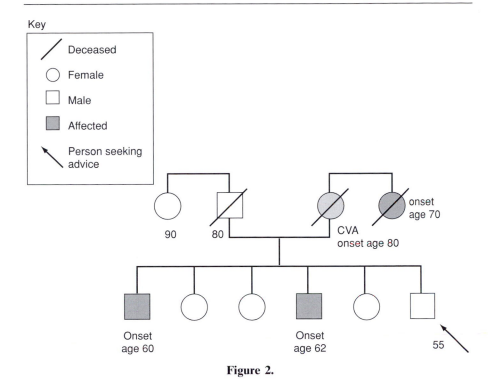

Figure 2.

and had obtained information from a helpline and from the Internet and believed that he came from an autosomal-dominant family because two brothers and an aunt were affected. However, because both parents were clearly free of dementia at the age of 80 he was reassured that this was not an autosomal-dominant picture and that his risk was no greater than that which would be expected for any other individual with an affected sibling.

Some families with clearly autosomal-dominant dementia, such as that shown in Figure 3, have presented to the clinic; many members of this individual's family have been seen. The family has considered mutation analysis which would be first performed on the affected individual but have decided, for the time being, not to proceed. However, DNA has been banked for future analysis if appropriate, and consent has been obtained for post-mortem examination in due course. Both measures will be important if other generations decide that genetic testing would be of use at some point in the future.

Finally a 54-year-old woman presented with only one affected family member (Figure 4). Because her father had an onset of dementia at the age of 50 she had become convinced that this was early-onset autosomal-dominant AD and that she, at the age of 54, was herself at real risk. She had become

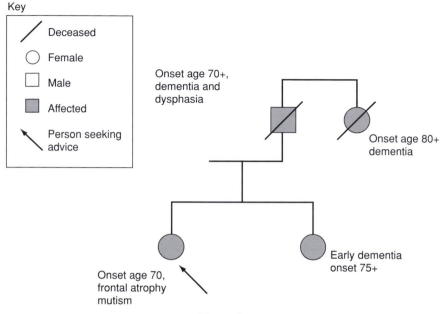

Figure 3.

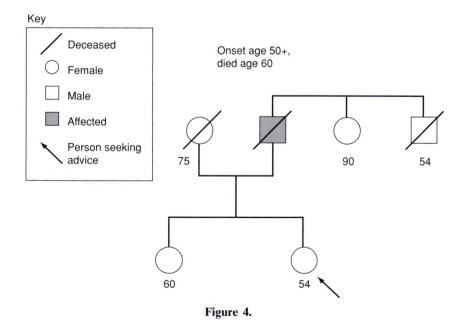

Figure 4.

so concerned about her own memory that she had had many referrals to secondary and, indeed, tertiary centres and had received extensive investigations, but was not reassured by consistently normal results. On examination in the clinic, she had evidence of a mild depressive episode with anhedonia, disturbed sleep and poor libido, and her work was affected. On discussion of her family history, it was pointed out that there was no evidence of autosomal-dominant AD and that, in fact, she was at no greater risk of suffering from dementia than anyone else in the population with an affected parent.

The experience of working with family members of those affected by dementia suggests that a percentage are extremely concerned about their own risk and often have sought advice in many different contexts. The information they have received has been variable and on a number of occasions investigations on themselves have been performed in an effort to reassure them. This rarely has the desired effect. A simple pedigree analysis is able to give individuals information in many cases and often an autosomal-dominant inheritance can be excluded. The premise of the AD genetics clinic is that information is empowering, although whether this has a lasting effect on reducing anxiety is not known. As AD genetics advances clinicians will have to respond. One model has been presented of a response by old age psychiatry working in collaboration with clinical geneticists. Undoubtedly other such models could be envisaged but it is almost certain that old age psychiatry as a profession will have an important role to play in the clinical consequences of these genetic advances.

REFERENCES

Adam, S., Wiggins, S., Whyte, P. *et al.* (1993). Five year study of prenatal testing for Huntington's disease: demand, attitudes, and psychological assessment. *J Med Genet* **30**, 549–556.

Alzheimer's Association and National Institute for Aging (1998). Consensus report of the Working Group on: 'Molecular and biochemical markers of Alzheimer's disease'. *Neurobiol Aging* **19**, 109–116.

Blacker, D. and Tanzi, R.E. (1998). The genetics of Alzheimer disease – current status and future prospects. *Arch Neurol* **55**, 294–296.

Bloch, M., Adam, S., Wiggins, S., Huggins, M. and Hayden, M.R. (1992). Predictive testing for Huntington disease in Canada: the experience of those receiving an increased risk. *Am J Med Genet* **42**, 499–507.

Cruts, M., van Duijn, C.M., Backhovens, H. *et al.* (1998). Estimation of the genetic contribution of presenilin-1 and -2 mutations in a population based study of presenile Alzheimer disease. *Hum Mol Genet* **7**, 43–51.

Decruyenaere, M., Evers Kiebooms, G., Boogaerts, A. *et al.* (1995). Predictive testing for Huntington's disease: risk perception, reasons for testing and psychological profile of test applicants. *Genet Couns* **6**, 1–13.

Farlow, M.R. (1997). Alzheimer's disease: clinical implications of the apolipoprotein E genotype. *Neurology* **48** (suppl 6), S30–S34.

Farlow, M.R., Lahiri, D.K., Poirier, J., Davignon, J., Schneider, L. and Hui, S.L. (1998). Treatment outcome of tacrine therapy depends on apolipoprotein genotype and gender of the subjects with Alzheimer's disease. *Neurology* **50**, 669–677.

Farrer, L.A., O'Sullivan, D.M., Cupples, L.A., Growdon, J.H. and Myers, R.H. (1989). Assessment of genetic risk for Alzheimer's disease among first-degree relatives. *Ann Neurol* **25**, 485–493.

Gray, F., Robert, F., Labrecque, R. *et al.* (1994). Autosomal dominant arteriopathic leuko-encephalopathy and Alzheimer's disease. *Neuropathol Appl Neurobiol* **20**, 22–30.

Growdon, J.H. (1998). Apolipoprotein E and Alzheimer disease. *Arch Neurol* **55**, 1053–1054.

Hardy, J. (1996). New insights into the genetics of Alzheimer's disease. *Ann Med* **28**, 255–258.

Harvey, R., Roques, P.K., Fox, N.C. and Rossor, M.N. (1998). CANDID – counselling and diagnosis in dementia: a national telemedicine service supporting the care of younger patients with dementia. *Int J Geriatr Psychiatry* **13**, 381–388.

Hayden, M.R., Bloch, M. and Wiggins, S. (1995). Psychological effects of predictive testing for Huntington's disease. *Adv Neurol* **65**, 201–210.

Higgins, J.J., Litvan, I., Pho, L.T., Li, W. and Nee, L.E. (1998). Progressive supranuclear gaze palsy is in linkage disequilibrium with the τ and not the α-synuclein gene. *Neurology* **50**, 270–273.

Huff, F.J., Auerbach, J., Chakravarti, A. and Boller, F. (1988). Risk of dementia in relatives of patients with Alzheimer's disease. *Neurology* **38**, 786–790.

Korten, A.E., Jorm, A.F., Henderson, A.S., Broe, G.A., Creasey, H. and McCusker, E. (1993). Assessing the risk of Alzheimer's disease in first-degree relatives of Alzheimer's disease cases. *Psychol Med* **23**, 915–923.

Lannfelt, L., Axelman, K., Lilius, L. and Basun, H. (1995). Genetic counseling in a Swedish Alzheimer family with amyloid precursor protein mutation [Letter]. *Am J Hum Genet* **56**, 332–335.

Lawson, K., Wiggins, S., Green, T., Adam, S., Bloch, M. and Hayden, M.R. (1996). Adverse psychological events occurring in the first year after predictive testing for Huntington's disease. *J Med Genet* **33**, 856–862.

Lovestone, S., Wilcock, G., Rossor, M., Cayton, H. and Ragan, I. (1996). Apolipoprotein E genotyping in Alzheimer's disease. *Lancet* **347**, 1775–1776.

Lovestone, S. (1998). Genetics consortiums can offer views facilitating best practice in Alzheimer's disease. *BMJ* **317**, 471.

Lovestone, S. and Harper, P. (1994). Genetic tests and Alzheimer's disease. *Psychiatr Bull* **18**, 645.

Martin, R.L., Gerteis, G. and Gabrielli, W.F. (1988). A family-genetic study of dementia of Alzheimer type. *Arch Gen Psychiatry* **45**, 894–900.

Mayeux, R., Saunders, A.M., Shea, S. *et al.* (1998). Utility of the apolipoprotein E genotype in the diagnosis of Alzheimer's disease. *N Engl J Med* **338**, 506–511.

Meyer, M.R., Tschanz, J.T., Norton, M.C. *et al.* (1998). APOE genotype predicts when – not whether – one is predisposed to develop Alzheimer disease. *Nat Genet* **19**, 321–322.

Neary, D., Snowden, J.S., Mann, D.M., Northen, B., Goulding, P.J. and Macdermott, N. (1990). Frontal lobe dementia and motor neuron disease. *J Neurol Neurosurg Psychiatry* **53**, 23–32.

Poirier, J., Delisle, M.C., Quirion, R. *et al.* (1995). Apolipoprotein E4 allele as a predictor of cholinergic deficits and treatment outcome in Alzheimer disease. *Proc Natl Acad Sci U S A* **92**, 12260–12264.

Polymeropoulos, M.H., Lavedan, C., Leroy, E. *et al.* (1997). Mutation in the α-synuclein gene identified in families with Parkinson's disease. *Science* **276**, 2045–2047.

Post, S.G., Whitehouse, P.J., Binstock, R.H. *et al.* (1997). The clinical introduction of genetic testing for Alzheimer disease. An ethical perspective. *JAMA* **227**, 832–836.

Relkin, N.R., Tanzi, R., Breitner, J. *et al.* (1996). Apolipoprotein E genotyping in Alzheimer's disease. *Lancet* **347**, 1091–1095.

Richard, F., Helbecque, N., Neuman, E., Guez, D., Levy, R. and Amouyel, P. (1997). APOE genotyping and response to drug treatment in Alzheimer's disease. *Lancet* **349**, 539.

Roses, A.D. (1996). The Alzheimer diseases. *Curr Opin Neurobiol* **6**, 644–650.

Roses, A.D. (1997). Genetics of the Alzheimer diseases. *Bibliogr Psychiatry* 115–118.

Rossor, M.N., Fox, N.C., Beck, J., Campbell, T.C. and Collinge, J. (1996). Incomplete penetrance of familial Alzheimer's disease in a pedigree with a novel presenilin-1 gene mutation. *Lancet* **347**, 1560.

Ruchoux, M.M. and Maurage, C.A. (1997). CADASIL: cerebral autosomal dominant arteriopathy with subcortical infarcts and leukoencephalopathy. *J Neuropathol Exp Neurol* **56**, 947–964.

Sadovnick, A.D., Irwin, M.E., Baird, P.A. and Beattie, B.L. (1989). Genetic studies on an Alzheimer clinic population. *Genet Epidemiol* **6**, 633–643.

Schellenberg, G.D., Anderson, L., O'dahl, S. *et al.* (1991). APP717, APP693, and PRIP gene mutations are rare in Alzheimer disease. *Am J Hum Genet* **49**, 511–517.

Scourfield, J., Soldan, J., Gray, J., Houlihan, G. and Harper, P.S. (1997). Huntington's disease: Psychiatric practice in molecular genetic prediction and diagnosis. *Br J Psychiatry* **170**, 146–149.

Seshadri, S., Drachman, D.A. and Lippa, C.F. (1995). Apolipoprotein E ε4 allele and the lifetime risk of Alzheimer's disease – what physicians know, and what they should know. *Arch Neurol* **52**, 1074–1079.

Simpson, S.A. and Harding, A.E. (1993). Predictive testing for Huntington's disease: after the gene. The United Kingdom Huntington's Disease Prediction Consortium. *J Med Genet* **30**, 1036–1038.

Slooter, A.J.C. and van Duijn, C.M. (1997). Genetic epidemiology of Alzheimer disease. *Epidemiol Rev* **19**, 107–119.

Small, G.W., Komo, S., La Rue, A. *et al.* (1996). Early detection of Alzheimer's disease by combining apolipoprotein E and neuroimaging. *Ann N Y Acad Sci* **802**, 70–78.

Spillantini, M.G., Bird, T.D. and Ghetti, B. (1998a). Frontotemporal dementia and parkinsonism linked to chromosome 17: a new group of tauopathies. *Brain Pathol* **8**, 387–402.

Spillantini, M.G., Murrell, J.R., Goedert, M., Farlow, M.R., Klug, A. and Ghetti, B. (1998b). Mutation in the tau gene in familial multiple system tauopathy with pre-senile dementia. *Proc Natl Acad Sci U S A* **95**, 7737–7741.

Strittmatter, W.J. and Roses, A.D. (1996). Apolipoprotein E and Alzheimer's disease. *Annu Rev Neurosci* **19**, 53–77.

Taylor, C.A. and Myers, R.H. (1997). Long-term impact of Huntington disease linkage testing. *Am J Med Genet* **70**, 365–370.

van Duijn, C.M., Clayton, D.G., Chandra, V. *et al.* (1994). Interaction between genetic and environmental risk factors for Alzheimer's disease: a reanalysis of case-control studies. *Genet Epidemiol* **11**, 539–551.

Wahlin, T.B.R., Lundin, A., Bäckman, L. *et al.* (1997). Reactions to predictive testing in Huntington disease: case reports of coping with a new genetic status. *Am J Med Genet* **73**, 356–365.

Wiggins, S., Whyte, P., Huggins, M. *et al.* (1992). The psychological consequences of predictive testing for Huntington's disease. Canadian Collaborative Study of Predictive Testing. *N Engl J Med* **327**, 1401–1405.

4

Dementia with Lewy Bodies: Recent Developments

E. JANE BYRNE

Department of Old Age Psychiatry, University of Manchester, Manchester, UK

Dementia with Lewy bodies (DLB), a term adopted in 1996 by the International Consensus Conference (McKeith *et al.*, 1996), while pragmatically bypassing the 'tower of Babel' (Hansen, 1996) of nosological terminology, nevertheless continues to provoke heated debate. While the focus has arguably been on whether DLB is a variant of Alzheimer's disease (AD), fascinating new data are emerging which enlarge upon the relationship between DLB and Parkinson's disease (PD). New clinical associations have been described, early validation data for clinical diagnosis are emerging and the first controlled treatment studies are under way.

GENETICS

A number of studies have found an increased frequency of the apolipoprotein $\epsilon 4$ allele in DLB (Pickering-Brown *et al.*, 1994; Harrington *et al.*, 1994; St Clair *et al.*, 1994; Galasko *et al.*, 1994). Because of its (albeit complex) association with AD these seem to support the hypothesis that DLB is a variant of AD (Hansen *et al.*, 1990). Harrington and colleagues' (1994) study showed that while DLB cases (named senile dementia of the Lewy body type by these authors) had similar frequencies of the $\epsilon 4$ allele to that found in AD cases, they had no significant tau pathology. A second group have confirmed this observation (Strong *et al.*, 1995). The link with AD was further strengthened by the finding of cortical and brainstem Lewy bodies in two members of a family with the 717 (Val to IIe) mutation of the amyloid precursor protein gene (Lantos *et al.*, 1994).

A number of studies suggest that genetic polymorphism of the cytochrome P450 CYP2D6 gene is associated with increased susceptibility to PD (Planté-Bordeneuve *et al.*, 1994; Smith *et al.*, 1992). Saitoh *et al.* (1995) were the first to report an overrepresentation of the mutant CYP2D6 B allele in DLB, an observation now confirmed by a further report (Tanaka *et al.*, 1998), but Rempfer *et al.*, (1994) did not confirm the association. In an intriguing study of predictors of dementia in PD, Hubble *et al.* (1998) report that exposure to pesticides and at least one copy of the CYP2D6 2aB+ allele had a 83% predicted probability of PD and dementia.

Familial autosomal-dominant DLB has now been reported by a Japanese group (Wakabayashi *et al.*, 1998) and Denson *et al.* (1997) have found DLB in the only autopsied case from a family affected by parkinsonism with dementia.

Alpha-synuclein

Alpha-synuclein was first discovered in 1993 by Uéda and colleagues (1993). It is a 35-amino acid peptide isolated from a preparation of Alzheimer's brain amyloid, different in sequence to β-amyloid. This group named it the non-Aβ component of Alzheimer amyloid (NAC). They also cloned a 140-amino acid precursor (NACP). The role of the synucleins remains to be established. Spillantini *et al.* (1997, 1998) have recently reported that Lewy bodies and Lewy neurites in both PD and DLB contain α-synuclein. These observations have been confirmed by others (Irizarry *et al.*, 1998; Baba *et al.*, 1998).

Polymeropoulos *et al.* (1997) have reported a mutation in the α-synuclein gene in an Italian family with PD. Others have found either no such association (Vaughan *et al.*, 1998) or very infrequent association in familial PD (Chan *et al.*, 1998). The interpretation of these genetic findings awaits further clarification.

CLINICAL SYMPTOMS

Despite the nosological debate the clinical symptoms of DLB continue to be relatively coherent. From early reports the combination of dementia (with or without specific features) and parkinsonism was recognized. The consensus criteria (McKeith *et al.*, 1996) are shown in Table 1. Early data from the Medical Research Council (MRC) study in Newcastle upon Tyne indicate satisfactory validity of the criteria, albeit in a selected series (Ballard, 1998).

Table 1. Consensus criteria for clinical diagnosis of probable and possible dementia with Lewy bodies (DLB).

1) The central feature required for a diagnosis of DLB is progressive cognitive decline of sufficient magnitude to interfere with normal social or occupational function. Prominent or persistent memory impairment may not necessarily occur in the early stages but is usually evident with progression. Deficits on tests of attention and of frontal-subcortical skills and visuospatial ability may be especially prominent.
2) Two of the following core features are essential for a diagnosis of probable DLB, and one is essential for possible DLB:
   a) Fluctuating cognition with pronounced variations in attention and alertness
   b) Recurrent visual hallucinations that are typically well formed and detailed
   c) Spontaneous motor features of parkinsonism
3) Features supportive of the diagnosis are:
   a) Repeated falls
   b) Syncope
   c) Transient loss of consciousness
   d) Neuroleptic sensitivity
   e) Systematized delusions
   f) Hallucinations in other modalities
4) A diagnosis of DLB is less likely in the presence of:
   a) Stroke disease, evident as focal neurologic signs or on brain imaging
   b) Evidence on physical examination and investigation of any physical illness or other brain disorder sufficient to account for the clinical picture

Source: McKeith *et al.*, 1996.

Parkinsonism

The European Study of Parkinsonism (de Rijk *et al.*, 1997) gives an indication of the prevalence of parkinsonism and PD in community elderly populations (two of the five studies screened total elderly populations) (Table 2). Only 5% of cases of parkinsonism were thought to be drug-induced while 9% arose in association with dementia and 14% were unspecified. It can

Table 2. Prevalence of parkinsonism and Parkinson's disease (per 100 000 population).

Age	Parkinsonism	Parkinson's disease
65–69	0.9	0.6
70–74	1.5	1.0
75–79	3.5	2.7
80–84	5.0	3.6
85–89	5.1	3.5

Source: de Rijk *et al.*, 1997.

reasonably be assumed that some of these cases are DLB and therefore that the prevalence of DLB does not exceed 14%.

The majority of cases of DLB develop parkinsonism at some point in the course of their illness (Lennox, 1992). Early studies (reviewed by Byrne, 1995) suggested that the parkinsonism was mild and not responsive to levodopa. In post-mortem-diagnosed cases of pure DLB (no evidence of Alzheimer neuritic pathology) Hely *et al.* (1996) found that five out of nine cases who presented with levodopa-responsive parkinsonism developed dementia within a mean of three years of presentation. Two cases of the nine presented with parkinsonism and dementia and the remaining two cases with dementia developed parkinsonism later.

In clinically diagnosed cases, Gnanalingham *et al.* (1997) found the motor features of DLB cases to be similar to PD and the neuropsychological features to be similar to AD (Table 3). Both Crystal *et al.* (1990) and Ala *et al.* (1997) suggest that extrapyramidal features early in the course of a dementia syndrome are more likely to be found in DLB cases. The disparity in the reports of extrapyramidal features in DLB (their severity and levodopa responsiveness) may lie in part in variability of the age of the patients (Hely and colleagues' (1996) cases were all under 70 years at presentation and Kosaka's (1990) type I cases (with levodopa-responsive parkinsonism) were all young), and in part on the degree of Alzheimer change in the brain. Weiner and colleagues' (1996) post-mortem study is an example. They looked at Lewy-body-variant AD cases (using Hansen *et al.'s* (1990) criteria) and compared them to 'pure' AD cases (using CERAD criteria). They found no difference in the extrapyramidal features between the two

Table 3. Motor and neuropsychological features in clinically diagnosed cases of dementia with Lewy bodies (DLB), Alzheimer's disease (AD), Parkinson's disease (PD) and normal controls.

Features (a)	Controls (n=20)	AD (n=22–25)	PD (n=15)	DLB (n=12–16)	F-ratio (f=68)
Total motor score (UPDRS)	1.0 (0.2)	5.9 (1)	29.5 (4)**††	38.3 (3)**‡‡	f=68 p < 0.001
Digit span:					
Forward	6.2 (0.3)	4.2 (0.4)**	6.1 (0.4)††	3.7 (0.5)**‡‡	f=11
Reverse	4.0 (0.3)	2.2 (0.4)**	4.2 (0.5)††	2.1 (0.4)**‡‡	p < 0.001
Verbal fluency	32.1 (3)	9.2 (2)**	21.0 (5)††**	8.3 (2)**‡‡	f=14 p > 0.0001

Note: Values are means (SEM). One-way ANCOVA, with Cornell Scale for Depression in Dementia scores as co-variates and *post hoc* Duncan's multiple range test.
Post hoc comparisons: *$p < 0.05$; **$p < 0.01$ vs controls; ††$p < 0.01$ vs AD, ‡‡$p < 0.01$ vs PD.
UPDRS, Unified Parkinson's Disease Rating Scale.
Source: Gnanalingham *et al.*, 1997.

groups. A further, but as yet speculative, explanation for the disparity in findings between groups is gender. In the literature on DLB (where gender is specified) there is a male preponderance; however, these are often highly selected series. Intriguingly Disshan and Dluzen (1997) have shown a dose-dependent modifying effect of oestradiol on MPTP-induced neurotoxicity. MPTP is metabolized to MPP+. When oestradiol (dose 300 nM) was infused with MPP+ into striatal tissue from ovariectomized rats the release of dopamine was significantly attenuated.

Gender has been recently reported as modifying phenotypic expression and the effects of treatment in other forms of dementia. Raghavan *et al.* (1994) reported on the phenotypic expression of Alzheimer's disease (at post-mortem) in people with Down's syndrome (trisomy 21) whose cognitive function had been prospectively assessed. They found that female Down's syndrome individuals had an earlier onset of dementia with higher neuro-cortical neurofibrillary tangle (NFT) counts rather than senile plaque (SP) density compared to males. Farlow *et al.* (1998) found that ApoE genotype (ε4) in women, but not in men, was significantly associated with poor response to treatment with tacrine in AD subjects.

Dementia

Previous reviews of the nature of the cognitive changes in DLB reflect the small case series and, as with extrapyramidal symptoms (EPS) in DLB, disparate findings (Byrne, 1996; Salmon and Galasko, 1996). Most comparisons have been made with AD cases, some earlier studies showing close similarities to neuropsychological function in DLB and AD and others clear differences. More recent studies are slightly less disparate in their findings and are larger, with clear methods of case identification. The rate of cognitive decline in DLB compared with AD has been carefully examined by Olichney *et al.* (1998). One hundred and forty-eight AD cases and 40 DLB cases were diagnosed according to the CERAD protocol. All had had serial Mini-Mental State Examination (MMSE) scores in life.

At baseline the mean MMSE scores were not significantly different, but intergroup differences were significant at one, two and three years later (1.8 points, 4.2 points and 5.6 points, respectively) with DLB cases declining more. Two studies have found significant differences between DLB cases and AD cases on the clock-drawing test (CDT) (Salmon and Galasko, 1996; Gnanalingham *et al.*, 1996). Using the Libon *et al.* (1993) version of the CDT, where subjects are first asked to draw a clock to command and then to copy a standard clock, both studies found the DLB subjects did not improve their scores on the 'copy' part of the test whereas both control subjects and AD cases did so.

Swanwick *et al.* (1996) found a similar pattern of 'copy' ≤ 'draw' in their clinically diagnosed AD cases. The proportion of cases with this pattern in this group (9%) is similar to reported rates of DLB in post-mortem studies of AD cases using the same diagnostic criteria (Burns *et al.*, 1990). While most recent autopsy-diagnosed case series comparing DLB and AD find no differences in overall dementia rating scale scores, all have found differences in subscale scores (Weiner *et al.*, 1996; Connor *et al.*, 1998). For example, Connor *et al.* (1998) found AD cases performed significantly worse on the memory subscale of the Mathis dementia rating scale than did DLB cases, whereas the DLB cases performed significantly worse on the Initiation/Perseveration subscale than the AD cases. The clinically diagnosed recent series (Walker *et al.*, 1997; Gnanalingham *et al.*, 1997) have disparate findings (although both series used the same diagnostic criteria for their clinical groups). These may, however, reflect the difference in neuropsychological tests which were used.

Walker *et al.* (1997) used the CAMCOG subscale scores to compare DLB and AD cases; they found significant differences in the visuospatial praxis subscale (AD > DLB) and recall subscale (AD < DLB). Gnanalingham *et al.* (1997) found no differences between DLB and AD cases on tests of verbal fluency, digit span, or the Nelson card sort test.

Noncognitive features

Noncognitive features in DLB are frequent and troublesome. There is a growing consensus that early (and, some say, persistent) hallucinations in the context of a dementia syndrome are predictive of post-mortem diagnosis of DLB. McShane *et al.* (1996) found that in 24 cases with dementia who had hallucinations (at any time in their course) and who had undergone autopsy, those with early-onset hallucinations were significantly more likely to have cortical Lewy bodies than those with late-onset hallucinations. In pure DLB seven of nine cases had hallucinations (Hely *et al.*, 1996), a figure similar to the frequency in the post-mortem study of Weiner *et al.* (1996) in which 64% of the DLB cases had hallucinations compared with 21% of the AD cases.

While depression and delusions are common in DLB, there is no clear evidence that either is more common or different in expression in DLB compared with AD.

Another noncognitive feature which is emerging as a probable distinctive feature of DLB is rapid eye movement sleep behaviour disorder (RBD). RBD is 'a parasomnia defined by intermittent loss of electromyographic atonia during REM sleep with emergence of complex and vigorous behaviours' (Schenck *et al.*, 1987).

A small number of case reports (Turner *et al.*, 1997; Schenck *et al.*, 1997) reported the association of RBD and the development of a dementia fulfilling clinical criteria for DLB. In one case (Schenck *et al.*, 1997) DLB was confirmed at autopsy. Boeve *et al.* (1998) report a series of 37 cases with

RBD in association with dementia, who were examined by polysomnography. Thirty-four (92%) of these cases fulfilled clinical diagnostic criteria for DLB and all three autopsied cases had cortical Lewy bodies. These patients are predominantly male. In Schenck and colleagues' (1987) series the RBD was successfully treated with clonazepam or desipramine. Sleep disorders are common in the author's prospective series of DLB cases (Byrne, 1996).

TREATMENT

The majority of treatment approaches in DLB are empirical (Byrne, 1999). Most clinicians are now aware of the hazards of conventional neuroleptics in dementia, especially in DLB. The 'novel' neuroleptics are not without hazard: while risperidone and clozapine have been used successfully in the treatment of DLB (Lee *et al.*, 1994; Geroldi *et al.*, 1997), adverse side-effects of both these drugs have been reported even in small doses (McKeith *et al.*, 1995; Burke *et al.*, 1998).

Similar problems are reported with the use of levodopa to treat the parkinsonian symptoms. While some patients have benefit, with improvement in EPS and no worsening of mental state (Williams *et al.*, 1993) others have no improvement in EPS and worsening of noncognitive features (Kuzuhara *et al.*, 1996). Low doses of levodopa with slow titration are likely to be the most successful treatment.

Other medications with reported benefit are chlormethiazole (Byrne, 1999) and carbamazepine (Lebert *et al.*, 1996). The first multicentre trial of the anticholinesterase rivastigmine is nearing completion. Eleven patients have entered the open phase of treatment with encouraging improvement in noncognitive symptoms and in parkinsonism.

CONCLUSION

The study of DLB continues to produce controversial findings but enhances our knowledge of two common neurodegenerative diseases, Alzheimer's disease and Parkinson's disease. The clinical challenges posed by relief of troublesome symptoms are likely to result in benefit for all dementia sufferers.

REFERENCES

Ala, T.A., Yang, K.-H., Sung, J.-H. and Frey, W.H. (1997). Hallucinations and signs of parkinsonism help distinguish patients with dementia and cortical Lewy bodies from patients with Alzheimer's disease at presentation: a clinicopathological study. *J Neurol Neurosurg Psychiatry* **62**, 16–21.

Baba, M., Nakajo, S., Tu, P.H. *et al.* (1998). Aggregation of alpha-synuclein in Lewy bodies of sporadic Parkinson's disease and dementia with Lewy bodies. *Am J Pathol* **152**, 879–884.

Ballard, C. (1998). Dementia with Lewy bodies commentary. *Adv Psychiatr Treatm* **4**, 366–368.

Boeve, B.F., Silber, M.H., Ferman, T.J. *et al.* (1998). REM sleep behaviour disorder and degenerative dementia: an association likely reflecting Lewy body disease. *Neurology* **51**, 363–370.

Burke, W.J., Pfeipfer, R.F. and McComb, R.D. (1998). Neuroleptic sensitivity to clozapine in dementia with Lewy bodies. *J Neuropsychiatry Clin Neurosci* **10**, 227–229.

Burns, A., Luthert, P., Levy, R., Jacoby, R. and Lantos, P. (1990). Accuracy of clinical diagnosis of Alzheimer's disease. *BMJ* **301**, 1026.

Byrne, E.J. (1995). Cortical Lewy body disease: an alternative view. In: Levy, R. and Howard, R. (eds), *Developments in Dementia and Functional Disorders in the Elderly*. Wrightson, Petersfield, pp. 21–30.

Byrne, E.J. (1996). The nature of the cognitive decline in Lewy body dementia. In: Perry, R., McKeith, I. and Perry, E. (eds), *Dementia with Lewy Bodies*. Cambridge University Press, Cambridge, pp. 57–66.

Byrne, E.J. (1999). Treatment of dementia with Lewy bodies. In: O'Brien, J., Ames, D. and Burns, A. (Eds), *Dementia*. Edward Arnold, London (in press).

Chan, P., Tanner, C.M., Jiang, X. and Langston, J.W. (1998). Failure to find the alpha-synuclein gene missense mutation (G209A) in 100 patients with younger onset Parkinson's disease. *Neurology* **50**, 513–514.

Connor, D.J., Salmon, D.P., Sandy, T.J., Galasko, D., Hansen, L.A. and Thal, L.J. (1998). Cognitive profiles of autopsy-confirmed Lewy body variant vs pure Alzheimer disease. *Arch Neurol* **55**, 994–1000.

Crystal, H.A., Dickson, D.W., Lizardi, J.E., Davies, P. and Wolfson, L.I. (1990). Antemortem diagnosis of diffuse Lewy body disease. *Neurology* **40**, 1523–1528.

de Rijk, M.C., Tzourio, C., Breteler, M.M.B. *et al.* (1997). Prevalence of parkinsonism and Parkinson's disease in Europe: the EUROPARKINSON collaborative study. *J Neurol Neurosurg Psychiatry* **62**, 10–15.

Denson, M.A., Wszolek, Z.K., Pfeiffer, R.F., Wszolek, E.K., Paschall, T.M. and McComb, R.D. (1997). Familial parkinsonism, dementia and Lewy body disease: study of family G. *Ann Neurol* **42**, 638–643.

Disshan, K.A. and Dluzen, D.E. (1997). Estragon as a neuromodulater of MPTP-induced neurotoxicity: effects upon striatal dopamine release. *Brain Res* **764**, 9–16.

Farlow, M.R., Lahiri, D.K., Poirier, J., Davignon, J., Schneider, L. and Hui, S.L. (1998). Treatment outcome of tacrine therapy depends on apolipoprotein genotype and gender of the subjects with Alzheimer's disease. *Neurology* **50**, 669–677.

Galasko, D., Hansen, L.A., Katzman, R. *et al.* (1994). Clinical-neuropathological correlations in Alzheimer's disease and related dementias. *Arch Neurol* **51**, 888–895.

Geroldi, C., Frisoni, G.B., Bianchetti, A. and Trabucchi, M. (1997). Drug treatment in Lewy body dementia. *Dement Geriatr Cogn Disord* **8**, 188–197.

Gnanalingham, K.K., Byrne, E.J. and Thornton, A. (1996). Clock-face drawing to differentiate Lewy body and Alzheimer type dementia syndrome. *Lancet* **347** 696–697.

Gnanalingham, K.K., Byrne, E.J., Thornton, A., Sambrook, M.A. and Bannester, P. (1997). Motor and cognitive function in Lewy body dementia: comparison with Alzheimer's and Parkinson's disease. *J Neurol Neurosurg Psychiatry* **62**, 243–252.

Hansen, L.A. (1996). Tautological tangles in neuropathologic criteria for dementias associated with Lewy bodies. In: Perry, R., McKeith, I. and Perry, E. (eds), *Dementia with Lewy Bodies*. Cambridge University Press, Cambridge, pp. 204–211.

Hansen, L.A., Salmon, D., Galasko, D. *et al.* (1990). The Lewy body variant of Alzheimer's disease: a clinical and pathologic entity. *Neurology* **40**, 1–8.

Harrington, C.R., Louwagie, J., Rossau, R. *et al.* (1994). Influence of apolipoprotein E genotype on senile dementia of the Alzheimer and Lewy body types. Significance for etiological theories of Alzheimer's disease. *Am J Pathol* **145**, 1472–1484.

Hely, M.A., Reid, W.G., Halliday, G.M. *et al.* (1996). Diffuse Lewy body disease: clinical features in nine cases without co-existent Alzheimer's disease. *J Neurol Neurosurg Psychiatry* **60**, 531–538.

Hubble, J.P., Kurth, J.H., Glatt, S.L. *et al.* (1998). Gene-toxin interaction as a putative risk factor for Parkinson's disease with dementia. *Neuroepidemiology* **17**, 96–104.

Irizarry, M.C., Growdon, W., Gomez-Isla, T. *et al.* (1998). Nigral and cortical Lewy bodies and dystrophic Lewy body disease contain alpha-synuclein immunoreactivity. *J Neuropath Exp Neurol* **57**, 334–337.

Kosaka, K. (1990). Diffuse Lewy body disease in Japan. *J Neurol* **237**, 197–204.

Kuzuhara, S., Yoshimura, M., Mizukani, T., Yamanouchi, H. and Ihara, Y. (1996). Clinical features of diffuse Lewy body disease in the elderly: analysis of 12 cases. In: Perry, R., McKeith, I. and Perry, E. (eds), *Dementia with Lewy Bodies*. Cambridge University Press, Cambridge, pp. 153–160.

Lantos, P.L., Ovenstane, I.M., Johnson, J., Clelland, C.A., Rogues, P. and Rossor, M.N. (1994). Lewy bodies in the brain of two members of a family with the 717 (Val to IIe) mutation of the amyloid precursor protein gene. *Neurosci Lett* **172**, 77–79.

Lebert, F., Souliez, L. and Pasquier, F. (1996). Tacrine and symptomatic treatment. In: Perry, R., McKeith, I. and Perry, E. (eds), *Dementia with Lewy Bodies*. Cambridge University Press, Cambridge, pp. 439–448.

Lee, H., Cooney, J.M. and Lawlor, B.A. (1994). Case report: the use of risperidone, an atypical neuroleptic in Lewy body disease. *Int J Geriatr Psychiatry* **9**, 415–417.

Lennox, G. (1992). Lewy body dementia. *Baillière's Clin Neurol* **1**, 653–676/

Libon, D.J., Swanson, R.A. and Baronski, E.J. (1993). Clock drawing as an assessment tool for dementia. *Arch Clin Neuropsychol* **8**, 405–415.

McKeith, I.G., Harrison, R.W.S. and Ballard, C.G. (1995). Neuroleptic sensitivity to risperidone in Lewy body dementia. *Lancet* **346**, 699.

McKeith, I.G., Galasko, D., Kosaka, K. *et al.* (1996). Consensus guidelines for the clinical and pathologic diagnosis of dementia with Lewy bodies (DLB): report of the consortium on DLB international workshop. *Neurology* **47**, 1113–1124.

McShane, R., Keene, J., Gedling, K. and Hope, T. (1996). Hallucinations, cortical Lewy body pathology, cognitive function and neuroleptic use in dementia. In: Perry, R., McKeith, I. and Perry, E. (eds), *Dementia with Lewy Bodies*. Cambridge University Press, Cambridge, pp. 85–98.

Olichney, J.M., Galasko, D., Salmon, D.P. *et al.* (1998). Cognitive decline is faster in Lewy body variant than in Alzheimer's disease. *Neurology* **51**, 351–357.

Pickering-Brown, S.M., Mann, D.M.A., Bourke, J.P. *et al.* (1994). Apolipoprotein E4 and Alzheimer's disease pathology in Lewy body diseases and in other β-amyloid forming diseases. *Lancet* **343**, 1155.

Planté-Bordeneuve, V., Davis, M.B., Maraganore, D.M., Marsden, C.M. and Harding, A.E. (1994). Debrisoquine hydroxylase gene polymorphism in familial Parkinson's disease. *J Neurol Neurosurg Psychiatry* **57**, 911–913.

Polymeropoulos, M.H., Lavedan, C., Leroy, E. *et al.* (1997). Mutation on the alpha-synuclein gene identified in families with Parkinson's disease. *Science* **276**, 2045–2047.

Raghavan, R., Khin-Nu, C., Brown, A.G. *et al.* (1994). Gender differences in the phenotypic expression of Alzheimer's disease in Down's syndrome (trisomy 21). *Neuroreport* **5**, 1393–1396.

Rempfer, R., Crook, R., Houlden, H. *et al.* (1994). Parkinson's disease but not Alzheimer's disease, Lewy body variant associated with mutant alleles at cytochrome Ph50 gene. *Lancet* **344**, 815.

Saitoh, T., Xia, Y., Chen, X. *et al.* (1995). The CYP2D6B mutant allele is overrepresented in the Lewy body variant. *Ann Neurol* **37**, 110–112.

Salmon, D.P. and Galasko, D. (1996). Neuropsychological aspects of Lewy body dementia. In: Perry, R., McKeith, I. and Perry, E. (eds), *Dementia with Lewy Bodies*. Cambridge University Press, Cambridge, pp. 99–113.

Schenck, C.H., Bundle, S.R., Patterson, A.L. and Mahowald, N.W. (1987). Rapid eye movement sleep behaviour disorder. *J Am Med Assoc* **257**, 1786–1789.

Schenck, C.H., Mahowald, M.W., Anderson, M.L., Silber, M.H., Boeve, B.F. and Parisi, J.E. (1997). Lewy body variant of Alzheimer's disease (AD) identified by post-mortem ubiquitin staining in a previously reported case of AD associated with REM sleep behaviour disorder. *Biol Psychiatry* **42**, 527–528.

Smith, C.A.D., Gough, A.C., Leigh, P.N. *et al.* (1992). Debrisoquine hydroxylase gene polymorphism and susceptibility to Parkinson's disease. *Lancet* **339**, 1375–1377.

Spillantini, M.G., Schmidt, M.L., Lee, V.M.-Y., Trofanowski, J.Q., Jakes, R. and Goedert, M. (1997). Synuclein in Lewy bodies. *Nature* **388**, 839–840.

Spillantini, M.G., Crowther, R.A., Jakes, R., Hasegara, M. and Goldert, M. (1998). Alpha-synuclein in filamentous inclusions of Lewy bodies from Parkinson's disease and dementia with Lewy bodies. *Proc Natl Acad Sci U S A* **95**, 6469–6473.

St Clair, D., Norman, J., Perry, R., Yates, C., Wilcock, G. and Brookes, A. (1994). Apolipoprotein E4 allele frequency in patients with Lewy body dementia, Alzheimer's disease and age matched controls. *Neurosci Lett* **176**, 45–46.

Strong, C., Anderton, B.H., Perry, R.H., Perry, E.K., Ince, P.G. and Lovestone, S. (1995). Abnormally phosphorylated tau protein in senile dementia of Lewy body type and Alzheimer's disease: evidence that the disorders are distinct. *Alzheimer Dis Assoc Disord* **9**, 218–222.

Swanwick, G.R.J., Coen, R.F., Maguire, C.P., Coakley, D. and Lawlor, B.A. (1996). Clock-face drawing to differentiate dementia syndrome. *Lancet* **347**, 1115.

Tanaka, S., Chen, X., Xia, Y. *et al.* (1998). Association of CYP2D microsatellite polymorphism with Lewy body variant of Alzheimer's disease. *Neurology* **50**, 1556–1562.

Turner, R.S., Chervin, R.D., Frey, K.A., Minoshima, S. and Kuhl, D.E. (1997). Probable diffuse Lewy body disease presenting as REM sleep behaviour disorder. *Neurology* **49**, 523–527.

Uéda, K., Fukushima, H., Masliah, E. *et al.* (1993). Molecular cloning of cDNA encoding an unrecognised component of amyloid in Alzheimer's disease. *Proc Natl Acad Sci U S A* **90**, 11282–11286.

Vaughan, J., Durr, A., Tassin, J. *et al.* (1998). The alpha synuclein Ala 53 Thr mutation is not a common cause of familial Parkinson's disease: a study of 230 European cases. *Ann Neurol* **44**, 270–273.

Wakabayashi, K., Hayashi, S., Ishikawa, A. *et al.* (1998). Autosomal dominant diffuse Lewy body disease. *Acta Neuropathol (Berl)* **96**, 207–210.

Walker, Z., Allen, R.L., Shergiel, S. and Katona, C.L.E. (1997). Neuropsychological performance in Lewy body dementia and Alzheimer's disease. *Br J Psychiatry* **170**, 156–158.

Weiner, M.F., Risser, R.C., Cullum, M. *et al.* (1996). Alzheimer's disease and its Lewy body variant: a clinical analysis of post-mortem verified cases. *Am J Psychiatry* **153**, 1269–1273.

Williams, S.W., Byrne, E.J. and Stokes, P. (1993). The treatment of diffuse Lewy body disease: a pilot study. *Int J Geriatr Psychiatry* **8**, 731–739.

5

Vascular Disease, Cognitive Impairment and Dementia

ROBERT STEWART

Section of Old Age Psychiatry, Institute of Psychiatry, London, UK

Accumulating epidemiological evidence suggests that conditions underlying cardiovascular and cerebrovascular disease may play an important role in the aetiology of late-life cognitive decline, raising important possibilities for prevention or treatment. Of 'environmental' risk factors for dementia, vascular disease is perhaps becoming the best understood thanks to large population-based studies, although the current conceptual systems underlying the classification of dementia *in vivo* are a hindrance to clear understanding of mechanisms which might be involved. Discussions of the relationship between vascular disease and dementia have tended to start with the diagnosis of 'vascular dementia' and describe the nature of the various syndromes subsumed under that heading. These do not, however, address the question of whether, to what extent and in what ways vascular disease and its principal risk factors affect the risk of developing dementia in later life, an issue which will be focused on in this chapter.

Important and often unacknowledged limitations due to inadequate or biased measurement of both exposure (vascular disease) and outcome (dementia/cognitive impairment) measures must be borne in mind before conclusions can be drawn from research findings. A substantial proportion of cardiovascular disease is undiagnosed and reliance on a history or not of a disorder may be an inadequate measure. The same applies to disorders which are risk factors for vascular disease (e.g. hypertension) but which often involve a somewhat arbitrary cut-off on a continuously distributed physiological parameter (e.g. recorded blood pressure), the issue here being not only whether to screen for the 'disorder' but also how extensively and invasively to investigate the physiological parameter (e.g. single or repeated blood pressure recordings, 24-hour ambulatory measures, orthostatic measures, etc.). An additional difficulty is that vascular risk factors are known to be closely associated and it may therefore be difficult to draw independent conclusions about the role of a specific disorder (e.g. of hypertension independent of glucose intolerance, lipid abnormalities, insulin resistance, etc.).

From a clinical perspective, what is most important as an outcome measure is the effect vascular disease or its risk factors may have on the chances of developing dementia. However, the use of dementia as an outcome has major drawbacks. The chief of these is that the classification system for dementia used in clinical and epidemiological research is underpinned (a) by a concept of vascular disease causing 'vascular dementia' (VaD) with inherent assumptions about mechanisms of causation; (b) by a concept of Alzheimer's disease (AD) as a diagnosis of exclusion, particularly with regard to vascular disease; and (c) by a dichotomous distinction between the two diagnoses, therefore introducing bias in aetiological research through categorizing, at least partly, by presumed aetiology. An aetiological study which uses VaD as an outcome is not only measuring factors associated with dementia but also those associated with cerebrovascular disease because both are part of the diagnosis. Similarly, a comparison using strictly defined AD may mask associations with vascular disease because these have been excluded as part of the diagnosis.

An additional drawback with dementia as an outcome measure is that it is a relatively late stage in an evolving process of cognitive decline where this has become severe enough to be associated with impaired function, and a study of potential risk factors, particularly those associated with increased mortality, may wish to examine earlier interactions. One alternative is to investigate effects of vascular disorders on cognitive function as estimated by psychometric assessment. This has the advantage of being relatively objective and feasible at ages where dementia is too rare an outcome to be picked up in adequate numbers but where opportunities may exist for preventative interventions and where mortality associated with vascular disorders has had less opportunity to dilute associations. However, performance on psychometric tests is heavily influenced by educational and social factors and large numbers are needed to allow adjustment for these. Prospective studies with repeated psychometric tests are advantageous in that individual cognitive change is measured rather than relative performance, thus minimizing educational confounding, but the cohort size and follow-up period still need to be adequate enough to see beyond random fluctuations over time to true cognitive decline, and it has to be established that observed effects on cognitive decline ultimately have some predictive value for a clinical outcome such as dementia.

EPIDEMIOLOGICAL FINDINGS

Stroke

One way of getting around the difficulties with 'vascular' dementia as a diagnosis and its aetiological assumptions has been to study subjects known to have cerebrovascular disease and examine the differences between those who do and do not develop dementia. Acute stroke has now been well established as a risk factor for subsequent dementia with studies assessing subjects three months after a stroke finding broadly consistent rates of dementia between 20 and 30%, representing an approximately ninefold increase in risk compared with controls (Tatemichi *et al.*, 1992; Loeb *et al.*, 1992; Kokmen *et al.*, 1996; Censori *et al.*, 1996; Pohjasvaara *et al.*, 1998). Risks of dementia after the three-month period have also been shown to remain significantly raised but to a lesser extent (Tatemichi *et al.*, 1994; Kokmen *et al.*, 1996). Co-morbid disorders as risk factors for poststroke dementia will be discussed in later sections of this chapter. With regard to features of the stroke episode, the follow-up studies of Tatemichi *et al.* (1993) and Pohjasvaara *et al.* (1998) both report dominant and supratentorial lesions to be associated with increased risk, although further breakdown into arterial territories affected has not yet produced consistent conclusions. Both studies also found previous cerebrovascular disease to be a risk factor and included subjects with one or more previous strokes. The study of Censori *et al.* (1996) of first-stroke-only cases reported subsequent dementia to be associated particularly with middle cerebral artery infarctions and with frontal lobe lesions on computerized tomography (CT).

While the impact of stroke on dementia incidence has been established, elucidating the type of dementia and underlying mechanisms becomes complicated by the system of classification mentioned earlier, with a history of stroke being an exclusion factor for 'probable AD' as a clinical diagnosis. However, it has been noted that a substantial proportion of dementia cases following acute stroke subsequently follow an AD-like clinical course (Kokmen *et al.*, 1996) and that dementia develops in the absence of further clinical stroke or depressive illness in approximately 75% of cases (Tatemichi *et al.*, 1994). Whether possible increased rates of AD are newly 'induced' disease or previous subclinical disease precipitated by stroke cannot yet be concluded. The Framingham Study reported that stroke cases had had previously worse Mini-Mental State Examination (MMSE) scores compared with non-cases but that the gap widened after the stroke episode and that the stroke itself was related to subsequent cognitive decline (Kase *et al.*, 1998), favouring a 'precipitation' mechanism but with common factors possibly underlying both the prestroke cognitive impairment and the stroke episode itself (White, 1996).

Atherosclerotic disease

Surprisingly little research has examined indices of systemic atherosclerotic disease in relation to cognitive impairment or dementia, most studies going no further than to ask about a history of ischaemic heart disease or myocardial infarction, vascular 'outcome' measures which do not provide an adequate reflection of underlying disease and whose associated mortality will result in underestimation of disease in age ranges of interest with respect to dementia. Electrocardiographic (ECG) ischaemia has been found to be associated with significant decline in performance on a memory test in subjects with a history of hypertension and with incident AD in the same population, the latter risk falling just outside conventional significance levels (Prince *et al.*, 1994). A more broad categorization of ECG abnormalities, however, did not predict incident dementia, either AD or VaD, in the prospective Hisayama Study (Yoshitake *et al.*, 1995). The Rotterdam Study quantified atherosclerotic disease using ankle–brachial blood pressure ratios and carotid ultrasound indices, reporting that increased disease was significantly associated with prevalent dementia and with both AD and VaD subtypes (Hofman *et al.*, 1997). This study also investigated atrial fibrillation as an exposure, finding significant associations with dementia, chiefly in women and stronger in younger subjects, although remaining significant in older groups when subjects with a history of stroke were excluded. The subtype of dementia most strongly associated with atrial fibrillation was AD with unrelated cerebrovascular disease rather than VaD (Ott *et al.*, 1997a).

Hypertension

Several large studies have now shown that raised blood pressure in mid-life is associated prospectively with worse cognitive function 20–25 years later (Elias *et al.*, 1993; Launer *et al.*, 1995; Kilander *et al.*, 1998) and that this effect is independent of other associated disease such as type 2 diabetes, although the two conditions appear to have a multiplicative interaction (Elias *et al.*, 1997). Cross-sectional associations of cognitive function with blood pressure levels have produced more conflicting findings and this appears to be because of a crossing-over of association from mid to late life, cognitive impairment being associated with raised blood pressure up to around age 75 and with lower blood pressure in older age groups. This has been suggested by the Framingham and Rotterdam studies (Farmer *et al.*, 1987; Breteler *et al.*, 1993b) and suggests that smaller studies with too broad an age range may fail to show an association between blood pressure and cognitive impairment because of opposing group effects. Interestingly, in a study of older subjects in good physical health, an association between raised blood pressure and cognitive impairment was still evident (Starr *et al.*, 1993) and the Rotterdam Study found that the association with low blood pressure in older subjects was principally in those with evidence of more severe atherosclerosis (Breteler *et al.*, 1993b). Co-morbid physical illness has been suggested as a confounding factor in the observed association between low blood pressure and increased mortality in later life (Boshuizen *et al.*, 1998) and the same may be true for cognitive impairment.

Case–control studies examining associations between hypertension and dementia are of limited generalizability because of the selected nature of cases and the classification bias discussed above. Considering population-based research, the prospective Hisayama Study reported an increased incidence of VaD over seven years associated with raised blood pressure at entry (Yoshitake *et al.*, 1995). However, the Kungsholmen Study found lower blood pressure cross-sectionally associated with VaD in over-75s (Guo *et al.*, 1996) and poststroke studies have either found no association with blood pressure and subsequent dementia (Censori *et al.*, 1996; Tatemichi *et al.*, 1993) or associations with *lower* blood pressure (Pohjasvaara *et al.*, 1998). Of cross-sectional population studies examining AD as an outcome, an association with raised blood pressure was reported by the Kuopio Study of 69–78-year-olds (Kuusisto *et al.*, 1997) and one with lower blood pressure by the Kungsholmen Study of 75–101-year-olds (Guo *et al.*, 1996). Two prospective studies with five- and seven-year follow-up periods found no association between blood pressure and AD incidence (Katzman *et al.*, 1989; Yoshitake *et al.*, 1995) although another suggested a raised risk associated with very high systolic blood pressure levels (>190 mmHg) in subjects without a family history of dementia (Prince *et al.*, 1994). The Göteborg Study, a 15-year follow-up study, however, reported that subjects who developed AD between the ages of 80 and 85 had had significantly higher systolic blood pressures at age 75 but had lower current blood pressures than those who did not develop dementia (Skoog *et al.*, 1996a), suggesting a crossing-over of association, similar to that seen in cognitive impairment studies.

What is apparent from epidemiological research is that raised blood pressure is a risk factor for future cognitive impairment and dementia in later life, large studies with long follow-up periods being required to demonstrate this association. The 'direction' of the later association of lower blood pressure with dementia cannot be concluded from epidemiological findings so far but possible mechanisms will be discussed later in this chapter. An important issue is whether iatrogenic lowering of blood pressure can worsen cognitive impairment – evidence so far points to little effect of antihypertensive medication on either cognitive decline or dementia (Prince *et al.*, 1996; Skoog *et al.*, 1996b) although adverse effects in 'at risk' subgroups cannot be ruled out. Similar questions are raised by research into the association between low blood pressure and increased mortality later in life

(Mattila *et al.*, 1988) and progress in this field of physical medicine may usefully inform a relatively neglected area of dementia research.

Type 2 diabetes

Case–control studies comparing subjects with and without diabetes have generally found relative impairment on psychometric tests but have been conflicting in their findings as to the extent of impairment or cognitive domains affected (Strachan *et al.*, 1997). Population-based studies have, on the whole, confirmed these findings using both global measures such as the MMSE and psychometric test batteries (Launer *et al.*, 1993; Kilander *et al.*, 1997; van Boxtel *et al.*, 1998). Relatively little attention, however, has been given to whether these associations are specific to diabetes or related to other co-morbid conditions. The Framingham Study found that a diagnosis of diabetes and duration of diabetes were both significantly associated with poor performance on memory and abstract reasoning tests 28–30 years later, independent of other risk factors for vascular disease, but that impairment on a test of visual memory and on composite scores derived from the psychometric test battery were only associated with diabetes in hypertensive subjects (Elias *et al.*, 1997), indicating potentially important interactions between these two common conditions in predicting cognitive impairment.

Cross-sectional population studies have reported a significant association between diabetes and 'dementia' (Ott *et al.*, 1996), a small association between diabetes and VaD (Lindsay *et al.*, 1997), and increased AD in type 2 diabetic subjects receiving insulin treatment (Ott *et al.*, 1996). Prospective results from the Hisayama and Rotterdam studies have in addition shown that subjects with type 2 diabetes have an increased risk of developing dementia, and findings from both suggest that this raised risk is for both VaD and AD (Yoshitake *et al.*, 1995; Ott *et al.*, 1997b), the Rotterdam Study reporting a particularly strong association in those subjects receiving insulin treatment and also that risks for AD were unaffected by adjustment for other vascular risk factors and indices of atherosclerosis indicating, perhaps, non-vascular mechanisms mediating this association (Ott *et al.*, 1997b). An important question, still unresolved, is the association between glycaemic control and dementia: in particular, whether it is prolonged hyperglycaemia, episodic hypoglycaemia, both, or neither which mediates the increased risk of dementia seen particularly in subjects on insulin treatment.

Cholesterol and dyslipidaemia

Evidence for a role of lipid levels in the aetiology of cognitive impairment has been conflicting. Hypercholesterolaemia was found to be associated with memory impairment in a cohort of 249 stroke-free volunteers, independent of other vascular risk factors (Desmond *et al.*, 1993). The Rotterdam Study, however, found no association between total cholesterol levels and MMSE scores in a much larger and population-based sample, but did find that HDL (high-density lipoprotein) cholesterol was positively related to cognitive function, particularly in women (Breteler *et al.*, 1993a). Raised triglyceride levels have been reported to be associated with impaired attentional function in subjects with type 2 diabetes, independent of glycaemic control (Perlmuter *et al.*, 1988), and with impaired composite scores from a cognitive test battery in one population study, although the latter effect fell below significance levels when subjects with stroke were excluded (Kilander *et al.*, 1997).

In research into dementia, dyslipidaemia has been principally assessed by cholesterol levels. Hypercholesterolaemia has not been found to be associated with vascular dementia in most case–control studies (Meyer *et al.*, 1988; Gorelick *et al.*, 1993; Shimano *et al.*, 1989; Mortel *et al.*, 1993), mirroring the uncertain role of cholesterol levels in the aetiology of stroke (Stoy, 1997). Studies examining lipid levels in AD have reported, if anything, lower cholesterol levels in cases (Hofman *et al.*, 1997; Kuusisto *et al.*, 1997). A problem with cross-sectional dementia studies in this respect is that cause and effect cannot be assumed, and metabolic changes in dementia may affect lipid levels. The prospective Hisayama study found that lipid levels did not predict incident dementia, either VaD or AD, in a cohort of 828 subjects over a seven-year follow-up period (Yoshitake *et al.*, 1995). However, the largest study to date examining dementia occurring after acute stroke reported an increased risk associated with hypercholesterolaemia (Pohjasvaara *et al.*, 1998). A recent longitudinal study found that AD cases had had previously raised cholesterol levels 20–30 years earlier, after adjusting for age and apoE genotype, although in men this had decreased prior to clinical manifestations of dementia (Notkola *et al.*, 1998), and the Rotterdam Study reported an increased risk of dementia associated with a diet high in saturated fat and decreased risks of both dementia and AD associated with fish consumption (Kalmijn *et al.*, 1997). What therefore may be emerging is a pattern of association between dyslipidaemia and dementia similar to that of hypertension with positive prospective risk but negative cross-sectional associations, possibly secondary to metabolic changes occurring during the development of dementia.

Smoking

The role of smoking in the aetiology of dementia remains controversial. Early studies examining this question were principally of case–control design using prevalent cases and are open to bias in selection of cases, in differential classification and through the mortality associated with smoking. More recent population-based studies have sought to address this issue. Current smoking has been reported to be associated cross-sectionally with worse cognitive function in one study (Kilander *et al.*, 1997) but not in others (Farmer *et al.*, 1987; Scherr *et al.*, 1988). The Zutphen Study found an increased risk of MMSE impairment at a three-year follow-up but only in subjects with vascular disease and not to a statistically significant extent (Launer *et al.*, 1996). However, the large Honolulu-Asia Aging Study found smoking in middle age to be associated with a significantly increased risk of cognitive impairment 20 years later (Galanis *et al.*, 1997).

Studies examining effects of smoking on dementia as an outcome have tended to focus on AD because of early reports of a protective effect. Findings with regard to VaD have largely been negative (Hébert and Brayne, 1995; Yoshitake *et al.*, 1995; Lindsay *et al.*, 1997) although current smoking was found to be associated with dementia in a group of subjects known to have multiple infarctions (Gorelick *et al.*, 1993) and with dementia following acute stroke in one study (Pohjasvaara *et al.*, 1998). Population-based research into the relationship between smoking and AD has not supported earlier reports (from smaller case–control studies) of the former being a protective factor and have, if anything, suggested the opposite. Prince *et al.* (1994), in a prospective study of hypertensive subjects, found smoking to be a factor associated with increased risk of incident AD and the Canadian Study of Health and Aging (1994) found that, while there was no significant association either way between AD and all smokers, heavy smokers had an increased risk and all smokers had a significantly reduced age of onset for the disease, even in 'familial' cases. The Rotterdam Study reported that current smokers had a greater than twofold increased incidence of AD although, interestingly, this appeared to be a risk factor only for subjects without an ApoE ϵ4 allele, suggesting a possible balancing of adverse and beneficial effects in subjects with genetic susceptibility (Ott *et al.*, 1998).

Gene–environment interactions

In addition to clarifying risks of cognitive impairment/dementia associated with vascular disease and its risk factors as 'environmental' effects, some population studies have also been of sufficient size to examine interactions with genetic factors. Possession of the apolipoprotein ϵ4 allele has been shown to be a risk factor for dementia – principally AD in this respect – although some reports have suggested that it may also be a risk factor for VaD (Noguchi *et al.*, 1993) and poststroke dementia (Slooter *et al.*, 1997). It has also been suggested that the ϵ4 allele may be a potential underlying factor for associations between cognitive impairment and vascular disease (Payne *et al.*, 1994). However, although carrying the ϵ4 allele is recognized to be associated with raised cholesterol levels, associations with vascular disease are still relatively tentative, if present at all to any important extent (van Duijn, 1998). Findings from the Rotterdam Study have suggested that the interaction between vascular disease and the ε4 allele in AD is one of parallel but mutually potentiating risk factors rather than one effect being mediated through the other: associations between indices of atherosclerosis and AD were seen to be much increased in subjects who carried an ε4 allele and, similarly, the association between the ε4 allele and AD was seen most strongly in subjects with more severe vascular disease (Hofman et al., 1997). Similar findings have been reported with other potential 'environmental' risk factors such as head injury (Tang et al., 1996) and herpes simplex virus exposure (Itzhaki et al., 1997), suggesting that apolipoprotein E genotype may mediate vulnerability to 'environmental' insults rather than being directly involved in AD neurodegenerative processes. Interestingly, some factors seem to interact in the opposite direction, being principally risk factors for ε4 non-carriers. Smoking has been discussed in this respect and may relate to a balance of damaging and protective effects. Insulin resistance (whose role is discussed below) also appears to be chiefly associated with AD in ε4 non-carriers (Kuusisto et al., 1997), possibly due to a pathological interaction between glucose intolerance and the ε4 allele leading to raised mortality (Ukkola et al., 1993) and therefore reduced likelihood of the two being found together in older subjects.

IS ALZHEIMER'S DISEASE A VASCULAR DEMENTIA?

An important number of epidemiological studies have suggested that vascular disorders are important in the aetiology not only of 'vascular' dementia but also of Alzheimer's disease (Stewart, 1998). What is less certain at present, however, is how this translates into pathological mechanisms. The problem with most work so far has been that the subclassification of dementia has relied on clinical estimates of cerebrovascular disease, albeit using established diagnostic criteria. In particular, imaging techniques have not been used to assess subclinical cerebrovascular disease and therefore it cannot be concluded that 'AD' groups did not include more 'mixed dementia' cases than earlier studies, accounting for the associations with vascular disorders. However, a problem with current in vivo diagnostic criteria is that they in effect dichotomize AD and VaD and do not reflect the high rates of mixed disease seen post-mortem. Poststroke studies suggest that a substantial proportion of subsequent dementia is gradually progressive and occurs in the absence of further clinical stroke (Tatemichi et al., 1994), arguing against a 'multi-infarct' mechanism as a common entity. This and evidence that cognitive impairment in stroke-free subjects is associated with an increased risk of subsequent stroke suggest either that cerebrovascular disease is associated with a gradually progressive dementia which looks like

AD, or that there is an interaction with Alzheimer processes. The relative rarity of cerebrovascular pathology seen associated with dementia post-mortem in the absence of Alzheimer pathology (Hulette *et al.*, 1997) supports the latter possibility.

If vascular disease is associated with increased AD, one possibility is that it acts to induce disease directly. Various plausible mechanisms may under-lie this and there is some support from post-mortem findings in nondemented subjects of increased senile plaque and neurofibrillary tangle counts in those with a history of hypertension and increased senile plaque counts in those with severe coronary artery disease (Sparks *et al.*, 1995). Increased activity of amyloid precursor protein and β-amyloid production has been described in the hippocampi of rodents following severe but transient ischaemia (Hall *et al.*, 1995). Although this is probably a nonspecific response to trauma, the question remains whether more mild but chronic ischaemia may result in similar sequelae, possibly through systemic disease interacting with pre-exist-ing abnormalities in the microvasculature, which have been described in association with AD (de la Torre and Mussivand, 1993), or through inflam-matory processes, increasingly recognized as important mediators of cerebral damage following ischaemic episodes, and with potential amyloidogenic interactions. Vascular amyloid deposition (cerebral amyloid angiopathy) is known to be a common finding in association with AD although its role in the disorder remains uncertain. It may, however, mediate interactions between systemic vascular disease and AD pathology as it has been reported to be increased in association with cerebral arteriosclerosis, cerebral infarc-tion and hypertension (Olichney *et al.*, 1995; Ellis *et al.*, 1996), possibly related to blood–brain barrier disturbances (Pluta *et al.*, 1996).

An alternative (and not mutually exclusive) possibility to that of direct induction of AD pathology is that vascular disease may interact with pre-exist-ing AD and precipitate the manifestation of clinical dementia at relatively mild stages of AD pathology. This has been suggested most recently by the 'nun study', which screened 678 female subjects over the age of 75, well matched for educational background with a cognitive test battery, and then reported on post-mortem findings on 102 subjects who died two to four years later (Snowdon *et al.*, 1997). Cerebral infarction was found to be common in those meeting neuropathological criteria for AD, was associated with an increased likelihood of having had clinical dementia and was associated with worse cognitive performance in those subjects with AD. Infarction was not associated with increased Alzheimer pathology but in those subjects with AD, neurofibrillary tangle counts were reduced if infarction was also present, suggesting that the latter may have precipitated dementia at relatively early stages of AD pathology rather than through a direct interaction.

The role of white matter abnormalities seen on magnetic resonance imaging remains uncertain in dementia but may be related to interactions with vascular disease. While the pathology underlying these abnormalities has not been conclusively demonstrated, vascular disorders (particularly hypertension) and increased age have been established to be principal factors in their aetiology (Breteler *et al.*, 1994). In population studies, white matter lesions have been found to be associated with relative cognitive impairment (Ylikoski *et al.*, 1993) but it is well recognized that severe abnormalities may exist without any adverse neuropsychological sequelae (Fein *et al.*, 1990), suggesting interactions with other processes. Periventricular lesions have been reported to be increased in AD although negative findings exist in this respect, principally in studies of younger age groups (Scheltens *et al.*, 1992) or those which have most rigorously excluded or controlled for co-morbid vascular disease. White matter abnormalities in AD may therefore be a marker for relatively mild co-morbid vascular pathology. Research into the effects of these abnormalities on the course of dementia has tended to show no significant effects (O'Brien *et al.*, 1996) but they may act to precipitate AD as discussed above, possibly through impairment of executive function – therefore increasing the chance of memory disturbance secondary to hippocampal cell loss in AD becoming clinically manifest.

Although mechanisms exist whereby vascular disease may influence either the pathogenesis or clinical expression of AD, the two processes may be (alternatively or additionally) related through common underlying factors. One possibility in this respect is insulin resistance – the relative resistance of membrane receptors to the action of insulin as manifested by raised circulating insulin levels measured in the fasting state or during a glucose tolerance test. Insulin resistance has been hypothesized as underlying a number of vascular risk factors such as hypertension, type 2 diabetes and dyslipidaemia – so-called 'Syndrome X' disorders – and explaining the observed close associations between these factors (Reaven, 1988). Relative insulin resistance has also been reported to be associated with cognitive impairment (Kuusisto *et al.*, 1993) and with AD in particular (Kuusisto *et al.*, 1997) although findings remain cross-sectional and it cannot yet be concluded that this is not an effect rather than a cause of the condition. Insulin receptors appear, however, to be particularly dense in the hippocampus (Unger *et al.*, 1989), and insulin itself has been reported to have adverse effects on hippocampal function (Palovcik *et al.*, 1984) and acetylcholine synthesis (Brass *et al.*, 1992) *in vitro*. Particularly interesting with respect to AD have been effects of insulin and insulin-related growth factor on the regulation of tau protein phosphorylation (Hong *et al.*, 1997), a key process in the formation of neurofibrillary tangles. Possibilities which require exploration in this respect include whether prolonged insulin resistance may affect neurofibrillary tangle development and directly increase the risk of AD or whether there may be common genetic factors which affect both processes independently.

PREVENTABLE DEMENTIA?

Evidence from prospective population-based studies has suggested increased rates of dementia associated with risk factors for vascular disease such as hypertension, type 2 diabetes, dyslipidaemia and smoking – all common in developed countries and rapidly assuming prominence in developing countries. Even though common underlying factors may underlie some of the associations, it is likely that a substantial effect on dementia is through direct causation and therefore open to preventative measures. It is also probable that this research field will identify avenues for treatment of dementia and some groups have already suggested that rigorous control of prevalent vascular risk factors may result in stabilization or improvement of cognition (Meyer *et al.*, 1986). However, treatment possibilities will also depend on further work to unravel some of the changes in patterns of association seen in older age groups. In particular, changes in blood pressure, lipid abnormalities and, possibly, glucose tolerance suggest a metabolic change which seems to predate the emergence of cognitive signs in dementia. Similar findings have been reported in other chronic late-life diseases (Ettinger and Harris, 1993) and it is possible that research into dementia may be excessively centred on changes occurring within the brain, ignoring systemic phenomena which, even if they are secondary to neurodegenerative processes, may at least be an early, possibly precognitive marker of disease.

THE FUTURE OF 'VASCULAR DEMENTIA'

While the issues surrounding the influences of vascular factors in AD require further elucidation, one important question arising from this field of research is the usefulness of 'vascular dementia' as an entity. The term itself subsumes a wide variety of potentially heterogeneous conditions where dementia is seen in association with vascular pathology. However, while the existence of dementia syndromes in association solely with vascular disease is in no doubt, the proportion of dementia secondary to vascular disease accounted for by these syndromes is more questionable. Differences of opinion with regard to whether or not vascular risk factors are associated with AD may well be due to different attitudes about how rigorously vascular disease is excluded as part of the diagnostic process; but this begs the question of how a classification based on presumed aetiology is appropriate for aetiological research – just as it might be questioned whether a study of life-events as risk factors for depression should divide the latter into endogenous and reactive categories. The term 'vascular dementia' implies a discrete mechanism of pathogenesis and a clearly identifiable single syndrome which are not supported by evidence so far and therefore should be abandoned

(Devasenapathy and Hachinski, 1997). However, it is also imperative that epidemiological research in this area works towards a more rigorous estimation of the extent of cerebral vascular disease before assuming that vascular factors have any direct influence on AD pathogenesis, exploiting increased availability of and advances in neuroimaging techniques to this end. An alternative system of measuring outcome arising from this would be to make a diagnosis simply of 'dementia' (possibly altering criteria to allow for detection at an earlier stage of cognitive decline), followed by an axial rather than categorical estimation of the extent of contributing pathologies (AD, cerebrovascular disease, Lewy body pathology, etc.), therefore better reflecting the mixture of pathology seen at post-mortem. Research into vascular disease as a risk factor for dementia may therefore be better served by a diagnostic system which keeps an open mind about mechanisms of pathogenesis rather than one which makes assumptions in this respect. The fact that 'vascular dementia' is a diagnosis with a long history behind it should not obscure the fact that it is still only an arbitrary concept which should be discarded if it fails to reflect increasing understanding of a complex risk–outcome relationship.

REFERENCES

Boshuizen, H.C., Izaks, G.J., van Buuren, S. *et al.* (1998). Blood pressure and mortality in elderly people aged 85 and older: community based study. *BMJ* **316**, 1780–1784.

Brass, B.J., Nonner, D. and Barrett, J.N. (1992). Differential effects of insulin on choline acetyltransferase and glutamic acid decarboxylase activities in neuron-rich striatal cultures. *J Neurochem* **59**, 415–424.

Breteler, M.M.B., Bots, M.L., Mosterd, A. *et al.* (1993a). Atherogenic and hemostatic factors and cognitive function in the elderly. The Rotterdam Study. In: Breteler, M.M.B. (Ed.), *Cognitive Decline in the Elderly. Epidemiologic Studies on Cognitive Function and Dementia*. Thesis, Erasmus University, Rotterdam, pp. 74–85.

Breteler, M.M.B., Grobbee, D.E. and Hofman, A. (1993b). Blood pressure, hypertension, orthostatic hypotension, and cognitive function in the elderly. The Rotterdam Study. In: Breteler, M.M.B. (Ed.), *Cognitive Decline in the Elderly. Epidemiologic Studies on Cognitive Function and Dementia*. Thesis, Erasmus University, Rotterdam, pp. 86–98.

Breteler, M.M.B., van Swieten, J.C., Bots, M.L. *et al.* (1994). Cerebral white matter lesions, vascular risk factors, and cognitive function in a population-based study: the Rotterdam Study. *Neurology* **44**, 1246–1252.

Canadian Study of Health and Aging (1994). Risk factors for Alzheimer's disease in Canada. *Neurology* **44**, 2073–2080.

Censori, B., Manara, O., Agostinis, C. *et al.* (1996). Dementia after first stroke. *Stroke* **27**, 1205–1210.

de la Torre, J.C. and Mussivand, T. (1993). Can disturbed microcirculation cause Alzheimer's disease? *Neurol Res* **15**, 146–153.

Desmond, D.W., Tatemichi, T.K., Paik, M. *et al.* (1993). Risk factors for cerebrovascular disease as correlates of cognitive function in a stroke-free cohort. *Arch Neurol* **50**, 162–166.

Devasenapathy, A. and Hachinski, V. (1997). Vascular cognitive impairment: a new approach. In: Holmes, C. and Howard, R. (Eds), *Advances in Old Age Psychiatry: Chromosomes to Community Care*. Wrightson Biomedical Publishing, Petersfield, pp. 79–95.

Elias, M.F., Wolf, P.A., D'Agostino, R.B. *et al.* (1993). Untreated blood pressure level is inversely related to cognitive functioning: the Framingham study. *Am J Epidemiol* **138**, 353–364.

Elias, P.K., Elias, M.F., D'Agostino, R.B. *et al.* (1997). NIDDM and blood pressure as risk factors for poor cognitive performance. *Diabetes Care* **20**, 1388–1395.

Ellis, R.J., Olichney, J.M., Thal, L.J. *et al.* (1996). Cerebral amyloid angiopathy in the brains of patients with Alzheimer's disease: the CERAD experience, part XV. *Neurology* **46**, 1592–1596.

Ettinger, W.H. and Harris, T. (1993). Causes of hypocholesterolemia. *Coron Artery Dis* **4**, 854–859.

Farmer, M.E., White, L.R., Abbott, R.D. *et al.* (1987). Blood pressure and cognitive performance: the Framingham Study. *Am J Epidemiol* **126**, 1103–1114.

Fein, G., Van Dyke, C., Davenport, L. *et al.* (1990). Preservation of normal cognitive functioning in elderly subjects with extensive white-matter lesions of long duration. *Arch Gen Psychiatry* **47**, 220–223.

Galanis, D.J., Petrovitch, H., Launer, L.J. *et al.* (1997). Smoking history in middle age and subsequent cognitive performance in elderly Japanese-American men. *Am J Epidemiol* **145**, 507–515.

Gorelick, P.B., Brody, J., Cohen, D. *et al.* (1993). Risk factors for dementia associated with multiple cerebral infarcts. *Arch Neurol* **50**, 714–720.

Guo, Z., Viitanen, M., Fratiglioni, L. *et al.* (1996). Low blood pressure and dementia in elderly people: the Kungsholmen project. *BMJ* **312**, 805–808.

Hall, E.D., Oostveen, J.A., Dunn, E. *et al.* (1995). Increased amyloid protein precursor and apolipoprotein E immunoreactivity in the selectively vulnerable hippocampus following transient forebrain ischemia in gerbils. *Exp Neurol* **135**, 17–27.

Hébert, R. and Brayne, C. (1995). Epidemiology of vascular dementia. *Neuroepidemiology* **14**, 240–257.

Hofman, A., Ott, A., Breteler, M.M.B. *et al.* (1997). Atherosclerosis, apolipoprotein E, and prevalence of dementia and Alzheimer's disease in the Rotterdam Study. *Lancet* **349**, 151–154.

Hong, M. and Lee, V.M.-Y. (1997). Insulin and insulin-like growth factor-1 regulate tau phosphorylation in cultured human neurons. *J Biol Chem* **272**, 19547–19553.

Hulette, C., Nochlin, D., McKeel, D. *et al.* (1997). Clinical-neuropathologic findings in multi-infarct dementia: a report of six autopsied cases. *Neurology* **48**, 668–672.

Itzhaki, R.F., Lin, W., Shang, D. *et al.* (1997). Herpes simplex virus type 1 in brain and risk of Alzheimer's disease. *Lancet* **349**, 241–244.

Kalmijn, S., Launer, L.J. and Ott, A. (1997). Dietary fat intake and the risk of incident dementia in the Rotterdam Study. *Ann Neurol* **42**, 776–782.

Kase, C.S., Wolf, P.A., Kelly-Hayes, M. *et al.* (1998). Intellectual decline after stroke. *Stroke* **29**, 805–812.

Katzman, R., Aronson, M., Fuld, P. *et al.* (1989). Development of dementing illness in an 80-year-old volunteer cohort. *Ann Neurol* **25**, 317–324.

Kilander, L., Nyman, H., Boberg, M. *et al.* (1997). Cognitive function, vascular risk factors and education. A cross-sectional study based on a cohort of 70-year-old men. *J Intern Med* **242**, 313–321.

Kilander, L., Nyman, H., Boberg, M. *et al.* (1998). Hypertension is related to cognitive impairment: a 20-year follow-up of 999 men. *Hypertension* **31**, 780–786.

Kokmen, E., Whistman, J.P., O'Fallon, W.M. *et al.* (1996). Dementia after ischemic stroke: a population-based study in Rochester, Minnesota (1960–1984). *Neurology* **19**, 154–159.

Kuusisto, J., Koivisto, K., Mykkänen, L. *et al.* (1993). Essential hypertension and cognitive function: the role of hyperinsulinemia. *Hypertension* **22**, 771–779.

Kuusisto, J., Koivisto, K., Mykkänen, L. *et al.* (1997). Association between features of the insulin resistance syndrome and Alzheimer's disease independently of apolipoprotein E4 phenotype: cross sectional population based study. *BMJ* **315**, 1045–1049.

Launer, L.J., Dinkgreve, M.A.H.M., Jonker, C. *et al.* (1993). Are age and education independent correlates of the mini-mental state exam performance of community-dwelling elderly? *J Gerontol* **48**, P271–P277.

Launer, L.J., Masaki, K., Petrovitch, H. *et al.* (1995). The association between midlife blood pressure levels and late-life cognitive function. *JAMA* **274**, 1846–1851.

Launer, L.J., Feskens, E.J.M., Kalmijn, S. *et al.* (1996). Smoking, drinking and thinking: the Zutphen Elderly Study. *Am J Epidemiol* **143**, 219–227.

Lindsay, J., Hébert, R. and Rockwood, K. (1997). The Canadian Study of Health and Aging: risk factors for vascular dementia. *Stroke* **28**, 526–530.

Loeb, C., Gandolfo, C., Croce, R. *et al.* (1992). Dementia associated with lacunar infarction. *Stroke* **23**, 1225–1229.

Mattila, K., Haavisto, M., Rajala, S. *et al.* (1988). Blood pressure and five year survival in the very old. *BMJ* **296**, 887–889.

Meyer, J.S., Judd, B.W. and Tawaklna, T. (1986). Improved cognition after control of risk factors for multi-infarct dementia. *JAMA* **256**, 2203–2309.

Meyer, J.S., McClintic, K.L., Rogers, R.L. *et al.* (1988). Aetiological considerations and risk factors for multi-infarct dementia. *J Neurol Neurosurg Psychiatry* **51**, 1489–1497.

Mortel, K.F., Wood, S., Pavol, M.A. *et al.* (1993). Analysis of familial and individual risk factors among patients with ischemic vascular dementia and Alzheimer's disease. *Angiology* **44**, 599–605.

Noguchi, S., Murakami, K. and Yamada, N. (1993). Apolipoprotein E genotype and Alzheimer's disease. *Lancet* **342**, 737.

Notkola, I., Sulkava, R. and Pekkanen, J. (1998). Serum total cholesterol, apolipoprotein E ε4 allele, and Alzheimer's disease. *Neuroepidemiology* **17**, 14–20.

O'Brien, J.T., Ames, D. and Schwietzer, I. (1996). White matter changes in depression and Alzheimer's disease: a review of magnetic resonance imaging studies. *Int J Geriatr Psychiatry* **11**, 681–694.

Olichney, J.M., Hansen, L.A., Hofstetter, C.R. *et al.* (1995). Cerebral infarction in Alzheimer's disease is associated with severe amyloid angiopathy and hypertension. *Arch Neurol* **52**, 702–708.

Ott, A., Stolk, R.P., Hofman, A. *et al.* (1996). Association of diabetes mellitus and dementia: the Rotterdam Study. *Diabetologia* **39**, 1392–1397.

Ott, A., Breteler, M.M.B., de Bruyne, M.C. *et al.* (1997a). Atrial fibrillation and dementia in a population-based study. *Stroke* **28**, 316–321.

Ott, A., Stolk, R.P., van Harskamp, F. *et al.* (1997b). Diabetes mellitus and the risk of dementia in an elderly population. In: Ott, A. (Ed.), *Risk of Dementia. The Rotterdam Study.* Judels en Brinkman, Delft, pp. 49–62.

Ott, A., Slooter, A.J.C. and Hofman, A. (1998). Smoking and risk of dementia and Alzheimer's disease in a population-based cohort study: the Rotterdam Study. *Lancet* **351**, 1840–1843.

Palovcik, R.A., Phillips, M.I., Kappy, M.S. *et al.* (1984). Insulin inhibits pyramidal neurons in hippocampal slices. *Brain Res* **309**, 187–191.

Payne, M.N., Jones, A.F., Murray, R.G. *et al.* (1994). Atherosclerotic disease and cognitive decline. *BMJ* **309**, 411.

Perlmuter, L.C., Nathan, D.M., Goldfinger, S.H. *et al.* (1988). Triglyceride levels affect cognitive function in noninsulin dependent diabetics. *J Diabetic Complications* **2**, 210–213.

Pluta, R., Barcikowska, M., Januszewski, S. *et al.* (1996). Evidence of blood-brain barrier permeability/leakage for circulating human Alzheimer's β-amyloid-(1-42)-peptide. *NeuroReport* **7**, 1261–1265.

Pohjasvaara, T., Erkinjuntti, T., Ylikoski, R. *et al.* (1998). Clinical determinants of poststroke dementia. *Stroke* **29**, 75–81.

Prince, M., Cullen, M. and Mann, A. (1994). Risk factors for Alzheimer's disease and dementia: a case-control study based on the MRC elderly hypertension trial. *Neurology* **44**, 97–104.

Prince, M., Bird, A.S., Blizard, R.A., *et al.* (1996). Is the cognitive function of older patients affected by antihypertensive treatment? Results from 54 months of the Medical Research Council's treatment trial of hypertension in older adults. *BMJ* **312**, 801–804.

Reaven, G.M. (1988). Role of insulin resistance in human disease. *Diabetes* **37**, 1595–1607.

Scheltens, P.H., Barkhof, F., Valk, J. *et al.* (1992). White matter lesions on magnetic resonance imaging in clinically diagnosed Alzheimer's disease. *Brain* **115**, 735–748.

Scherr, P.A., Albert, M.S., Funkenstein, H.H. *et al.* (1988). Correlates of cognitive function in an elderly community population. *Am J Epidemiol* **128**, 1084–1101.

Shimano, H., Ishibashi, S., Murase, T. *et al.* (1989). Plasma apolipoproteins in patients with multi-infarct dementia. *Atherosclerosis* **79**, 257–260.

Skoog, I., Lernfelt, B., Landahl, S. *et al.* (1996a). 15-year longitudinal study of blood pressure and dementia. *Lancet* **347**, 1141–1145.

Skoog, I., Landahl, S. and Lernfelt, B. (1996b). *Lancet* **348**, 66.

Slooter, A.J.C., Tang, M.X., van Duijn, C.M. *et al.* (1997). Apolipoprotein E epsilon 4 and the risk of dementia with stroke: a population-based investigation. *JAMA* **277**, 818–821.

Snowdon, D.A., Greiner, L.H., Mortimer, J.A. *et al.* (1997). Brain infarction and the clinical expression of Alzheimer disease. *JAMA* **277**, 813–817

Sparks, D.L., Scheff, S.W., Liu, H. *et al.* (1995). Increased incidence of neurofibrillary tangles in non-demented individuals with hypertension. *J Neurol Sci* **131**, 162–169.

Starr, J.M., Whalley, L.J., Inch, S. *et al.* (1993). Blood pressure and cognitive function in healthy old people. *J Am Geriatr Soc* **41**, 753–756.

Stewart, R. (1998). Cardiovascular factors in Alzheimer's disease. *J Neurol Neurosurg Psychiatry* **65**, 143–147.

Stoy, N.S. (1997). Stroke and cholesterol: 'enigma variations'? *J R Coll Phys Lond* **31**, 521–526.

Strachan, M.W.J., Deary, I.J., Ewing, F.M.E. *et al.* (1997). Is type II diabetes associated with an increased risk of cognitive dysfunction? *Diabetes Care* **20**, 438–445.

Tang, M.X., Maestre, G., Tsai, W.Y. *et al.* (1996). Effect of age, ethnicity, and head injury on the association between APOE genotypes and Alzheimer's disease. *Ann N Y Acad Sci* **802**, 6–15.

Tatemichi, T.K., Desmond, D.W., Mayeux, R. *et al.* (1992). Dementia after stroke: baseline frequency, risks and clinical features in a hospitalised cohort. *Neurology* **42**, 1185–1193.

Tatemichi, T.K., Desmond, D.W., Paik, M. *et al.* (1993). Clinical determinants of dementia related to stroke. *Ann Neurol* **33**, 568–575.

Tatemichi, T.K., Paik, M., Bagiella, E. *et al.* (1994). Risk of dementia after stroke in a hospitalised cohort: results of a longitudinal study. *Neurology* **44**, 1885–1891.

Ukkola, O., Kervinen, K., Salmela, P.I. *et al.* (1993). Apolipoprotein E phenotype is related to macro- and microangiopathy in patients with non-insulin-dependent diabetes mellitus. *Atherosclerosis* **101**, 9–15.

Unger, J., McNeill, T.H., Moxley R.T. III *et al.* (1989). Distribution of insulin receptor-like immunoreactivity in the rat forebrain. *Neuroscience* **31**, 143–157.

van Boxtel, M.P.J., Buntinx, F., Houx, P.J. *et al.* (1998). The relation between morbidity and cognitive performance in a normal aging population. *J Gerontol* **53**, M147–M154.

van Duijn, C.M. (1998). Genetic and environmental factors and the incidence of Alzheimer's disease. *Neurobiol Aging* **19** (suppl 4), S227.

White, L. (1996). Is silent cerebrovascular disease an important cause of late-life cognitive decline ? *J Am Geriatr Soc* **44**, 328–330.

Ylikoski, R., Ylikoski, A., Erkinjuntti, T. *et al.* (1993). White matter changes in healthy elderly persons correlate with attention and speed of mental processing. *Arch Neurol* **50**, 818–824.

Yoshitake, T., Kiyohara, Y., Kato, I. *et al.* (1995). Incidence and risk factors of vascular dementia and Alzheimer's disease in a defined elderly Japanese population: the Hisayama Study. *Neurology* **45**, 1161–1168.

Everything You Need to Know About Old Age Psychiatry . . .
Edited by Robert Howard
©1999 Wrightson Biomedical Publishing Ltd

6

Prions

GLENN C. TELLING

*MRC Prion Diseases Unit, Imperial College School of Medicine at St Mary's,
London, UK*

The prion diseases, or transmissible spongiform encephalopathies (TSEs), are a group of fatal neurologic conditions of humans and animals with the unique properties of being both inherited and infectious diseases. Prion diseases have taken centre stage with the emergence of bovine spongiform encephalopathy (BSE) in Europe, and more recently with the appearance of a new variant of Creutzfeldt–Jakob disease (vCJD) in humans which appears to be caused by exposure to BSE. However, these and similar transmissible neurodegenerative diseases of the central nervous system (CNS), including scrapie of sheep and goats and the human disease kuru, have been studied for many years because of their extraordinary biology and the unique properties of the infectious agent.

THE PRION PROTEIN AND PRION REPLICATION

Because it can only be assayed in experimental animals, and the time between inoculation and disease is extremely long, characterization of the infectious agent has been enormously difficult. The molecular structure of the causative agent remained enigmatic for many decades and still eludes definitive identification. Since they hold many features in common with conventional viral diseases (for instance, they are transmissible, the agent is filterable and there are multiple strains of the agent), it was widely believed that TSEs were caused by viruses or unconventional infectious agents containing a nucleic acid genome. However, Alper and colleagues demonstrated in UV irradiation studies that the target size of the agent was considerably smaller than a virus and suggested that a nucleic acid might not be involved (Alper *et al.*, 1966, 1967). Prusiner and colleagues succeeded in purifying scrapie infectivity from hamster brains and demonstrated characteristics that were typical of proteins and inconsistent with the agent containing nucleic acids (Prusiner *et al.*, 1982; Prusiner, 1982). To distinguish these 'proteinaceous infectious' agents from conventional pathogens, Prusiner coined the term 'prion' which was defined as a small proteinaceous infectious particle that resists inactivation by procedures that modify nucleic acids (Prusiner, 1982). During prion purification, Prusiner and co-workers found an extremely good correlation between infectivity and enrichment of an insoluble, partially protease-resistant protein of relative molecular mass in SDS-PAGE of 27–30 kDa, which they referred to as prion protein, or PrP (Bolton *et al.*, 1982; McKinley *et al.*, 1983)

The determination of the amino-terminal amino acid sequence of purified PrP27–30 (Prusiner *et al.*, 1984) led to the recovery of PrP-encoding cDNA clones from libraries derived from the brains of scrapie-infected Syrian hamster (Oesch *et al.*, 1985) and mouse (Chesebro *et al.*, 1985). Surprisingly, PrP mRNA proved to be the product of a host cell gene that was expressed at the same levels in the brains of infected and uninfected animals, and PrP primary structure was shown to be identical in normal and infected animals (Basler *et al.*, 1986). These studies gave the first indication that PrP exists in at least two conformational states with different physicochemical properties; these were termed PrP^C for the cellular form of the prion protein, which is present in infected and uninfected brains, is soluble in detergents and sensitive to protease treatment, and PrP^{Sc}, the disease-associated isoform which is found only in infected brains, is insoluble and partially resistant to protease treatment. Protease treatment of PrP^{Sc} gives rise to PrP27–30 kDa as a result of protease cleavage of the amino-terminal 66, or so, amino acids (Figure 1). Structural analysis of purified PrP^C and PrP27–30 shows that PrP^C has a high α-helical content and is virtually devoid of β-sheet while PrP^{Sc} has a high β-sheet content (Pan *et al.*, 1993). The three-dimensional structures of bacterially expressed recombinant mouse PrP (residues 121–231) (Riek *et al.*, 1996) and Syrian hamster PrP (residues 29-231) (James *et al.*, 1997), which is assumed to approximate to PrP^C, have been determined by nuclear magnetic resonance (NMR) spectroscopy. These studies show that the structured globular carboxy-terminal portion of PrP consists of three α-helices, designated H1, H2 and H3, interspersed with two short sections which form a short β-pleated sheet, while the amino-terminal region is largely unstructured (Figure 1).

PrP is synthesized as a precursor which is processed by removal of a 22-amino acid amino-terminal signal peptide and 23 amino acids from the carboxyl terminus to which a glycophosphatidyl inositol (GPI) moiety is attached (Stahl *et al.*, 1987) and which anchors the protein to the external surface of cells. The resulting protein is glycosylated at two asparagine residues and has a molecular weight 33–35 kDa (Figure 1).

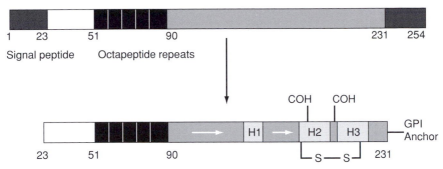

Figure 1. Structural features of the prion protein. The mouse PrP gene encodes a 254 amino acid residue translation product which is processed by removal of an amino-terminal signal peptide of 22 amino acids and a carboxyl-terminal hydrophobic peptide of 23 amino acids, both shown in dark grey. After cleavage of the carboxyl-terminal peptide a glycosyl phosphatidylinositol (GPI) anchor is added. The three α-helices (designated H1, H2 and H3) and two short sections forming a β-pleated sheet (represented as arrows) which have been identified by nuclear magnetic resonance (NMR) spectroscopy of recombinant mouse PrP are shown in light grey. H1 extends from amino acid residue 143 to amino acid residue 153, H2 from amino acid residue 175 to amino acid residue 192 and H3 from amino acid residue 199 to amino acid residue 218; the two regions making up the β-pleated sheet extend from amino acid residues 127 to 130 and amino acid residues 160 to 163 (numbering of amino acid residues is related to human PrP). The amino-terminal portion of the molecule appears to be largely unstructured and contains a tandem array of five octapeptide repeats between codons 51 and 90 which are represented by solid black boxes. Asn-linked oligosaccharides are attached at residues 180 and 196 and H2 and H3 are connected by a disulphide bond that joins codons 178 and 213. Protease cleavage of the amino-terminal 66, or so, amino acids of PrPSc gives rise to a protease-resistant core represented by PrP27-30 which is shown in mid grey.

During the disease process, PrPC is converted to PrPSc by a post-translational process (Borchelt *et al.*, 1990). Whereas no covalent modifications have been found that distinguish PrPC from PrPSc (Stahl *et al.*, 1993), considerable evidence argues that prion diseases are disorders of protein conformation and that prion replication involves the conformational conversion of host-encoded PrPC into PrPSc. The central event in the protein-only model of prion propagation is the coercion of normal PrP by PrPSc to adopt to the infectivity-associated conformation (Figure 2) (Cohen *et al.*, 1994). It has been proposed that PrPC exists in equilibrium with PrP* (Cohen *et al.*, 1994) and that it is bound to an ancillary factor, referred to as 'protein X' (Telling *et al.*, 1995). The PrP*-protein X complex interacts with PrPSc which induces a conformational change in PrP*, the end result being two molecules of PrP with the infectious PrPSc conformation which are free to induce conformational changes in additional PrP* molecules during the infectious cycle. This

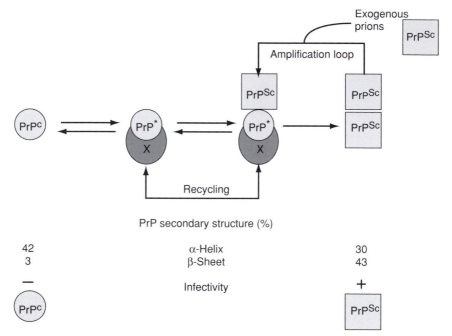

Figure 2. Prion replication. The prion protein (PrP) exists in at least two different conformational states: PrP^C which has a high content of α-helix and PrP^{Sc} which is rich in β-pleated sheet. It has been proposed that PrP^C exists in equilibrium with PrP* that is bound to an ancillary factor, referred to as 'protein X' and that the PrP*-protein X complex interacts with PrP^{Sc} which induces a conformational change in PrP*. The end result is two molecules of PrP with the infectious PrP^{Sc} conformation which are free to induce conformational changes in additional PrP* molecules during the infectious cycle.

model predicts that, since PrP^C is the source of PrP^{Sc}, elimination of PrP^C would result in the abolition of prion replication. Indeed, homozygous *Prnp$^{0/0}$*, which express no PrP^C, fail to develop the characteristic clinical and neuropathological symptoms of scrapie after inoculation with mouse prions and do not propagate prion infectivity (Bueler *et al.*, 1993).

Mice in which the gene for PrP has been ablated have also been studied to probe the normal function of PrP^C. Two independently generated lines of gene-targeted *Prnp$^{0/0}$* developed normally and appeared to suffer no gross phenotypic defects (Bueler *et al.*, 1992; Manson *et al.*, 1994). The relative normality of these PrP-null mice could result from effective adaptive changes during development. However, cerebellar Purkinje cell degeneration has been reported in a third line of *Prnp$^{0/0}$* mice (Sakaguchi *et al.*, 1996) and several other phenotypic defects are being investigated in *Prnp$^{0/0}$* mice including altered circadian rhythms and sleep patterns (Tobler *et al.*, 1996), alterations in superoxide dismutase activity (SOD-1) (Brown *et al.*, 1997a) and defects in copper metabolism (Brown *et al.*, 1997b). Electrophysiological studies have demonstrated that $GABA_A$-receptor-mediated fast inhibition and long-term potentiation were impaired in hippocampal slices from *Prnp⁰/⁰* mice (Collinge *et al.*, 1994; Whittington *et al.*, 1995) and calcium-activated potassium currents were disrupted (Colling *et al.*, 1996).

ANIMAL PRION DISEASES

Scrapie is the prototypic prion disease (Table 1) which has long been recognized as a disease of sheep and goats. While the aetiology of natural scrapie remained the subject of intense debate for many years it is now clear that it is an infectious disease in which susceptibility is genetically modulated by the host. Other prion diseases of animals include a transmissible encephalopathy in captive populations of mink (TME) which, although the origin of infection is unclear, has been attributed to prion-infected foodstuffs, and chronic wasting disease (CWD) in mule deer and elk in western regions of the USA. Epidemiological studies suggest intraspecific lateral transmission as the most plausible explanation for the spread of CWD in captive populations of Rocky Mountain elk. CWD has also been diagnosed in free-ranging mule deer, Rocky Mountain elk and white-tailed deer from north-central Colorado (Spraker *et al.*, 1997).

Table 1.   Animal prion diseases.

Disease	Host	Aetiology
Scrapie	Sheep and goats	Thought to involve both horizontal and vertical transmission.
Transmissible mink encephalopathy (TME)	Captive mink	Probably food-borne although the origin of infectious prions is uncertain.
Chronic wasting disease (CWD)	Captive and free-ranging mule deer and Rocky Mountain elk	Possibly food-borne although there is evidence for horizontal transmission
Bovine spongiform encephalopathy	Cattle	Food-borne in the form of contaminated meat and bonemeal.
Feline spongiform encephalopathy	Domestic and zoo cats	BSE-contaminated feed
Exotic ungulate encephalopathy	Captive bovidae	BSE-contaminated feed

Since its discovery in 1985, BSE has reached epidemic proportions, affecting over 170 000 cattle in the UK and to a lesser extent in certain other European countries. It has been estimated that up to one million cattle were infected with BSE in the UK (Anderson *et al.*, 1996). Epidemiological studies point to contaminated offal used in the manufacture of meat and bonemeal (MBM) and fed to cattle as the source of prions responsible for BSE (Wilesmith *et al.*, 1988). BSE-contaminated foodstuffs had caused disease in several other animal species in Great Britain, including feline spongiform encephalopathy (FSE) in domestic cats and exotic ungulates and captive cats in zoos. In addition, BSE has been experimentally transmitted to a wide variety of species.

It was hypothesized that scrapie-contaminated sheep offal was the initial source of BSE. However, the alternative view that BSE prions originated spontaneously in cattle with subsequent amplification of infection by recycling infected cattle with subclinical disease cannot be excluded. When it was realized that BSE was caused by feeding prion-contaminated foodstuffs to cattle, a ban on feeding ruminant-derived protein to other ruminants was

Table 2. Annual incidence of confirmed cases of BSE and vCJD in Great Britain.

Year	BSE[a]	vCJD[b]
1988	2 184	–
1989	7 137	–
1990	14 181	–
1991	25 032	–
1992	36 682	–
1993	34 370	–
1994	23 945	–
1995	14 300	3
1996	8 016	10
1997	4 311	10
1998[c]	1 680	6

[a]Figures represent the total number of suspect cases of BSE that were slaughtered and the diagnosis of BSE confirmed after removal and examination of brain tissue. Figures for 1998 are current until 30 October.
[b]Figures include definite vCJD cases still alive which are cases where the diagnosis has been pathologically confirmed (by brain biopsy) and probable vCJD in which post-mortem (or brain biopsy) has not been carried out but which fulfil preliminary criteria for the clinical diagnosis of vCJD.
[c]To 30 September 1998. Total number of definite and probable cases of vCJD = 30 (including one death since 30 September 1998).
BSE, bovine spongiform encephalopathy; vCJD, new variant Creutzfeldt–Jakob disease.

introduced in July 1988 to break the cycle of infection via feed. The specified bovine offals (SBO) ban was introduced in the UK in 1989 to prevent inclusion in the human food chain of bovine tissues thought to contain the highest titre of prions, including tissues from the lymphoreticular system (LRS) and CNS. Since the announcement in March 1996 that BSE and vCJD may be linked, more than 1.35 million cattle over 30 months old have been culled in the UK in a further attempt to limit human exposure to BSE. As a result of these measures, the BSE epidemic reached its peak in 1992 and has since steadily declined (Table 2).

Since BSE infectivity has also been detected in dorsal root ganglia, which may on occasion be included in meat for human consumption, the British Government also introduced a controversial ban on the sale of 'beef on the bone' in 1997. Although there is no evidence that disease can be transmitted via blood or blood products, the long incubation period of prion diseases and the possibility of increased numbers of future cases of CJD as a result of exposure to BSE has raised the issue of blood as a possible vehicle for iatrogenic disease. As a protective measure against this theoretical risk, the British Government recently decided on leucodepletion of all blood donations.

HUMAN PRION DISEASES

The human prion diseases are unique in biology in that they are manifest as sporadic, genetic and infectious diseases (Table 3). The majority of cases of human prion disease occur sporadically as CJD at a rate of roughly one per million population across the world. The aetiology of sporadic CJD is unknown, although hypotheses include somatic mutation of the PrP gene (referred to as *PRNP*), and the spontaneous conversion of PrP^C into PrP^{Sc} as a rare stochastic event. Approximately 10–20% of human prion diseases are inherited, with an autosomal-dominant mode of inheritance. To date, 20 different missense and insertion *PRNP* mutations that segregate with dominantly inherited neurodegenerative disorders have been identified (Figure 3). Five of these mutations are genetically linked to loci controlling familial CJD, Gerstmann–Sträussler–Scheinker (GSS) syndrome and fatal familial insomnia (FFI) which are inherited human prion diseases that can be transmitted to experimental animals (Collinge, 1997). Analysis of mutations in the coding sequence of the prion protein gene (Figure 2) may be used for presymptomatic diagnosis in affected families (Collinge *et al.*, 1991a). In addition to these pathogeneic mutations, there are several benign polymorphisms of *PRNP*, the most common being at codon 129 which encodes either methionine or valine (Figure 2). Homozygosity at this position predisposes individuals to developing sporadic and iatrogenic CJD (Palmer *et al.*, 1991; Collinge *et al.*, 1991b).

Table 3. Human prion diseases.

Disease	Incidence	Aetiology	Age of onset/incubation period and duration of illness
Sporadic CJD	One per million population	Unknown but hypotheses include somatic mutation or spontaneous conversion of PrPc into PrPsc	Age of onset is usually in the 45–75 year age group with peak onset between 60–65 years. 70% of cases die in under 6 months.
Familial CJD, GSS, FFI	10–20% of human prion disease cases	Autosomal-dominant *PRNP* mutation	Average age of onset for GSS is 45 years with a 5-year mean duration of illness.
Kuru (1957–1982)	>2500 cases among the Fore in Papua New Guinea	Infection through ritualistic cannibalism	Incubation periods range from 60 to 360 months with duration of illness between 3 and 12 months.
Iatrogenic CJD	About 80 cases to date	Infection from contaminated human growth hormone (HGH), human gonadotrophin, depth electrodes, corneal transplants, dura mater grafts, neurosurgical procedures	Incubation periods of HGH cases range from 4 to 30 years with a duration of illness between 6 and 18 months
New variant CJD	31 young adults in the UK and France	Infection by BSE prions	Mean age of onset is 26 years with a mean duration of illness of 14 months

CJD, Creutzfeldt–Jakob disease; GSS, Gerstmann–Sträussler–Scheinker syndrome; FFI, fatal familial insomnia.

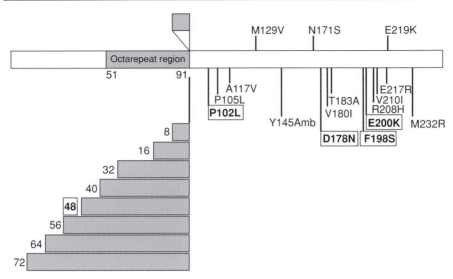

Figure 3. Pathogenic mutations and polymorphisms in the human prion protein gene. The 253 amino acid residue coding sequence of the human PrP gene (*PRNP*) is represented as an extended rectangle. The pathogenic mutations associated with the human prion diseases CJD, GSS and FFI are shown below. These consist of 8, 16, 32, 40, 48, 56, 64 and 72 amino acids insertions within the octarepeat region between codons 51 and 91, and point mutations causing nonconservative missense amino acid substitutions. Point mutations are designated by the wild-type amino acid preceding the codon number, followed by the mutant residue, using single-letter amino acid conventions. The mutations for which genetic linkage with familial CJD, GSS and FFI has been established are shown in boxes. Deletion of a single octapeptide repeat is not associated with disease. Other nonpathogenic polymorphisms found at codons 129, 171 and 219 are also shown above the coding sequence.

To model how a mutation in the PrP gene could result in a disease that was both inherited and infectious, transgenic mice were engineered to express a PrP gene mutation associated with GSS. These mice spontaneously developed clinical and neuropathological symptoms similar to mouse scrapie at between 150 and 300 days of age (Hsiao *et al.*, 1990; Telling *et al.*, 1996a). Importantly, the serial propagation of infectivity from the brains of these spontaneously sick mice to indicator mice expressing low levels of mutant protein which otherwise do not get sick demonstrated that infectious prions had been produced *de novo* in the brains of these spontaneously sick mice (Hsiao *et al.*, 1994; Telling *et al.*, 1996a).

While the human prion diseases are experimentally transmissible, the acquired forms have, until recently, been confined to rare and unusual situations. For example, kuru is thought to have been spread by ritualistic cannibalism among the Fore linguistic group in Papua New Guinea (Gajdusek,

1977). Since the cessation of cannibalistic practices around 1956, the disease has all but died out, with only a handful of cases currently occurring in older individuals who were presumably exposed to kuru as young children. Other examples of acquired human prion diseases have occurred as a result of accidental transmission of CJD during corneal transplantation, contaminated electroencephalographic electrode implantation and surgical operations using contaminated instruments or apparatus. In addition, iatrogenic CJD has occurred as a result of implantation of dura mater grafts and treatment with human cadaveric pituitary-derived growth hormone or gonadotrophin (Brown *et al.*, 1992). The replacement of human cadaveric pituitary-derived growth hormone with recombinant growth hormone was implemented to avoid the continued iatrogenic transmission of CJD to young children with growth hormone deficiency. Similarly, since CJD has resulted from the use of prion-contaminated surgical instruments or apparatus after neurosurgical or ophthalmic procedures, it is advised that surgical instruments be inciner- ated in cases where CJD is suspected to avoid future iatrogenic transmission of prion disease.

The appearance of CJD cases in teenagers and young adults in the UK at the height of the BSE epidemic prompted considerable concern that they might be acquired by exposure to bovine prions. By March 1996 it became clear that the unusual clinical presentation and neuropathology in these new cases was remarkably consistent (Will *et al.*, 1996). To date, 30 cases of vCJD have been reported in the UK (Table 3) and a single case of vCJD in France. Molecular strain typing, which focuses on the biochemical properties of PrP^{Sc} from the brains of BSE-infected cattle and patients with CJD, has demon- strated that vCJD is different from sporadic CJD but similar to BSE (Collinge *et al.*, 1996; Hill *et al.*, 1997). Moreover, the incubation times and profile of neuropathological lesions of vCJD and BSE prions are indistin- guishable in inbred lines of mice (Bruce *et al.*, 1997). These data argue convincingly that BSE and vCJD are the same strain.

CHARACTERISTICS OF THE PRION DISEASES

Clinical features

The prion disorders of animals and humans share a number of features in common. The incubation times of the prion diseases are long and range from months to decades (Table 3). While incubation times are long, once clinical symptoms have appeared the progression to death is inevitable and rapid, with a duration of illness usually lasting no more than 6–12 months. In scrapie, affected animals exhibit behavioural changes which are character- ized by anxiousness and hypersensitivity, followed by intense pruritus. In fact, the term scrapie derives from the tendency of affected animals to rub themselves against walls and fences, thus removing much of their fleece. Later stages of the disease are characterized by unsteady gait, eventually resulting in severe ataxia, with animals becoming recumbent in the terminal phase of the disease. The clinical features of BSE are also well described and include temperament changes, postural abnormalities, co-ordination problems and terminal recumbence.

Classical CJD is a rapidly progressive dementia accompanied by myoclonus. Decline to akinetic mutism and death is rapid and often occurs within three to four months. Cerebellar ataxia, extrapyramidal and pyramidal features, and cortical blindness are also frequently seen. These clinical symptoms are usually accompanied by pseudocharacteristic periodic sharp wave complexes (PSWCs) on electroencephalography (EEG). Atypical cases of CJD are, however, well recognized and can present diagnostic difficulties. The clinical features of kuru consist of a progressive cerebellar ataxia accompanied by dementia in the later stages and death which usually occurs within nine months. The clinical presentation of vCJD resembles kuru more than classical CJD and is characterized clinically by a progressive neuropsychiatric disorder, peripheral sensory disturbance, early cerebellar ataxia, dementia and myoclonus (or chorea) without the typical EEG appearance of CJD. The duration of disease is longer in vCJD, with mean patient survival times of about 14 months compared to about four months for sporadic CJD. Moreover, whereas classical CJD is predominantly a late-onset disease with a peak onset between 60 and 65 years, the median age of onset of vCJD is 26 years (Table 3).

Neuropathological features

Perhaps the most consistent and characteristic features of the prion diseases are the neuropathological changes that accompany disease in the CNS. While the brains of patients or animals with prion disease frequently show no recognizable abnormalities on gross examination, microscopic examination of the CNS typically reveals a characteristic triad of histopathological changes which are required to confirm diagnosis of prion disease by brain biopsy or at necropsy. These features consist of neuronal vacuolation and degeneration which confers a microvacuolated or 'spongiform' appearance upon any part of the cerebral grey matter, and a reactive proliferation of astroglial cells which is often out of all proportion to the degree of nerve cell loss. Although it is frequently detected, spongiform degeneration is not an obligatory neuropathological feature of prion disease and astrocytic gliosis, while not specific to the prion diseases, is more constantly seen. The lack of an inflammatory response is also an important characteristic. While by no means a constant feature, some examples of prion disease are characterized by deposition of amyloid plaques composed of insoluble aggregates of PrP. Amyloid plaques are a notable feature of kuru and GSS syndrome but are infrequently found in the brains of patients with sporadic CJD.

While there is wide variation in the neuropathological profiles of different forms of human prion disease, the histopathological features of vCJD are remarkably constant and distinguish it from other human prion diseases. Large numbers of PrP-positive amyloid plaques are a constant feature of vCJD but they differ in morphology from kuru and GSS plaques in that the surrounding tissue takes on a microvacuolated appearance, giving the plaques a florid appearance (Will *et al.*, 1996). Of note, transmission of BSE to three macaques produced disease with neuropathological features similar to those reported for cases of vCJD in humans (Lasmézas *et al.*, 1996a).

Detection of PrP^{Sc} in brain material by immunohistochemical or immunoblotting techniques is considered to be diagnostic of prion disease. However, certain examples of natural and experimental prion disease occur without accumulation of detectable protease resistant PrP^{Sc} (Telling *et al.*, 1996a; Collinge *et al.*, 1995; Medori *et al.*, 1992) and the time course of neurodegeneration is not equivalent to the time course of PrP^{Sc} accumulation in mice expressing lower than normal levels of PrP^{C} (Bueler *et al.*, 1995). Moreover, PrP^{Sc} is not toxic to cells that do not express PrP^{C} (Brandner *et al.* 1996). Thus, it appears that accumulation of PrP^{Sc} may not be the sole cause of pathology in prion diseases. An alternative mechanism of PrP-induced neuronal degeneration has been suggested from recent studies of mutant forms of PrP that disrupt the regulation of PrP biogenesis in the endoplasmic reticulum (Hegde *et al.*, 1998).

Although the pathological consequences of prion infection occur in the CNS and experimental transmission of these diseases is most efficiently accomplished by intracerebral inoculation, most natural infections do not occur by these means. Indeed, administration to sites other than the CNS is known to be associated with much longer incubation periods, which may extend to 20 years or more. Experimental evidence suggests that this latent period is associated with clinically silent prion replication in the lymphoreticular tissue, while neuroinvasion may take place later (Blattler *et al.*, 1997). Mice with severe combined immune deficiency (SCID) are largely resistant to disease after extracerebral inoculation with prions (Kitamoto *et al.*, 1991; Lasmézas *et al.*, 1996b), and steroid treatment substantially delays disease in mice intraperitoneally challenged with scrapie prions (Outram *et al.*, 1974). Recent studies have indicated that differentiated B lymphocytes may be crucial for prion neuroinvasion (Klein *et al.*, 1997). Because of the involvement of the LRS in prion disease, treatments that inhibit prion replication in lymphoid organs may represent a viable strategy for rational secondary prophylaxis after accidental exposure (Aguzzi and Collinge, 1997). Future studies on the peripheral pathogenesis of prion disease should identify the crucial steps in the spread of prions from the periphery that may be amenable to pharmacological intervention.

PRION VARIATION: SPECIES BARRIERS AND STRAINS

Two features of the biology of these diseases account for prion variation. The 'species barrier' describes the difficulty with which prions from one species can cause disease in another. The initial passage of prions between species is associated with a prolonged incubation time with only a few animals developing illness. Subsequent passage in the same species is characterized by all the animals becoming ill after greatly shortened incubation times. Prion species barriers have been successfully overcome by expressing PrP genes from other species, or artificially engineered hybrid PrP genes in transgenic mice. For instance, wild-type mice are normally resistant to infection with Syrian hamster prions. However, by expression of Syrian hamster PrPc in transgenic mice, referred to as Tg(SHaPrP) mice, the species barrier to Syrian hamster prion infectivity was abrogated (Scott *et al.*, 1989). These, and subsequent studies (Prusiner *et al.*, 1990), indicated that disease transmission is facilitated when elements of the primary structure of host-encoded PrPc and PrPsc in the inoculum are identical.

The infrequent transmission of human prion disease to rodents has also been cited as an example of the species barrier. Based on the results with Tg(SHaPrP) mice, it was expected that the species barrier to human prion propagation would similarly be abrogated in transgenic mice expressing human PrP. However, transmission of human prion disease was generally no more efficient in Tg(HuPrP) transgenic mice expressing human PrPc on a wild-type background than in nontransgenic mice (Telling *et al.*, 1994). In contrast, propagation of human prions was highly efficient in transgenic mice expressing a chimeric mouse–human PrP gene, referred to as Tg(MHu2M) (Telling *et al.*, 1994; Telling *et al.*, 1995). The barrier to CJD transmission in Tg(HuPrP) mice was abolished by expressing HuPrP on a *Prnp*$^{0/0}$ background, demonstrating that mouse PrPc inhibited the transmission of prions to Tg mice expressing human PrPc but not to those expressing chimeric PrP (Telling *et al.*, 1995). To explain these and other data, it was proposed that the most likely mediator of this inhibition is an auxiliary non-PrP molecule, provisionally designated protein X, that participates in the formation of prions by interacting with the carboxy-terminal region of PrPc to facilitate conversion to PrPsc (Telling *et al.*, 1995).

Like other infectious agents, prions exist as different strains with well defined, heritable properties of incubation time and CNS pathology in inbred strains of mice. In the face of convincing evidence that vCJD is caused by human exposure to BSE, the issue of prion strains has acquired very practical consequences. Recent developments indicate that prion strain information is enciphered within the conformation of PrP^{Sc}, providing a mechanism for both the generation and propagation of prion strains. Two strains of prion disease in mink (transmissible mink encephalopathy), referred to as hyper (HY) and drowsy (DY), which produced different clinical symptoms and incubation periods in Syrian hamsters, showed different resistance to proteinase K digestion and altered amino-terminal proteinase K cleavage sites (Bessen and Marsh, 1992), suggesting that different strains might represent different conformational states of PrP^{Sc}. Evidence supporting the concept that the conformation of PrP^{Sc} functions as a template in directing the formation of nascent PrP^{Sc} emerged from transmission studies of inherited human prion diseases in transgenic mice. Expression of different mutant prion proteins in patients with FFI and fCJD(E200K) results in variations in PrP conformation, reflected in altered proteinase K cleavage sites which generate PrP^{Sc} molecules with molecular weights of 19 kDa in FFI and 21 kDa in other inherited and sporadic diseases (Monari *et al.*, 1994). Extracts from the brains of FFI and CJD patients transmit disease to transgenic mice and induce the formation of the 19 kDa PrP^{Sc} and 21 kDa PrP^{Sc}, respectively (Telling *et al.*, 1996b). On subsequent passage, these characteristic molecular sizes remain constant but the incubation times for FFI and fCJD(E200K) prions diverge (Telling and Prusiner, unpublished observations) suggesting that mutant prion proteins with different primary structures produce distinct prion strains and that different tertiary structures of PrP^{Sc} can be imparted upon a single PrP^{C} by conformational templating. Studies of established mouse and Syrian hamster prion strains in transgenic mice suggest that the diversity of prion strains may be limited to a finite constellation of PrP^{Sc} conformations that can be adopted by the primary structure of PrP in the host (Scott *et al.*, 1997).

REFERENCES

Aguzzi, A. and Collinge, J. (1997). Post-exposure prophylaxis after accidental prion inoculation. *Lancet* **350**,1519–1520.

Alper, T., Haig, D.A. and Clarke, M.C. (1966). The exceptionally small size of the scrapie agent. *Biochem Biophys Res Commun* **22**, 278–284.

Alper, T., Cramp, W.A., Haig, D.A. and Clarke, M.C. (1967). Does the agent of scrapie replicate without nucleic acid? *Nature* **214**, 764–766.

Anderson, R.M., Donnelly, C.A., Ferguson, N.M. *et al.* (1996). Transmission dynamics and epidemiology of BSE in British cattle. *Nature* **382**, 779–788.

Basler, K., Oesch, B., Scott, M. *et al.* (1986). Scrapie and cellular PrP isoforms are encoded by the same chromosomal gene. *Cell* **46**, 417–428.

Bessen, R.A. and Marsh, R.F. (1992). Biochemical and physical properties of the prion protein from two strains of the transmissible mink encephalopathy agent. *J Virol* **66**, 2096–2101.

Blattler, T., Brandner, S., Raeber, A.J. *et al.* (1997). PrP-expressing tissue required for transfer of scrapie infectivity from spleen to brain. *Nature* **389**, 69–73.

Bolton, D.C., McKinley, M.P. and Prusiner, S.B. (1982). Identification of a protein that purifies with the scrapie prion. *Science* **218**, 1309–1311.

Borchelt, D.R., Scott, M., Taraboulos, A., Stahl, N. and Prusiner, S.B. (1990). Scrapie and cellular prion proteins differ in their kinetics of synthesis and topology in cultured cells. *J Cell Biol* **110**, 743–752.

Brandner, S., Isenmann, S., Raeber, A. *et al.* (1996). Normal host prion protein necessary for scrapie-induced neurotoxicity. *Nature* **379**, 339–343.

Brown, D.R., Schulz-Schaeffer, W.J., Schmidt, B. and Kretzschmar, H.A. (1997a). Prion protein-deficient cells show altered response to oxidative stress due to decreased SOD-1 activity. *Exp Neurol* **146**, 104–112.

Brown, D.R., Qin, K., Herms, J.W. *et al.* (1997b). The cellular prion protein binds copper *in vivo*. *Nature* **390**, 684–687.

Brown, P., Preece, M.A. and Will, R.G. (1992). 'Friendly fire' in medicine: hormones, homografts, and Creutzfeldt–Jakob disease. *Lancet* **340**, 24–27.

Bruce, M.E., Will, R.G., Ironside, J.W. *et al.* (1997). Transmissions to mice indicate that 'new variant' CJD is caused by the BSE agent. *Nature* **389**, 498–501.

Bueler, H., Fischer, M., Lang, Y. *et al.* (1992). Normal development and behaviour of mice lacking the neuronal cell-surface PrP protein. *Nature* **356**, 577–582.

Bueler, H., Aguzzi, A., Sailer, A. *et al.* (1993). Mice devoid of PrP are resistant to scrapie. *Cell* **73**, 1339–1347.

Bueler, H., Raeber, A., Sailer, A., Fischer, M., Aguzzi, A. and Weissmann, C. (1995). High prion and PrPSc levels but delayed onset of disease in scrapie-inoculated mice heterozygous for a disrupted PrP gene. *Mol Med* **1**, 19–30.

Chesebro, B., Race, R., Wehrly, K. *et al.* (1985). Identification of scrapie prion protein-specific mRNA in scrapie-infected and uninfected brain. *Nature* **315**, 331–333.

Cohen, F.E., Pan, K.-M., Huang, Z., Baldwin, M., Fletterick, R.J. and Prusiner, S.B. (1994). Structural clues to prion replication. *Science* **264**, 530–531.

Colling, S.B., Collinge, J. and Jefferys, J.G.R. (1996). Hippocampal slices from prion protein null mice: disrupted CA2+-activated K+ currents. *Neurosci Lett* **209**, 49–52.

Collinge, J. (1997). Human prion diseases and bovine spongiform encephalopathy (BSE). *Hum Mol Genet* **6**, 1699–1705.

Collinge, J., Poulter, M., Davis, M.B. *et al.* (1991a). Presymptomatic detection or exclusion of prion protein gene defects in families with inherited prion diseases. *Am J Hum Genet* **49**, 1351–1354.

Collinge, J., Palmer, M.S. and Dryden, A.J. (1991b). Genetic predisposition to iatrogenic Creutzfeldt–Jakob disease. *Lancet* **337**, 1441–1442.

Collinge, J., Whittington, M.A., Sidle, K.C.L. *et al.* (1994). Prion protein is necessary for normal synaptic function. *Nature* **370**, 295–297.

Collinge, J., Palmer, M.S., Sidle, K.C.L. *et al.* (1995). Transmission of fatal familial insomnia to laboratory animals. *Lancet* **346**, 569–570.

Collinge, J., Sidle, K.C.L., Meads, J., Ironside, J. and Hill, A.F. (1996). Molecular analysis of prion strain variation and the aetiology of 'new variant' CJD. *Nature* **383**, 685–690.

Gajdusek, D.C. (1977). Unconventional viruses and the origin and disappearance of kuru. *Science* **197**, 943–960.

Hegde, R.S., Mastrianni, J.A., Scott, M.R. *et al.* (1998). A transmembrane form of the prion protein in neurodegenerative disease. *Science* **279**, 827–834.

Hill, A.F., Desbruslais, M., Joiner, S., Sidle, K.C.L., Gowland, I. and Collinge, J. (1997). The same prion strain causes vCJD and BSE. *Nature* **389**, 448–450.

Hsiao, K.K., Scott, M., Foster, D., Groth, D.F., DeArmond, S.J. and Prusiner, S.B. (1990). Spontaneous neurodegeneration in transgenic mice with mutant prion protein. *Science* **250**, 1587–1590.

Hsiao, K.K., Groth, D., Scott, M. *et al.* (1994). Serial transmission in rodents of neurodegeneration from transgenic mice expressing mutant prion protein. *Proc Natl Acad Sci U S A* **91**, 9126–9130.

James, T.L., Liu, H., Ulyanov, N.B. *et al.* (1997). Solution structure of a 142-residue recombinant prion protein corresponding to the infectious fragment of the scrapie isoform. *Proc Natl Acad Sci U S A* **94**, 10086–10091.

Kitamoto, T., Muramoto, T., Mohri, S., Doh-ura, K. and Tateishi, J. (1991). Abnormal isoform of prion protein accumulates in follicular dendritic cells in mice with Creutzfeldt–Jakob disease. *J Virol* **65**, 6292–6295.

Klein, M.A., Frigg, R., Flechsig, E. *et al.* (1997). A crucial role for B cells in neuro-invasive scrapie. *Nature* **390**, 687–690.

Lasmézas, C.I., Deslys, J.-P., Demaimay, R. *et al.* (1996a). BSE transmission to macaques. *Nature* **381**, 743–744.

Lasmézas, C.I., Cesbron, J.Y., Deslys, J.P. *et al.* (1996b). Immune system-dependent and -independent replication of the scrapie agent. *J Virol* **70**, 1292–1295.

Manson, J.C., Clarke, A.R., Hooper, M.L., Aitchison, L., McConnell, I. and Hope, J. (1994). 129/Ola mice carrying a null mutation in PrP that abolishes mRNA production are developmentally normal. *Mol Neurobiol* **8**, 121–127.

McKinley, M.P., Bolton, D.C. and Prusiner, S.B. (1983). A protease-resistant protein is a structural component of the scrapie prion. *Cell* **35**, 57–62.

Medori, R., Montagna, P., Tritschler, H.J. *et al.* (1992). Fatal familial insomnia: A second kindred with mutation of prion protein gene at codon 178. *Neurology* **42**, 669–670.

Monari, L., Chen, S.G., Brown, P. *et al.* (1994). Fatal familial insomnia and familial Creutzfeldt–Jakob disease: different prion proteins determined by a DNA polymorphism. *Proc Natl Acad Sci U S A* **91**, 2839–2842.

Oesch, B., Westaway, D., Walchli, M. *et al.* (1985). A cellular gene encodes scrapie PrP 27-30 protein. *Cell* **40**, 735–746.

Outram, G.W., Dickinson, A.G. and Fraser, H. (1974). Reduced susceptibility to scrapie in mice after steroid administration. *Nature* **249**, 855–856.

Palmer, M.S., Dryden, A.J., Hughes, J.T. and Collinge, J. (1991). Homozygous prion protein genotype predisposes to sporadic Creutzfeldt-Jakob disease. *Nature* **352**, 340–342.

Pan, K., Baldwin, M.A., Nguyen, J. *et al.* (1993). Conversion of a-helices into b-sheets features in the formation of the scrapie prion proteins. *Proc Natl Acad Sci U S A* **90**, 10962–10966.

Prusiner, S.B. (1982). Novel proteinaceous infectious particles cause scrapie. *Science* **216**, 136–144.

Prusiner, S.B., Bolton, D.C., Groth, D.F., Bowman, K., Cochran, S.P. and McKinley, M.P. (1982). Further purification and characterization of scrapie prions. *Biochemistry* **21**, 6942–6950.

Prusiner, S.B., Groth, D.F., Bolton, D.C., Kent, S.B. and Hood, L.E. (1984). Purification and structural studies of a major scrapie prion protein. *Cell* **38**, 127–134.

Prusiner, S.B., Scott, M., Foster, D. *et al.* (1990). Transgenetic studies implicate interactions between homologous PrP isoforms in scrapie prion replication. *Cell* **63**, 673–686.

Riek, R., Hornemann, S., Wider, G., Billeter, M., Glockshuber, R. and Wuthrich, K. (1996). NMR structure of the mouse prion protein domain PrP (121-231). *Nature* **382**, 180–182.

Sakaguchi, S., Katamine, S., Nishida, N. *et al.* (1996). Loss of cerebellar Purkinje cells in aged mice homozygous for a disrupted PrP gene. *Nature* **380**, 528–531.

Scott, M., Foster, D., Mirenda, C. *et al.* (1989). Transgenic mice expressing hamster prion protein produce species-specific scrapie infectivity and amyloid plaques. *Cell* **59**, 847–857.

Scott, M.R., Groth, D., Tatzelt, J. *et al.* (1997). Propagation of prion strains through specific conformers of the prion protein. *J Virol* **71**, 9032–9044.

Spraker, T.R., Miller, M.W., Williams, E.S. *et al.* (1997). Spongiform encephalopathy in free-ranging mule deer (*Odocoileus hemionus*), white-tailed deer (*Odocoileus virginianus*) and Rocky Mountain elk (*Cervus elaphus nelsoni*) in northcentral Colorado. *J Wildl Dis* **33**, 1–6.

Stahl, N., Borchelt, D.R., Hsiao, K. and Prusiner, S.B. (1987). Scrapie prion protein contains a phosphatidylinositol glycolipid. *Cell* **51**, 229–240.

Stahl, N., Baldwin, M.A., Teplow, D.B. *et al.* (1993). Structural studies of the scrapie prion protein using mass spectrometry and amino acid sequencing. *Biochemistry* **32**, 1991–2002.

Telling, G.C., Scott, M., Hsiao, K.K. *et al.* (1994). Transmission of Creutzfeldt–Jakob disease from humans to transgenic mice expressing chimeric human-mouse prion protein. *Proc Natl Acad Sci U S A* **91**, 9936–9940.

Telling, G.C., Scott, M., Mastrianni, J. *et al.* (1995). Prion propagation in mice expressing human and chimeric PrP transgenes implicates the interaction of cellular PrP with another protein. *Cell* **83**, 79–90.

Telling, G.C., Haga, T., Torchia, M., Tremblay, P., DeArmond, S.J. and Prusiner, S.B. (1996a). Interactions between wild-type and mutant prion proteins modulate neurodegeneration transgenic mice. *Genes Dev* **10**, 1736–1750.

Telling, G.C., Parchi, P., DeArmond, S.J. *et al.* (1996b). Evidence for the conformation of the pathologic isoform of the prion protein enciphering and propagating prion diversity. *Science* **274**, 2079–2082.

Tobler, I., Gaus, S.E., Deboer, T. *et al.* (1996). Altered circadian activity rhythms and sleep in mice devoid of prion protein. *Nature* **380**, 639–642.

Whittington, M.A., Sidle, K.C.L., Gowland, I. *et al.* (1995). Rescue of neurophysiological phenotype seen in PrP null mice by transgene encoding human prion protein. *Nat Genet* **9**, 197–201.

Wilesmith, J.W., Wells, G.A., Cranwell, M.P. and Ryan, J.B. (1988). Bovine spongiform encephalopathy: epidemiological studies. *Vet Rec* **123**, 638–644.

Will, R.G., Ironside, J.W., Zeidler, M. *et al.* (1996). A new variant of Creutzfeldt–Jakob disease in the UK. *Lancet* **347**, 921–925.

II

The Dementias:
Treatments and Ethical
Considerations

Everything You Need to Know About Old Age Psychiatry . . .
Edited by Robert Howard
©1999 Wrightson Biomedical Publishing Ltd

7

Drug Treatments for the Cognitive Symptoms of Dementia

IAN G. McKEITH

Professor of Old Age Psychiatry, Institute for the Health of the Elderly, Newcastle General Hospital, Newcastle upon Tyne, UK

INTRODUCTION

The recent appearance of anti-dementia drugs in the British National Formulary has profoundly altered attitudes about the treatment of Alzheimer's disease (AD), by instilling some cause for hope into what was previously a gloomy therapeutic area. Sadly, this optimism has been tainted by generalized professional and public dissatisfaction, in response to the financial restrictions which have led to widespread and continuing unavailability of the new drugs within the NHS. Their potential impact within UK clinical services, therefore remains largely untested.

The modest effects of the current generation of anti-dementia drugs were originally demonstrated in clinical trials which were designed for regulatory submission. These trials invariably recorded improvements in the patient's cognitive performance and the clinician's personal assessment of change in the patient's global function, before and during treatment. Those responsible for introducing the new drugs to national and local formularies, and for commissioning service developments, have been understandably uncertain how to interpret these measures. The clinical relevance of small improvements in cognition has been questioned and requests made for additional evidence of significant improvements in activities of daily living and quality of life. A positive, or at least neutral, cost/benefit analysis of the new treatments is also considered desirable to justify their introduction into clinical practice (O'Brien, 1998).

This chapter will consider some of the reasons for the discrepancy between what we have so far learned about the effects of anti-dementia drugs and what we would really like to know. The interpretation of effects upon cognitive performance will be used to illustrate some of the difficulties.

THE CURRENT/NEW WAVE OF ANTI-DEMENTIA DRUGS

A great deal has been said and written about novel approaches to the treatment of dementia, particularly about neuroprotective strategies with the potential to slow or even prevent disease progression, e.g. anti-inflammatories, antioxidants, nerve growth factors and oestrogens (McGeer *et al.*, 1996; Tang *et al.*, 1996; Sano *et al.*, 1997). In reality, randomized trials have to date only demonstrated symptomatic (as opposed to disease modifying) treatment effects in AD and most drugs which have been assessed as showing satisfactory risk:benefit assessment come from within the class of cholinesterase inhibitors.

The impetus to develop cholinergic treatments for AD was based on observations of loss of cholinergic neurones in the nucleus basalis of Meynert and decline in basal–cortical projections (Whitehouse *et al.*, 1981), with a reduction in cortical acetyltransferase, the enzyme responsible for the synthesis of acetylcholine from choline and acetyl coenzyme-A. Volunteer studies showed that normal subjects given scopolamine developed memory deficits similar to those of AD, and post mortem studies of AD patients found the cortical (particularly hippocampal) cholinergic deficit to be positively correlated with both the severity of cognitive impairment and the density of plaque and tangle pathology (Perry *et al.*, 1978). Although the cholinergic hypothesis of AD as originally stated may now seem rather oversimplistic, there is no doubt that cholinesterase inhibition remains a rationally based treatment strategy and improvement in cognitive performance an equally rational target symptom.

The cholinesterase inhibitors currently available or in the late stages of development prior to regulatory submission are listed in Table 1. Although they share class effects and probably operate by broadly similar mechanisms, there are differences between them which may be important in determining efficacy, tolerability and ease of use. The ideal cholinesterase inhibitor might be characterized as follows.

Central nervous system selectivity

The original cholinergic hypothesis of AD stressed the functional importance of acetyl- rather than butyrylcholinesterase within the central nervous system (CNS) and selective acetylcholinesterase (AcChE) inhibition was predicted as therapeutically desirable. More recently butyrylcholinesterase (BuChE),

Table 1. Cholinesterase inhibitors licensed for treatment of AD or in the late phase of development.

Drug name: Generic (Proprietary)	Compound type	Selectivity of enzyme inhibition	Competitive or non-competitive inhibition	Reversible or irreversible inhibition	Dose and frequency of administration
Tacrine (Cognex)	Aminoacridine	AcChE selective	Non-competitive	Reversible	20–30 mg four times daily
Donepezil (Aricept)	Piperidine	AcChE selective	Non-competitive	Reversible	5–10 mg once daily
Rivastigmine (Exelon)	Carbamate	AcChE and BuChE (with some selectivity for CNS AcChE G1)	Non-competitive	Pseudo-irreversible	3–6 mg twice daily
Metrifonate (Memobay)	Organophosphate	AcChE and BuChE	Competitive	Irreversible	60–80 mg once daily
Galantamine (Reminyl)	Tertiary alkaloid	AcChE and BuChE (with nicotinic agonist activity)	Competitive	Reversible	12–16 mg twice daily

which is preserved in AD brain, has been proposed to participate in the transformation of benign, diffuse β-amyloid into malignant neurotoxic plaques (Mesulam, 1994), suggesting that BuChE inhibition may well be an advantageous feature. Many of the side effects of cholinesterase inhibition are mediated by stimulation of peripheral muscarinic and nicotinic receptors, e.g. increased gastrointestinal motility, muscle fasciculation and bradycardia, and these side effects will be reduced if CNS situated enzyme only is inhibited. Within the CNS there are several isoforms of AcChE which are differentially distributed. The globular tetrameric G4 form is most common in brain and is selectively lost in AD, particularly in hippocampus and neocortex. Levels of the monomeric G1 form are not reduced in AD and it has been suggested that selective inhibition of this remaining active moiety is particularly important.

Competitive inhibition

A competitive inhibitor will be maximally effective in brain regions where endogenous cholinergic activity is most reduced, thereby producing a disease targeting effect.

Reversible inhibition

Cholinergic neurotransmission is so important in regulating vital functions, e.g. level of consciousness, cardiovascular function and muscle tone, that irreversible enzyme inhibition may be inconvenient or hazardous, e.g. if a depolarizing muscle relaxant is used during general anaesthesia or in the event of a cholinesterase inhibitor overdose.

Low toxicity

Side effects related to increased cholinergic tone appear to be related to the rate of enzyme inhibition rather than the absolute level of inhibition which is typically 70–80% at therapeutic doses. There appear to be minor differences between drugs which necessitate slower dose titration with some. Other side effects may be related to the class of compound, e.g. the aminoacridine molecule of tacrine produced reversible hepatoxicity which is not shared by the other non-acridine drugs.

Few drug interactions

Most cholinesterase inhibitors have relatively low protein binding and limited metabolism by hepatic microsomal oxidases.

Long active half-life

Infrequent dosing regimes are a potential benefit particularly for patients living at home alone and reliant upon carers visiting to supervise the taking of medication. The drugs listed in Table 1 all differ in their pharmacodynamic and pharmacokinetic characteristics and this is reflected in their clinical profiles. Metrifonate, with its long half-life and slow onset of enzyme inhibition can be given once daily or less, in a fixed dose requiring no titration. The irreversible and non-selective inhibition of both acetyl- and butyryl-cholinesterase do however raise potential concerns about overdose, anaesthesia and long-term side effects. Rivastigmine and galantamine require twice daily dosing with a relatively extended dose titration phase to reduce cholinergic side effects – typically a minimum of six weeks to reach the maximum recommended daily dose. Donepezil is given once daily and a one-stage dose titration reaches maximum dose after four weeks.

WHY USE COGNITION AS AN OUTCOME MEASURE?

Cognitive failure is central to all definitions of dementia, with deterioration in personal and social function usually being considered as secondary consequences of the patient's intellectual failure. Memory impairment in particular is emphasized as an early symptom of AD, consistent with the early pathological and radiological involvement of the medial temporal lobes. The correlations between cognitive test score, pathological lesions and the severity of the cholinergic deficit have already been referred to. Cognitive function can for these reasons be regarded as an obvious outcome measure to be used in clinical trials. Not only would an improvement in cognitive performance have high face validity for a putative anti-dementia drug effect, but it would also be consistent with the cholinergic hypothesis of AD. A rather more pragmatic reason for the selection of cognition as a primary treatment target is the fact that it is relatively easy to measure compared with other variables, and a wide variety of assessment tools already exist.

It was similar logic which prompted the US Food and Drink Administration (FDA) CNS drugs group to conclude that in order to meet regulatory requirements for the granting of a licence for the treatment of AD, a drug should show a statistically significant effect upon cognition (Leber, 1990). It was recognised that if the treatment effect was only small, it might have little or no clinical relevance and although such an effect might provide proof in principle of the cholinergic hypothesis, it would not be sufficient to justify a drug's clinical use. The additional requirement was therefore introduced, for a measure of clinical effect size, to take the form either of an activities of daily living (ADL) scale or a clinician's global impression of change. Although superficially appealing, this approach simply displaces the question about the relevance of the size of change in cognitive score on to the other items. In practice, ADL scores have proved to be very unreliable instruments in most trials and onus of proof of clinical relevance has therefore fallen upon the clinical global score.

Clinical Global Assessment of Change

The CIBIC (clinical interview based impression of change) is the semi-structured instrument which has been devised entirely for this purpose and is intended to capture a holistic view of cognitive abilities and functional performance via repeated semi-structured interviews. Assessing the effects of a drug by systematically interviewing carer then patient and comparing all available information with baseline performance is intuitively plausible and probably should be adopted as a model of good practice in anti-dementia drug treatment clinics. CIBIC quantifies changes from baseline (pre-treatment) to endpoint (post-treatment) on a seven point visual analogue scale with the midpoint (4) representing no change. Proponents of CIBIC (there are now several versions on the market: Rockwood and Morris, 1996) claim that the interview's inherent insensitivity is an advantage in this situation and that the effects of a drug must be clinically relevant if CIBIC can detect them. CIBIC data are most useful when used in a responder frequency analysis which compares the proportions of drug treated and placebo patients who experience similar clinical global outcomes. All categories of positive response (minimal, moderate and marked improvement) tend to be lumped together in such analyses. Typical CIBIC responder rates are; donepezil 25% vs placebo 11% (Rogers et al., 1998) and rivastigmine 24% vs placebo 16% (Corey-Bloom et al., 1998). This means that 25% of patients treated with these drugs are considered by an experienced clinician to show clinical improvement but that up to two-thirds (16/24) of these responses may be attributable to placebo and other halo effects. Clinically relevant improvement can therefore be attributed to the pharmacological effects of cholinesterase inhibition in 8–14% of all AD patients who are treated with active medication, figures which are worth bearing in mind when explaining the likely benefits of treatment to patients and when later trying to assess their responder status in the clinic.

CIBIC data are harder to interpret when averaged across groups of individuals. Most cholinesterase inhibitor trials show a mean CIBIC treatment effect size of 0.3–0.5, when active treatment and placebo groups are compared (Knapp et al., 1994; Rogers et al., 1998; Corey-Bloom et al., 1998; Cummings et al., 1998). This is on a scale in which one full point of change indicates only a minimal degree of improvement or worsening. Although this may fulfil the requirement for an independent measure of clinical effect size for regulatory purposes, a mean 0.3 point improvement in CIBIC is a very abstract concept and its clinical relevance is almost certainly more difficult to interpret than a change in cognitive score. Measures of cognitive change endure as the most robust and understandable data which have emerged from treatment studies and cognitive improvement is the yardstick by which such trials tend to be assessed and compared, one with another.

The disadvantages of using cognitive scores as outcome measures in anti-dementia drug trials

Cognitive function in dementia is a broad concept. Aspects of intellectual function such as short term memory, attention and executive function may be affected differentially, even within one disease category such as AD. Performance on cognitive testing is dependent upon the 'match' between items within the test procedure and the profile of intellectual and other deficits present in the subject. Poor eyesight and hearing, low educational attainment and test anxiety are obvious confounders in elderly demented subjects. Cognitive testing is particularly susceptible to practice effects and these must be controlled for, before assuming that an improved score on retesting is attributable to a drug treatment.

Author's comment: I recently compared the baseline (pre-treatment) mini-mental state examination (MMSE) scores of 14 consecutive AD patients attending our treatment clinic, with their scores repeated under similar conditions, 12 weeks after reaching their maximum tolerated dose of either donepezil or rivastigmine (mean MMSE post treatment = 19.6, range 14–30). A paired sample t-test showed this within-group improvement to be statistically significant; t=–2.424, df=13, p<0.05. Only one patient scored worse than baseline (by two points), two patients scored the same as baseline and the other 11 patients increased their scores, eight of them (57% of all patients treated) by four MMSE points or more. These changes cannot all be accounted for by pharmacological effects and suggest that the particular circumstances of an anti-dementia drug clinic can substantially affect the test–retest reliability of a well established instrument such as the MMSE. Likely factors include traditional practice and learning effects, genuine improvement due to the halo effects of therapeutic activity and, probably of particular significance, greater efforts by patient (and clinician?) on the second test administration in order to obtain the plaudit of 'drug responder' in order to be offered continuing medication. This experience suggests to me that an improvement, even of four points or more, in MMSE score, is not by itself sufficient evidence of a true cholinesterase inhibitor treatment response.

Cognitive scales

We are still uncertain which aspects of cognition are most responsive to cholinergic enhancement. Recent evidence suggests that the largest effects of procholinergics are upon attention, vigilance and speed of information processing. These effects may underlie many of the improvements seen in other cognitive domains, e.g. recall and recognition memory, and also manifest themselves in clinically observable behavioural changes such as increased alertness and decreased apathy.

Computer based cognitive test batteries are particularly sensitive to changes in attention and psychomotor speed and probably are the best tools for investigating the real effects of psychoactive drugs on cognitive performance (Simpson *et al.*, 1991). Such systems are not however designed to generate a single numerical score which is what most clinicians seem to prefer. Cognitive test batteries used in anti-dementia trials have tended therefore to be of the extended MMSE variety, which may not directly measure those aspects of cognition related to cholinergic dysfunction, but which can express a patient's global cognitive performance as a summative score. The cognitive part of the Alzheimer's Disease Assessment Scale (ADAScog: Mohs *et al.*, 1983) is the outcome scale which has found favour with most pharmaceutical sponsors of anti-dementia drug trials, despite it taking up to an hour to administer and omitting to assess some important aspects of cognition, including working memory, delayed recall, attention, agnosia and executive function. Because ADAScog is not used in routine UK clinical practice and is therefore unfamiliar to most clinicians experienced in dementia care, difficulties occur when they are confronted with ADAScog findings from clinical trials. Whether or not a four point improvement on the ADAScog (a figure often quoted in scientific papers and by pharmaceutical company promotional material) is of any clinical significance, is not a question which most UK trained old age psychiatrists, neurologists or geriatricians can readily answer, on the basis of their clinical training and experience. Fortunately a large volume of data is available about rates of cognitive decline in AD, as measured by ADAScog. This allows the change in ADAScog scores (for better or worse) which occur during treatment to be converted into a 'disease equivalent', which is an estimate of the time period over which an untreated patient's cognitive performance would have declined by that same number of ADAScog points. Disease equivalence is increasingly being used in the discussion of effect size in anti-dementia drug trials (e.g. Rogers *et al.*, 1998) and although this may be legitimate, the conversion of change in test score into months' worth of disease is liable to produce some apparently inconsistent findings which will be considered in the final part of the chapter.

Aside from the problems inherent in measuring cognitive performance, there are two perhaps more fundamental reasons why cognition may not always be the most appropriate outcome measure for anti-dementia drug trials. First, mental test scores are not highly correlated with functional disability, particularly in mild to moderately demented AD patients with MMSE scores of 10–26, and who are generally considered eligible for cholinesterase inhibitor trials or clinical treatment. Secondly, it is the non-cognitive features of dementia which are increasingly being recognized as the major determinants of care burden and need for treatment and care. The concept of non-cognitive features embraces mood disorders, personality change and other neuropsychiatric features such as hallucinations, delusions, agitation, apathy and disturbances of sleep and appetite. Recent cholinesterase inhibitor trials have started to include and assess such features with appropriate measures such as the Neuropsychiatric Inventory (NPI: Cummings *et al.*, 1994). Initial results suggest that non-cognitive symptoms such as apathy, delusions, hallucinations and agitation do indeed improve, and that such improvements may be relatively independent of cognitive change (Kaufer *et al.*, 1996; Morris *et al.*, 1998).

Using cognitive performance data to interpret the effects of anti-dementia drug trials

Figure 1 shows the way in which cognitive performance data from anti-dementia drug trials are usually presented. The most often quoted cognitive outcome measure is the change in ADAScog scores (ΔADAScog) before and after **c** weeks of treatment. The mean $\Delta ADAScog_{(placebo)}$ in Figure 1 is (+**b**) points, the increase in ADAScog score indicating cognitive decline, whereas $\Delta ADAScog_{(drug)}$ is (–**a**) points, indicating that on average, drug treated subjects are performing slightly better after treatment than they were at baseline. The difference between ΔADAScog scores for placebo and active drug treated patients (**a** – **b**) is usually taken as a measure of effect size. Table 2 shows typical data from two hypothetical trials using drugs X and Y and expressed in the same terms as in Figure 1.

There are statistically significant differences between active and placebo groups at week 26 for both treatments, the ADAScog treatment effect size for drug X being 4.5 points, and 3.25 points for drug Y. Drug X is by this analysis more effective than drug Y but how can the clinical significance of either of these symptomatic improvements be judged? Since the ADAScog scale has a 70 point range, the relative effects of drugs X and Y could be converted into 6.5% and 4.6%, respectively, of total score but this does not convey much additional clinical meaning. An alternative is to convert the change in cognitive performance into a period of disease equivalence.

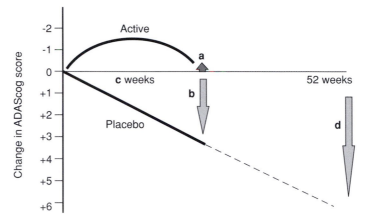

Figure 1. Presentation of cognitive performance results from a typical Alzheimer's disease symptomatic treatment study: treatment effect size = (**a–b**) ADAScog points.

Table 2. Results of two hypothetical trials comparing cholinesterase inhibitors X and Y in an identical design lasting 26 weeks. Cognitive outcomes are presented either as a change in points score (ΔADAScog) or as an estimated equivalent of disease progression (letters in parentheses refer to Figure 1). Although drug X produces the larger change in points score (4.5 ADAScog points), the disease progression equivalent of drug Y is almost twice as large as that for drug X. The reasons for this apparent discrepancy are explained in the text.

| | $\Delta ADAScog_{(drug)}$ | $\Delta ADAScog_{(placebo)}$ | ADAScog treatment effect size (in points) | Annualized rate of placebo decline | Disease progression equivalent (in months) |
	(a)	*(b)*	*(a–b)*	*(d)*	*12(a–b)/d*
DRUG X	–0.5	+4.0	–4.5	+8.0	6.75
DRUG Y	–1.5	+1.75	–3.25	+3.5	11.14

Disease equivalence as a measure of effect size

The first calculations of disease equivalence were based on literature reports that typical AD patients deteriorate an average of 9 ADAScog points per annum. Thus the active drug/placebo difference of 4.5 points achieved by drug X would be regarded as equivalent to the reversal of 6 months of disease progression and the 3.25 points of drug Y, to 4.3 months. Unfortunately such calculations are based on two fallacies, the first being that patients in separate trials have similar placebo deterioration rates, and, the second, that patients in trials deteriorate at the same rate as AD patients

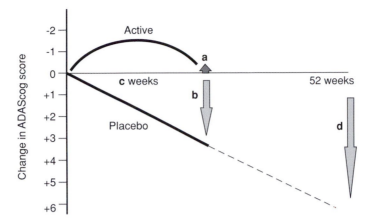

Figure 2. ADAScog treatment effect expressed with respect to annualized rate of placebo decline is the Disease Progression Equivalent = **(a–b)**/**d** ADAScog points.

who are seen in typical clinical practice. Close inspection of Table 2 shows that the placebo patients in trial X do in fact deteriorate by 4.0 points over 26 weeks, equivalent to 8.0 points in a year. Trial Y is much more representative of most published trials, the rate of placebo decline being only 1.75 points over 26 weeks, or 3.5 points per annum. If disease equivalence is calculated using the formula **(a–b)**/**d**, i.e. ADAScog effect/annualized rate of placebo decline *in the given study* (see Figure 2), the effect size in trial X is 4.5/8 = 0.56 years (6.75 months) and in trial Y is 3.25/3.5 = 0.93 years (11.14 months). The relative effectiveness of the two treatments is reversed by this calculation, drug Y now appearing superior to drug X. Disease progression equivalent, referenced to the correct placebo decline rate can be calculated for any trial using the general formula

$$12 \; \frac{(\mathbf{a-b})\mathbf{c,}}{52\mathbf{b/c}} \quad \text{months}$$

if three simple pieces of information are known: **a**, the change in cognitive test score in the group receiving active drug; **b**, the change in cognitive test score in the group receiving placebo; and **c** the length of the trial in weeks. Cognitive test scores can be measured using any scale and do not have to be in ADAScog points.

Although the data presented for drugs X and Y are truly hypothetical, one does not have to look far to find parallels in the real clinical trial literature. The 24 week donepezil study of Rogers *et al.* (1998) produced an ADAScog treatment effect size of 2.9 points, with an annualized rate of placebo decline of 3.9 points and a disease progression equivalent of 8.9 months. Similar calculations for the rivastigmine study of Corey-Bloom *et al.* (1998) find a

3.9 ADAScog treatment effect, 8.2 points annual placebo decline and 5.6 months of disease progression equivalent. It is apparent that the cognitive effect size in such trials is highly dependent upon the rate of cognitive decline in the placebo group. Rapid placebo decline, as in trial X, produces relatively large test score differences between active and placebo groups, whereas slow placebo decline (trial Y) produces longer estimates of disease progression equivalence.

CONCLUSIONS

Cognition is neither a necessary, nor indeed a sufficient measure of anti-dementia drug efficacy and a drug might have very substantial benefits, e.g. upon aspects of behaviour or ADL function without markedly improving cognitive performance. Nevertheless, cognitive failure is a central feature of dementia and when treatments intended to enhance cholinergic neurotransmission are used in AD patients, cognition is centrally important and should be evaluated. Unfortunately the cognitive measures used in clinical trials are not easily transferred to clinical practice and simple tools, such as MMSE, which clinicians routinely use to measure change in performance may be confounded by practice effects and unrealistic expectations of treatment. Presentation of the results of anti-dementia drug trials must pay central attention to the important issue of placebo deterioration rates because they have a major influence upon the interpretation of effect size. The cognitive effects of different drugs cannot be directly compared across studies, despite apparently similar trial designs having been used. Clinicians need to be aware of these issues, not only for their own practice but to help them advise formulary pharmacists and healthcare purchasers.

REFERENCES

Corey-Bloom, J., Anand, R. and Veach, J., for the ENA 713 B352 Study Group. (1998). A randomized trial evaluating the efficacy and safety of ENA 713 (rivastigmine tartrate), a new acetylcholinesterase inhibitor, in patients with mild to moderately severe Alzheimer's disease. *Int J Geriatr Psychopharmacol* **1**, 55–65.

Cummings, J.L., Mega, M., Gray, K., Rosenburg-Thompson, G., Carusi, D.A. and Gornbein, J. (1994). The Neuropsychiatric Inventory: comprehensive assessment of psychopathology in dementia. *Neurology* **44**, 2308–2314.

Cummings, J.L., Cyrus, P.A., Mas, J., Orazem, J., Gulanski, B. and the Metrifonate Study Group (1998). Metrifonate treatment of the cognitive deficits of Alzheimer's disease. *Neurology* **50**, 1214–1221.

Kaufer, D.I., Cummings, J.L. and Christine, D. (1996). Effect of tacrine on behavioural symptoms in Alzheimer's disease: an open label study. *J Geriatr Psychiatry Neurol* **9**, 1–6.

Knapp, M.J, Knopman, D.S. and Solomon, P.R. (1994). A 30 week randomised controlled trial of high-dose tacrine in patients with Alzheimer's disease. *JAMA* **271**, 985–991.

Leber, P. (1990). *Guidelines for Clinical Evaluation of Antidementia Drugs*, US Food and Drug Administration, Washington DC.

McGeer, P.L., Schulzer, M. and McGeer, E.G. (1996). Arthritis and anti-inflammatory agents as possible protective factors for Alzheimer's disease: a review of 17 epidemiological studies. *Neurology* **47**, 425-432.

Mesulam, M.M. (1994). In: Giacobini, E. and Becker, R.E. (Eds), *Cholinergic Basis for Alzheimer Therapy*, Birkhauser, Boston, pp. 79–83.

Mohs, R.C., Rosen, W.G. and Davies, K.L. (1983). The Alzheimer's Disease Assessment Scale: an instrument of assessing treatment efficacy. *Psychopharmacol Bull* **6**, 87–94.

Morris, J.C., Cyrus, P.A., Orazem, J. *et al.* (1998). Metrifonate benefits cognitive, behavioural and global function in patients with Alzheimer's disease. *Neurology* **50**, 1222–1230.

O'Brien, B.J. (1998). Pharmacoeconomic evaluation of new treatments for Alzheimer's disease. In: Gauthier, S. (Ed.), *Pharmacotherapy of Alzheimer's disease*, Martin Dunitz, London, pp. 101–112.

Perry, E.K., Tomlinson, B.E., Blessed, G., Bergmann, K., Gibson, P. and Perry, R. (1978). Correlation of cholinergic abnormalities with senile plaques and mental test scores in senile dementia. *Br Med J* **2**, 1457–1459.

Rockwood, K. and Morris, J.C. (1996). Global staging measures in dementia. In: Gauthier, S. (Ed.). *Clinical Diagnosis and Management of Alzheimer's Disease*, Martin Dunitz, London, pp. 141–150.

Rogers, S.L., Farlow, M.R., Doody, R.S., Mohs, R., Friedhoff, L.T. and the Donepezil Study Group (1998). A 24 week double blind, placebo-controlled trial of donepezil in patients with Alzheimer's disease. *Neurology* **50**, 136–145.

Sano, M., Ernesto, C., Thomas, R.G. *et al.* (1997). A controlled trial of selegiline, α-tocopherol, or both as treatment for Alzheimer's disease. *New England Journal of Medicine* **336**, 1216–1222.

Simpson, P.M., Surmon, D.J., Wesnes, K.A. and Wilcock, C.G. (1991). The Cognitive Drug Research computerised assessment system for demented patients: a validation study. *Int J Geriatr Psychiatry* **6**, 95–102.

Tang, M.-X., Jacobs, D., Stern, Y. *et al.* (1996). Effect of oestrogen during menopause on lifetime risk and age of onset of Alzheimer's disease. *Lancet* **348**, 429–432.

Whitehouse, P.J., Price, D.L., Clark, A.W., Coyle, J.T. and DeLong, M.R. (1981). Alzheimer's disease: evidence for selective loss of cholinergic neurons in the nucleus basalis. *Ann Neurol* **10**, 122–126.

Everything You Need to Know About Old Age Psychiatry . . .
Edited by Robert Howard
©1999 Wrightson Biomedical Publishing Ltd

8

The Importance of Being an Old Age Psychiatrist

DAVID JOLLEY

Professor of Old Age Psychiatry, Penn Hospital, Wolverhampton, UK

The arguments for the development of the specialty of old age psychiatry within the British National Health Service (NHS) can be identified among weaknesses and difficulties in past provision of services for a particularly vulnerable group of patients: older people suffering from mental illnesses (Carse *et al.*, 1958). These weaknesses had continued after the creation of the Health Service in 1948 and had persisted through the 1950s and into the 1960s (Brothwood, 1971). But, from then on, the ideas of pioneer individuals who had found either the study or the development of services for older people a satisfactory area of work were brought together in a discipline based on the public health vision of a systematic, organized attack upon identifiable unmet need.

There are still those who find it difficult to comprehend what it is that makes old age psychiatry anything other than the exhibition of good practice in mental health among patients who happen to be elderly. They pursue their arguments to suggest that good practice can best be guaranteed and ageism avoided if all general psychiatrists simply take on to their caseloads any patients presenting to them irrespective of age. More successful and persistent similar arguments within the area of physical health have arguably led to irreparable damage to geriatric medicine (Mann, 1995).

Old age psychiatry is a discipline for patients, for their families and for all those professionals and volunteers who give their time and talent to older people with mental illnesses.

THE SCOPE OF OLD AGE PSYCHIATRY

From the onset, the main condition of interest in old age psychiatry has been dementia. It was dementia, with its characteristic of irreversible, often progressive decline, which contaminated people's views of mental illness in late life to such an extent that older people with mental illness became almost 'untouchables' (Isaac, 1969; Isaac and Neville, 1976). Some services have restricted their interests to the dementias, through most have found it appropriate and rewarding to take on older people suffering from other late-onset illnesses, including depression, paranoid states and other disorders. In doing so, it has been usual to identify an age threshold for entry into services and this has been most usually the age of 65, though there have been variations on this by which people with dementia have been accepted over the age of 65, whereas people with other disorders have not been accepted unless their age of onset was over 70 or 75. These variations were almost always determined by the availability of consultant manpower within the old age service to cope with predictable workloads. Many services now work to much more flexible entry criteria and will take on patients of whatever diagnostic group who share the characteristics of late life with or without physical dependency and progressive deterioration. Thus, many services now include older chronic psychotics, previously cared for within the orbit of general adult psychiatry (Jolley et al., 1998), and others who have psychiatric disorders complicating chronic or progressive physical illnesses, for instance parkinsonism, stroke disorder and even respiratory or cardiovascular disorders, even if they are not yet 65 years old. It has been a feature of the specialty that as experience and knowledge have expanded it has remained flexible and responsive to new challenges and opportunities.

THE ORIENTATION OF OLD AGE PSYCHIATRY

As many of the disorders of late life have links with biological change within the brain or other organs of the body, the discipline has always had its attractions, and these are perhaps stronger than ever now for psychiatrists of a 'biological' orientation. Nevertheless, the strongest theme within the discipline is that of social, community-orientated psychiatry, not forgetting the general-hospital equivalent of these – liaison psychiatry (Arie, 1970; Arie and Jolley, 1982, 1998). Psychotherapeutic approaches have always been an integral part of thinking among practitioners in contrast to the received wisdom that psychotherapy had little to offer the older patient. In recent years there has been a considerable increase in writing about psychotherapeutic approaches to older people, both individually and in groups (Ong et al., 1987; Benbow, 1988; Moffatt et al., 1995).

THE RANGE OF OLD AGE PSYCHIATRY

It is common to most services that older people are often best seen in the place where they are living. This takes psychiatrists into people's own homes, into residential homes and into nursing homes. There the older person is seen alongside their personal history and alongside the strengths or apparent weaknesses of support available to them. There are variations in emphasis between services as to who carries out home visits and whether they are restricted to initial contacts or follow-ups, but most will accept that knowledge gained by interactions at home serves as a major strength for therapy in the future. The practice gives confidence for patients and their carers in the commitment of the service to understand their needs and to give them all appropriate respect.

Further assessment away from home, or the alternative home setting, may be arranged in a traditional outpatients' or general practitioner's surgery and one important development within this mode is the 'memory clinic' (Wright and Lindesay, 1995). The advantage of such clinics is that they allow a more detailed investigation and assessment in a controlled environment and can make use of the expertise of a number of different staff and types of equipment, both conveniently and efficiently. Thus, they complement the advantages of home visits.

Day hospitals may also be used to further investigations and assessments and allow the exhibition of treatments over a planned programme of sessions linked to monitoring of their effects (Arie, 1974; Jolley, 1994). They also have potential for relieving strain upon carers and opening up the opportunity for the patient to become involved in activities that life at home has had to restrict or deny. The grading between a therapeutic day hospital and a therapeutic day centre is not clear-cut and can give rise to some uncertainties as regards best uses of resources (Fasey, 1994). There are various ways of dealing with this but, whatever is done, it is clear that there should be a close relationship between the NHS day hospital and day care provided by all other agencies (Jolley, 1994).

Inpatient care is required for the assessment, investigation and treatment of people who present problems that are too complicated or too hazardous to be managed elsewhere. It is understood that the number of such beds required is relatively modest but increases as the scope of services expands (Royal College of Psychiatrists, 1995). Life with continued disability or the prospect of frequent relapse remains the lot of many patients suffering from mental illness in late life, certainly including the dementias but also other conditions. Thus, old age psychiatry has always had and will always have an interest and responsibility for continuing care. In many instances this involves seeing patients through, with their families, in their own homes. Other patients will move on to residential homes or nursing homes and very few will require continuing care within an NHS hospital. Nevertheless, it is clearly the case that some patients benefit from such care and it is a blessing that after periods of some difficulty the need for this mode of care has been confirmed and will be provided (Department of Health, 1995). 'Seeing patients through' often means seeing them through to death, for death is part of late life and particularly a part of the psychiatric disorders of late life. Sometimes this is because those disorders are complications of other illnesses, which in themselves are terminal. Dementia itself can be looked on as a progressive terminal illness and, indeed, statistics on the cause of death are now collected in a way that reflects this (Jolley and Baxter, 1997). Mood disorders of late life also carry a raised death rate, as does schizophrenia (Harris and Barraclough, 1998). Thus, management of death and its aftermath for families and staff is part of the work of old age psychiatry.

The range of old age psychiatry spreads from early recognition of disorders through assessment and treatment, rehabilitation and maintenance, decline and death.

ROLES OF THE OLD AGE PSYCHIATRIST

Advocate

There are many competing claims for people's interests and resources. There are now a number of pressure groups, notably the Alzheimer's Disease Society, which have taken up the cause of older people with mental illness but these were pre-dated by the early psychogeriatricians, and indeed most receive considerable support from the new generation of psychogeriatricians. Within the local politics of the NHS and, indeed, other organizations and sources of funding the old age psychiatrist is still required to identify and fight his or her corner.

Teacher

Academic posts have come only fairly recently but teaching for medical students was taken on very early by enthusiasts with NHS contracts and the majority of teaching continues to be in their hands. Almost all medical students are appropriately exposed to good teaching on not only the biology of psychiatric disorders of late life but also the related clinical and service aspects. Beyond medicine and medical students, old age psychiatrists and their teams have contributed to teaching and training for nurses, social workers, occupational therapists, physiotherapists and many other professionals. These disciplines have much to contribute to special services for older people with mental illnesses and many of their patients who come from other sources have emotional and other psychiatric disorders, an understanding of which improves their therapeutic potential, approach and outcomes.

There has been increasing interest among the lay public eager to know about health matters of all sorts so that schools and colleges include topics related to emotional and other problems including dementia in late life, and are pleased to have input from the special services. The media have certainly taken on board Alzheimer's disease and encourage discussion of the issues relating to the emergence of a very large population of older people. Anxiety and antipathy towards this population of elders is not uncommon and it is important to help everyone view the opportunities of later life more positively and indeed more realistically.

Much of the interest and pressure for information comes because many people understand that they themselves may become patients suffering from disorders in late life or are already finding themselves part of a family where one or more members is experiencing these difficulties. Pressure for information from families and patients increases as they quite properly wish to remain in control of their own destinies, getting the best out of available resources.

Health educationalist/health promoter

Just beginning to emerge from all this thirst for information is the prospect of old age psychiatry contributing to the health and well-being of populations by the avoidance of illness as well as the modification and minimization of problems arising from illnesses that have developed.

Student

The knowledge-base necessary to provide an optimal response to patients' needs is great and, thankfully, growing. There is a good deal to be known about the psychiatry of late life, both its history and its current best practice. New developments in the medicine of late life continue to emerge, both in terms of specific therapies for particular conditions and the best way of bringing these therapies into practice. Appreciations of older people through gerontological studies aimed at psychology, sociology, history and geography are often on the periphery of the knowledge of most practising old age psychiatrists but are available as additional delights to those who will turn their attention to these matters.

Within medicine, the discipline of clinical audit has been encompassed over the last 10 years, providing a framework within which clinicians and their teams can both monitor and evaluate the effectiveness and consequences of their practice.

Opportunities for research and development remain open and extensive. It is a criticism of our work that much innovation has been undertaken without rigorous evaluation. This is a criticism perhaps to be accepted as a challenge but not to be allowed to paralyse confidence and vision.

Innovator

The very concept of a special service for older people with mental illness was, of course, in itself an innovation and within this framework a satisfying and stimulating range of alternatives have been explored. It has been one of the attractions of the discipline in its early years that a considerable freedom has been experienced for individuals to be creative and most have treated these opportunities with respect and responsibility. While there is an understandable concern that all parts of our population should be provided with services and responses of equal quality, that should not imply that everything is reduced to a sterile uniformity. It is through the initiatives of enthusiasts that developments and progress have been made.

Point of reference

Most referrals into specialist old age psychiatry come from primary care or from geriatric medicine or other specialist health services. In addition, the old age psychiatry service and its consultants are identifiable as places to refer to for information and help from other agencies, including social services, voluntary sector and private sector organizations, and individuals. Some services have made a point of accepting or even encouraging direct referrals from sources outside medicine, but within the discipline of the NHS it is clearly wise that primary health care is always involved and informed when patients become subject to specialist service interventions.

Team player

The consultant old age psychiatrist finds himself or herself involved in a number of teams: the community mental health team for older people within the community; the day hospital team; the ward team in the assessment unit; the liaison team within the hospital; the audit team; the research team; the teaching unit. Within all of these, he or she must find and play the appropriate role. There has been some heat generated by discussion of the most appropriate role for the consultant within the community mental health team for older people (Figures 1 and 2), some being keen to see the team as made up of equipotent, equable practitioners, much in the model of total football that had some popularity in the 1970s and 1980s. While it is clear that certain individuals referred to services are likely to benefit

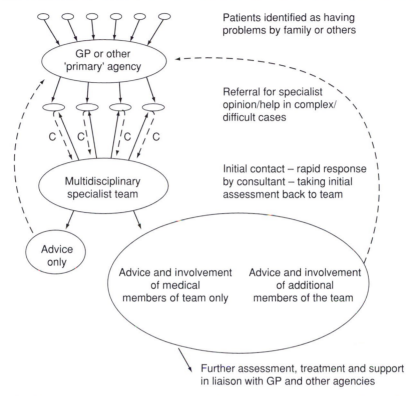

Figure 1. Model of responses from a team with early consultant contact (C, consultant).

most particularly from the skills of particular specialists, including the occupational therapist, perhaps the speech therapist, perhaps the clinical psychologist or community psychiatric nurse, it is probable that best functioning for the total team as well as best service to individual patients can be achieved by initial referral to one of the generalist professionals within the team, i.e. the consultant or a community psychiatric nurse. Where there is an expectation that the specialist team is to take responsibility for formal assessment, including investigation and diagnosis, in association with altered treatment, it is almost always appropriate for the patient to be seen early by the consultant. There is clearly advantage in detached evaluation of best strategies espoused by enthusiasts. For the moment, all that is available in the literature are the accounts of enthusiasts, and indeed experts, in particular modes of practice, together with their evaluations of outcome (Herzberg, 1995).

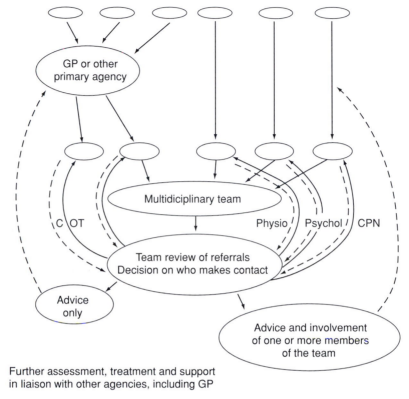

Figure 2. Model of a team using 'multidisciplinary' first contact (C, consultant; OT, occupational therapist; Physio, physiotherapist; Psychol, psychologist; CPN, community psychiatric nurse).

Missionary

The concept and practice of specialist old age psychiatry services came from England and has been taken around the world by the pioneers who visited Australia, Canada, the USA and parts of Europe. Again, Professor Arie played a particular role in conducting a series of courses at Nottingham under the auspices of the British Council and this led to a rapid spread of the principles to a number of underdeveloped countries as well as to the developed world. International organizations including the International Psychogeriatric Association, the European Association of Geriatric Psychiatry and the World Psychiatry Association's Section on Old Age Psychiatry have been spawned by these initiatives.

Perhaps the most important missionary work, however, has occurred within Great Britain itself, with a progressive spread through the regions and smaller administrative units of the recurrently reorganized NHS, so that by 1998 most parts of England, Wales, Scotland and Northern Ireland have a recognizable specialist old age psychiatry service; Ireland is beginning to follow suit.

The model of a successful and strong discipline of old age psychiatry is now looked on as helpful to the rest of psychiatry. Most of the specialist sections can claim to be successful and strong, in contrast to general psychiatry which is perhaps belatedly beginning to learn the lessons (Milton, 1998).

Other parts of medicine have experienced similar consequences of specialization, i.e. that specialist services have grown and prospered, sometimes to the disbenefit of overall service provision. Older people are faced with the dilemma that, whereas it is clearly desirable that no one is denied access to the skills of experts in particular organ pathologies simply because they are older, many people who get into difficulties in late life do so not as a consequence of one failing organ but because of the interaction of several organs failing in disharmony and played against the background of social circumstances which may not be sustaining. Optimal management in this situation requires the broad-based skills of geriatric medicine or geriatric psychiatry.

THE IMPORTANCE OF BEING AN OLD AGE PSYCHIATRIST

While old age psychiatry has gained strength from being able to give to others, there is a very real sense that membership of the group of old age psychiatrists is a source of mutual support. There has been increasing interest in stress among doctors and psychiatrists and the ways in which stress weakens people, encourages them to early retirement, and occasionally brings forward death (Kendall and Pearce, 1998; Benbow and Jolley, 1998a). There is little doubt that, at the moment, old age psychiatrists find themselves members of a pleasant group of people, open-hearted and generous in their approach to patients and each other, brave and strong in standing their ground and encouraged by four decades of progressive success. This cohesion in itself is probably our strongest guarantee of further successes but we must be aware of the ravages that self-interest and disorganization have visited upon others. We will need to continue to recruit and train into the discipline and to care for each other locally, within regional groups, or in subregional groups as the numbers increase, nationally and internationally (Jolley and Benbow, 1997; Benbow and Jolley, 1998b; Wattis, 1998).

REFERENCES

Arie, T. (1970). The first year of the Goodmayes psychiatric service for old people. *Lancet* **ii**, 1179–1182.
Arie, T. (1974). Day care in geriatric psychiatry. *Gerontol Clin* **17**, 31–39.

Arie, T. and Jolley, D. (1982). Making services work: organisation and style of psychogeriatric services. In: Levy, R. and Post, F. (Eds), *The Psychiatry of Late Life*. Blackwell Scientific, Oxford, pp. 222–251.

Arie, T. and Jolley, D. (1998). Psychogeriatric services. In: Tallis, R., Fillit, H. and Brocklehurst, J. (Eds), *Brocklehurst's Textbook of Gerontology and Geriatric Medicine*, fifth edition. Churchill Livingstone, Edinburgh, pp. 1567–1574.

Benbow, S.M. (1988). Family therapy in the elderly. In: *Current Approaches to Affective Disorders in the Elderly*. Duphas, Southampton, pp. 44–46.

Benbow, S.M. and Jolley, D.J. (1998a). Psychiatrists under stress. *Psychiatr Bull* **22**, 1–2.

Benbow, S.M. and Jolley, D. (1998b). Gender, isolation, work patterns and stress among old age psychiatrists. *Int J Geriatr Psychiatry* **10**, 37–40.

Brothwood, J. (1971). The organisation and development of services for the aged, with special reference to the mentally ill. In: Kay, D.W.K. and Walk, A. (Eds), *Recent Developments in Psycho-Geriatrics*. British Journal of Psychiatry, London, pp. 99–112.

Carse, J., Parton, N. and Watt, A. (1958). A district mental health service: the Worthing experiment. *Lancet* **i**, 39–42.

Department of Health (1995). *NHS Responsibilities for Meeting Continuing Health Care Needs*. HSG(95) 8. LAC(95)5. HMSO, London.

Fasey, C. (1994). The day hospital in old age psychiatry: the case against. *Int J Geriatr Psychiatry* **9**, 519–523.

Harris, E.C. and Barraclough, B. (1998). Excess mortality of mental disorder. *Br J Psychiatry* **173**, 11–53.

Herzberg, J. (1995). Can multidisciplinary teams carry out competent and safe psychogeriatric assessments in the community? *Int J Geriatr Psychiatry* **10**, 1073–1077.

Isaac, B. (1969). Some characteristics of geriatric patients. *Scot Med J* **14**, 243–252.

Isaac, B. and Neville, Y. (1976). The needs of old people. *Br J Prevent Soc Med* **30**, 79–85.

Jolley, D. (1994). The development of day hospitals and day hospital care. In: Copeland, J.R.M., Abou-Saleh, M. and Blazer, D. (Eds), *Principles and Practice of Geriatric Psychiatry*. John Wiley, Chichester, pp. 905–910.

Jolley, D. and Baxter, D. (1997). Life expectation in organic brain disease. *Adv Psychiatr Treat* **3**, 211–218.

Jolley, D. and Benbow, S.M. (1997). The everyday work of geriatric psychiatrists. *Int J Geriatr Psychiatry* **12**, 109–113.

Jolley, D., Russell, E. and Lennon, S. (1998). The organisation of services in geriatric psychiatry. In: Pathy, J.S.M. (Ed.), *Principles and Practice of Geriatric Medicine*, third edition. John Wiley, Chichester, pp. 1055–1068.

Kendall, R.E. and Pearce, A. (1998). Consultant psychiatrists who retire prematurely. *Psychiatr Bull* **21**, 741–745.

Mann, A.H. (1995). Future directions for the speciality of old age psychiatry. *Int J Geriatr Psychiatry* **1**, 87–91.

Milton, J. (1998). So who wants to be a consultant general psychiatrist? *Psychiatr Bull* **22**, 345–347.

Moffatt, F., Mohr, C, and Ames, D. (1995). A group therapy programme for depressed and anxious elderly patients. *Int J Geriatr Psychiatry* **10**, 37–40.

Ong, Y., Martineau, F., Lloyd, C. and Robbins, I. (1987). A support group for the depressed elderly. *Int J Geriatr Psychiatry* **2**, 119–123.

Royal College of Psychiatrists (1995). *Caring for a community: the community care policy of the Royal College of Psychiatrists*. Royal College of Psychiatrists, London.

Wattis, J. (1998). The state of the nation. The 1996 survey of old age psychiatry. *Old Age Psychiatrist* **11**, 1.

Wright, N. and Lindesay, J. (1995). A survey of memory clinics in the British Isles. *Int J Geriatr Psychiatry* **10**, 379–385.

Everything You Need to Know About Old Age Psychiatry . . .
Edited by Robert Howard
©1999 Wrightson Biomedical Publishing Ltd

9

Residential Care: Quality and Costs

JUSTINE SCHNEIDER

Centre for Applied Social Studies, University of Durham, Durham, UK

INTRODUCTION

Defining quality

Quality is an elusive concept. Like 'truth' or 'goodness', it is something which people think they know instinctively. However, our understanding of quality is inseparable from our experience. If someone has never stayed in a five-star hotel, it may be difficult for them to conceive how it might differ from the three-star accommodation with which they are familiar. But if they have never even visited a hotel, much less stayed in one, the criteria of quality that they may be tempted to apply may be limited, if not wholly unsuitable. Analogously, it is quite common for older people and their close relatives to be faced with the task of assessing the quality of a small number of residential homes, despite the fact that they have never visited one, much less stayed in one. This task usually arises when admission is urgent, emotions are mixed and financial resources are limited. For older people and their families, as well as for the professionals who care for them, reliable measures of the quality of residential care are vitally important.

In our commercial society we can often place a material value on quality, as the example of hotel rooms shows: the higher the quality, the higher the cost. It seems reasonable to expect the same to apply in purchasing residential care. However, until we define quality we cannot demonstrate the relationship between costs and quality, and it would be simplistic to assume that there is a linear association between the two. In this chapter it is hoped to show that not all aspects of quality have an identifiable cost although some things which might be taken as indicators of quality have clear cost implications.

Defining costs

When we talk about costs in the context of health or social care we are not usually talking about prices. Economists use the term 'opportunity cost' in measuring the costs of health and social care. 'Opportunity' means that costs are seen as opportunities foregone, not money spent. The opportunity cost is therefore meant to reflect the true social value of a thing. This is a notional value, not a price. 'Opportunity' cost can be applied to labour, resources or services in their best alternative use. The opportunity cost of taking your dog for a walk is not merely the amount you could earn in those 20 minutes. It is this amount, less the tax and overheads you would have incurred, and the benefits you and the dog derive from walking. That is one way of calculating the cost to you, which is only one possible perspective. There are three different perspectives that are commonly taken in calculating economic costs, according to who might be responsible for meeting the costs. This can be calculated from the perspective of the individual person or dog-owner, from that of the body of taxpayers (cost to the Exchequer) or from the point of view of society as a whole. The cost to the taxpayer might also need to take into account clearing up after your dog, if you are an irresponsible dog-owner. The cost to society at large would include the nuisance caused by your dog barking at pigeons in the park, and so on.

Clearly, the calculation of opportunity costs is an art, and it employs many judgements about which elements should be included in estimations, and how to place a value on these elements. In costing health and social care, conventions have been developed. By convention, what should be measured is in fact long-run marginal opportunity cost. This is the opportunity cost of adding one more client to a service, taking into account the costs of setting up a new service if required. In practice, short-run average revenue costs plus capital and overhead elements are most frequently used to estimate opportunity costs. A full discussion of this approach is given by Netten and Beecham (1993).

Residential care and its costs

An understanding of the costs of residential care requires knowledge of historical background. Part III of the 1948 National Assistance Act gave local authorities a duty to provide accommodation for needy older people who did not require the health care provided under the new National Health Service (NHS). The homes which were set up still carried the stigma of the workhouse. Local authorities were empowered to charge according to residents' ability to pay, so they were means-tested to make financial contributions to the costs of care. In 1979, social security introduced a Residential Care Allowance, which permitted anyone living at about subsistence level and therefore entitled to Supplementary Benefit (Income Support) to enter residential care without further ado. A rapid growth in demand for residential home placements ensued. This was fuelled by the policy of long-term hospital bed closures and discharge of long-stay patients into community settings. About the same time, a boom in the property market fostered a huge increase in the supply of private residential places to meet the growing demand for such care. Between 1979 and 1989 the number of places in private residential homes alone rose by 323% in England, from 32 000 to 135 000. Public expenditure on residential care rose 100-fold, from £10 million in 1970 to £1000 million in 1989. By 1989, private providers had overtaken local authorities in terms of residential care bed numbers. However, it should be noted that in total no more than 5–6% of people aged over 70 were accommodated in any form of residential care (Challis, 1992; Hugman, 1994).

The Audit Commission (1986) drew attention to the fact that state funding for people entitled to social security who wished to enter residential care was a perverse incentive which increased the demand for beds. This was a key force behind the White Paper *Caring for People: Community Care in the Next Decade and Beyond* (Department of Health, 1989) and the National Health Service and Community Care Act 1990. Together, these policy initiatives represented far-reaching reforms. Here, only those changes directly affecting residential care will be noted. Local authorities were given the responsibility for assessment of people wishing to enter residential care. They were also given the budget for care through the transfer, in 1993, of about £500 million from the social security budget to local authorities, to fund new residential placements and alternative forms of caring for people in their own homes. To protect the private sector and promote the 'mixed economy' of provision, the funds came with the condition that no more than 20% should be spent on services provided by the local authority.

In this way, the local authority entered the market for residential care as a key purchaser, in addition to its pre-existing duty to inspect and register residential homes. Freed from the obligation to maintain its own provision, the local authority was faced with the problem of comparing the quality of care in different settings in order both to ensure that value for money was obtained and to satisfy its moral duty towards dependent residents.

So far, nursing care has not been mentioned. The growth in nursing beds has occurred over the same period, similarly influenced by hospital closures and the community care reforms, funded by social security budget and latterly by the NHS, which has the responsibility for inspection and registration of nursing homes. Since 1993, the funding source is probably the most important difference between nursing and residential care, with nursing home places being mostly funded by the health service. There is a predictable hierarchy of levels of dependency in different settings: sheltered housing, very sheltered housing, voluntary residential homes, private residential homes, local authority residential homes, nursing homes and hospital wards (Darton, 1994). However, there is also considerable overlap. Average levels of dependency in local authority residential homes increased in the 1980s, but equivalent information over time for nursing homes is difficult to find. Moreover, it is important to assess both mental and physical dependency, since patients in psychiatric and psychogeriatric wards seem to be less physically disabled than patients in geriatric wards or nursing homes.

A redefinition of long-term care responsibilities between health and social services has been stimulated by the directive on continuing care (Department of Health, 1996). This has required health authorities and local authorities to define precisely their financial responsibilities for care of different types in different settings. It has forced the recognition that some of the care provided in nursing homes may be categorized as 'social care', while even some of the care provided in domiciliary settings may be classed properly as 'health care'. It has generated huge debates and is far from settled. In practice there seems to have been recent growth in dually-registered homes. This can be seen as a response both to the ageing of the resident population and to stricter admission criteria being operated by local authorities or the health service, as more home-based care has become available. In short, the distinction between residential and nursing care is not clear-cut. The criteria of quality in nursing homes seem likely to include all those which apply in residential settings, plus additional criteria related to health care and health needs. In some areas joint registration teams are operating and there is a move towards a single registration system of residential and nursing homes following the publication of a Department of Health review on regulation and inspection in 1996 (Burgner, 1996). Taking all long-stay care places together (residential, nursing and long-stay hospital beds) a useful rule of thumb is that there were about half a million people accommodated in this way in 1994 (Dalley, 1997). Issues of quality apply to any care setting, and while most of the illustrations given below come from a study of residential homes, they will have relevance for almost any setting.

Residential care and its quality

Quality of residential care cannot be separated entirely from quality of life in residential care. Quality of life measurement has become an industry in itself in health care evaluation. Numerous instruments exist, both to measure generic quality of life (subjective or objective) and to assess disease-specific quality of life (Bowling, 1991). Some of them have applications in the evaluation of the quality of residential care (Barry et al., 1993; Oliver et al., 1995). In order to understand the distinction between quality of care and quality of life, it may be helpful to differentiate between process and outcome (Donabedian, 1980). In this sense, residential care is a process whose features may be assessed, and one of its outcomes for the individual may be described as quality of life. To the extent that the opinion of the individual resident is the final arbiter on all judgements of quality, quality of care and quality of life are closely associated. One reason for addressing the issue of quality of care is that we assume that the process of care is directly amenable to intervention. If we can understand what is good or bad about the process, this can be improved by taking appropriate steps.

Any evaluation of residential settings for elderly people inevitably encounters the difficulty that a high proportion have dementia and, although some information can be gleaned from most people with dementia, this may not be comparable with data gathered from people without cognitive impairment. This fact may tend to favour more 'objective' methods in evaluating residential care. I would argue that neither dimension alone is sufficient to measure quality of residential care. To demonstrate this point, it is possible to imagine a home which performs well on process indicators but where the residents are all unhappy, or a home where the residents are all happy, but the process indicators are poor. Few people would argue that either home is an example of high-quality residential care. For this to be true, both subjective and objective measures need to show good ratings.

To sum up the introductory comments, this chapter is concerned with the quality of the care process. Quality is a rather nebulous concept, but it seems to have at least two principal dimensions: objective quality, measurable by means of verifiable data; and subjective quality, which depends upon the experience of the individual recipient of care or people close to them. Economists and accountants do not necessarily see costs the same way. Opportunity costs may vary according to whose perspective is adopted. In judging the costs of residential care, an attempt should be made to quantify social effects (benefits or harm). Residential care costs are of great interest not just because a growing proportion of the population is having recourse to this type of provision, but also because the value for money achieved in residential settings has a direct impact on the resources available for health and social welfare. In the section which follows, standards for residential care which have been set by authoritative sources (specifically, the Centre for Policy on Ageing) are introduced and tested empirically with reference to one study, not to prove or disprove their reliability and validity, but mainly to illustrate their application in practice.

DEFINING QUALITY OF CARE

In the health care context, several definitions have been put forward to elucidate the concept of quality. Criteria, which have been applied by commentators (Black, 1990; Higginson, 1994) include, in no particular order:

- effectiveness – the impact of interventions on patients' expected health outcomes;
- acceptability – humanity and consideration for patients' preferences and rights;
- efficiency – value for money of health outcomes;
- access – availability of services when or where patients need them;
- equity – fair treatment of patients; and
- relevance – match of services to needs and wants.

Although developed in the context of health care quality assessment, all of these can be applied to some extent to quality of residential care.

Effectiveness is usually applied to treatment interventions, and in relation to residential care it begs the question 'to what effect?' It might seem that long-term care has no obvious outcome except death. Nevertheless, since people are now only admitted to residential care if their needs cannot be met in their own homes, the extent to which the residential setting satisfies these needs (for protection, care or treatment) can be judged as its effectiveness. Indeed, as found in the study described below, there can be wide variation in the extent to which health needs are met in different settings.

Acceptability introduces the consumer viewpoint, and may be applied to the resident, their close relatives, inspectors or visitors to the home. The environment of the home, menus, rules and attitudes may be judged differently by different people. Even within one group, for example local authority inspectors, consistency is difficult to achieve (Gibbs and Sinclair, 1992). Questions of acceptability raise questions of cultural values and norms, and these can be analysed from the perspective of rights or from that of cultural awareness. Variations in lifestyle pose a challenge in long-term settings where people are unavoidably made aware of their co-residents' preferences. In such settings, risks taken by one person may have repercussions for other residents. Therefore, some 'rights' are likely to be defended more vigorously than others. For instance, the right to practise one's religion will be more popular than the right to imbibe large quantities of alcohol. Hence, acceptability may be an area of rights and restrictions which is constantly being renegotiated, and against which established norms are subject to change over time.

Equity is an important issue in all group living arrangements, where consideration for the individual's wishes may need to be weighed against the interests of other residents. The criterion of equity can be applied by asking what share of the home's resources (space, care-staff time, entertainment, food) each resident enjoys. Issues of equity commonly arise in residential settings where demented and nondemented residents are cared for together. As in rationing health care, the patient or resident's 'ability to benefit' may be used as a means of rationing resources within homes.

Access may not seem to be a problem for those people already in residential care, but physical disability can prevent people from fully utilizing a building and its facilities, while the accessibility of personal care from staff may encounter barriers of communication and staff availability, for example. Cultural accessibility is another consideration: for people living in settings which are entirely geared to a culture other than their own, access to familiar pastimes, food or social organizations may be restricted.

Relevance can be seen as the match of services to needs and wants. A closely related concept in residential care might be targeting; ensuring that people receive adequate and appropriate support, without inducing dependency or making unrealistic demands on residents or staff. The accuracy of such targeting may sometimes be closely associated with efficiency in evaluations of residential care.

Setting standards

Home Life: A Code of Practice for Residential Care (Avebury, 1984), and *A Better Home Life: A Code of Practice for Residential and Nursing Care* (Avebury, 1996) are, respectively, the report of a working party sponsored by the Department of Health and Social Security, and the report of an advisory group, both convened by the Centre for Policy on Ageing and chaired by Lady Avebury. These reports provide detailed and comprehensive guidelines of best practice in care. The later publication, *A Better Home Life*, brings in the community care reforms, and extends the scope of the guidelines in relation to older people, particularly those people who have dementia. In recognition of the diversification of types of care, this report covers nursing homes, long-stay hospital wards and sheltered housing:

> The boundaries between social, personal and nursing care are notoriously hard to define ... More important, in our view, is the holistic approach to care of people in residential settings where all the different aspects are linked by a commitment to offer the best possible quality of life. (Avebury, 1996, xi)

The basic rights of residents underpinning the first report, *Home Life*, which was written for all groups of people in residential care were:

- fulfillment – enabling a person to achieve their physical, emotional, social and intellectual potential
- dignity – preserving self-respect, privacy and recognition of sensitivities and talents
- autonomy – a basic right to self-determination in the context of a communal setting; no rigid regimentation
- individuality – responsiveness to the needs and cultural requirements of residents

- esteem – respect for the life and knowledge of the individual
- quality of experience – availability of the widest possible range of 'normal' experiences
- emotional needs – freedom for emotional expression, including intimate relations
- risk and choice – responsible risk-taking should be regarded as normal. (Avebury, 1984, pp. 15–17)

Home Life contains 218 recommendations, so it would be impossible to examine them all here. However, the following (numbers 134–138) specifically pertain to older people:

- The right of elderly people to autonomy and choice should always be respected.
- The layout, décor and furnishing of the home should be designed to minimize confusion.
- Staff should be trained to understand the needs of mentally and physically frail old people.
- Community support and treatment services should be consulted in the care of mentally ill elderly people.
- Physical restraint and control by sedation should not be used. (Avebury, 1984, p. 70)

The sequel, *A Better Home Life*, reformulates the basic principles, adding as desirable goals 'choice' and 'control', 'expression of beliefs', 'safety', 'citizens' rights' and 'opportunities for leisure activities' (Avebury, 1996, pp. 8–11). This book states even more strongly that the misapplication of drugs constitutes abuse:

> The use of drugs to control or restrain a resident is unacceptable unless medically required. The overuse and misuse of sedatives, and other medications, which too often happens in homes, should be regarded as evidence of bad practice (Avebury, 1996, p. 106).

A Better Home Life underlines the importance of care plans as 'essential', and says that these should be comprehensive, and should be reviewed every three to six months. It also addresses the need for leisure activities, both within and outside the residential home.

Testing standards

In 1995/96, a study funded by the UK Department of Health looked in detail at 17 residential homes distributed throughout England. These homes were selected to include eight which had participated in the staff development module of the Department of Health-sponsored Caring in Homes Initiative (Youll and McCourt-Perring, 1993), a programme aimed at improving quality of care in homes. Each home was matched with another in terms of size, geographical location and sector (private, voluntary or Local Authority). Due to a high number of vacancies, two homes had to be matched with one, resulting in a sample of 17 homes. This sample, while not statistically representative of all residential homes in England, is nevertheless fairly typical of average or superior homes. It comprised four homes run by voluntary organizations, four privately-run homes and nine Local Authority homes. It proved difficult to recruit more private homes to the study, although this would have yielded a sample that better reflected the current supply of residential care places. Here, selected criteria of quality nominated by *Home Life* and *A Better Home Life* are considered in relation to the data collected by this study. Full details are reported in Schneider *et al.* (1997, 1998).

Staff training

The study found that, while there may have been extensive on-the-job and vocational training, particularly National Vocational Qualifications, very few staff had formal nursing or social work qualifications. On average, fewer than two members of staff per home had training at a level which local authorities would accept for management posts (DipSW, CQSW, CSS, CRSW, SRN, RMN, RGN, CPN or SEN).

Community services

Of the 300 residents in the study, 63% had seen a general practitioner in the previous three months and 35% had been visited by a district nurse. Only 12% had been to the dentist, however, and fewer than 30% of residents had seen a geriatrician, physiotherapist or occupational therapist. No resident's notes recorded that they had seen a community psychiatric nurse (CPN), although about 40% of the people in this sample had a severe degree of dementia.

Physical restraint

This was not witnessed by researchers, and restraint by medication is difficult to judge. Nineteen per cent of the residents were taking major tranquillizers, with 23% taking hypnotic medication. Therefore, roughly one-fifth of residents were being given sedative medication of some kind. However, whether control by sedation applies depends somewhat on knowledge about a person's prior mental health. While some former residents of psychiatric hospitals may have been on maintenance doses of major tranquillizers, the numbers to whom this applies do not account for all those people taking sedative medication.

Care plans

Care plans for the residents were scrutinized. If they had been reviewed within the past six months they were rated according to whether four areas were covered: physical care, emotional care, social care and cultural requirements. There was considerable variation in the extent to which care plans met these simple criteria. The following table shows the distribution of the ratings for the 17 homes in the study. While they were not a representative sample of all homes, these findings illustrate the variability in standards that exists. This variability, in turn, indicates that quality is not consistent between homes (Table 1).

Table 1.   Proportion of care plans up to date and acceptable in 17 homes (%).

Care plans subject	Mean	Minimum	Maximum
Physical care	28	0	96
Emotional care	16	0	91
Social care	23	0	100
Cultural needs	16	0	100

These findings, therefore, illustrate that the standards set by *Home Life*, even 10 years on, still posed a challenge in residential care, and that some of the criteria of *A Better Home Life* were being observed only by a minority of homes.

Social interactions

As indicated above, value judgements are implicit in many measures of quality, and where social relationships are the focus, such judgements may vary widely. This can be illustrated by looking in detail at one instrument which is used to measure the social climate in homes, the Sheltered Care Environment Scale of Moos and Lemke (1984). This is an instrument with 60 questions which can be completed by residents or staff. It has seven subscales: cohesion, independence, self-disclosure, organization, resident influence, physical comfort and conflict. The conflict indicators reflect a high level of what could be called emotional expressiveness:

- residents sometimes start arguments;
- it is not unusual for residents to express their anger;
- residents sometimes criticize this place;
- residents seldom keep their disagreements to themselves;
- it is not unusual for residents to complain about each other;
- it is not always peaceful and quiet here;
- residents often get impatient with each other;
- residents complain a lot; and
- residents criticize each other a lot.

The maximum score of 100% therefore represents agreement with all nine statements. When about 250 staff in 17 homes were surveyed, the mean conflict score was 48%. However, the 95% confidence interval ranged from 28 to 76%. Which end of this distribution represents a desirable atmosphere? The question is, how should we weight high conflict scores: as permitting open expression and ventilation of feelings, or as reflecting hostility and even violence? Is high emotional expression acceptable in homes for older people and bad in homes for people with functional mental health problems? Or could it be that each home has its conflict 'norm', and deviations from this in response to other changes are of interest?

Effective health care

This is not explicitly emphasized by *Home Life* or *A Better Home Life*, but it is stressed by the quality guidelines generated by the health care tradition, more than by the residential care standards. This is understandable in the light of the divisions that still exist between social care and health care, but it is an area which long-term care needs to address because of the high levels of dependency in all settings. The study described above interviewed the key worker of each resident about their perception of the health needs of residents and how they responded to these. It found that common health needs such as immobility, instability, hearing loss and visual impairment were not always properly treated. Hearing loss is a good example. Thirty-nine percent of the residents interviewed were assessed by the research nurses as having significant hearing loss. Key workers were judged to respond well (a) if they were aware of this impairment, (b) if steps were taken to remedy it, such as provision of a hearing aid or assessment by an audiologist, and (c) if aids were in working order. Key workers for just over half of the hearing-impaired residents (55%) satisfied the research nurses that they were responding appropriately, while 37% of key workers were rated as giving poor or inappropriate responses. However, when such physical needs as these were met, residents were significantly less likely to suffer from depression. One of the most important outcomes of the study was this finding of an association between physical and psychological well-being (Schneider *et al.*, 1998).

QUALITY OF CARE AND COSTS

A report by Tim Watkins and Nich Pearson (1996) of the Welsh Consumer Council breaks down the concept of quality into four aspects:

- **quality of the environment** in which people live (thickness of carpets, state of décor, availability of telephones, space and access to amenities)
- **quality of services received** (help given, adequacy of meals, heating, cleaning, toilet facilities)
- **quality of service delivery** (how staff address residents, whether they knock before entering rooms, choice available to residents, staff–resident interactions in general)
- **quality of each resident's life experience** (social network, interests, activities, sense of meaning, belonging, self-esteem)

These can be combined with the health care criteria discussed above, and with the spirit of the standards set in *Home Life* (see Table 2).

One advantage of this conceptualization is that it makes it clearer which aspects of quality are most likely to be associated with costs. Clearly, a price can be attached to material comfort in residential homes, just as it is in hotels: thick carpets cost more than bare boards and a town centre location has higher capital costs than one out of town. Cost is also likely to be directly linked to the services received; since staffing costs are one of the biggest overheads in residential care, the availability of staff to provide services which are effective, relevant and responsive is crucial. Of course, there are costs incurred through training, not least because staff need to be replaced while they go on training courses. By contrast, the way in which services are delivered may have more to do with staff attitudes and morale than with staff

Table 2. Four dimensions of quality.

A *Environment* Access to services, comfort	B *Services received* Effectiveness, relevance
D *Service delivery* Efficiency, acceptability respect	C *Individual experience* Control, dignity, privacy choice, atmosphere

numbers. And while residents' experience of choice, control and the atmosphere in the home will be conditioned by cost-related dimensions of décor and space, it may equally be influenced by relationships between staff and residents, contact with visitors and the extent to which the local community is involved in the home. These latter factors are likely to depend more on organizational factors and the mix of personalities in a home than on the material surroundings and the services provided.

Evidence of associations between quality and costs

In the study described above, no association was found between costs and a composite measure of quality of care based on 25 criteria. Given the complex interweaving of cost-related and non-cost-related elements in definitions of quality, it is hardly surprising that it is difficult to demonstrate a statistical association between the costs of residential care and the quality found therein. Whether this holds may depend upon the way in which definitions of quality are operationalized: if the emphasis is on factors in boxes A and B (Table 2), an association with costs may well be found. By contrast, if the definition of quality stresses boxes C and D, this is less likely. Of course, there may be indirect effects, whereby investment in the cost-related elements does impact on non-cost-related elements. For example, better-paid staff might treat residents with greater respect because they themselves have higher self-esteem. It would be interesting to design an experiment to test this hypothesis. However, the message which the author wishes to convey is that it seems that better quality can often be achieved without increasing costs. This can be done by focusing on the elements that are also stressed by the Centre for Policy on Ageing: respect for residents as individuals, and attention to the manner in which care is delivered.

REFERENCES

Audit Commission (1986). *Making a Reality of Community Care*. HMSO, London.

Avebury, K. (1984). *Home Life: A Code of Practice for Residential Care*. Report of a working party, Centre for Policy on Ageing, London.

Avebury, K. (1996). *A Better Home Life: A Code of Good Practice for Residential and Nursing Home Care*. Centre for Policy on Ageing, London.

Barry, M., Crosby, C. and Bogg, J. (1993). Methodological issues in evaluating quality of life of long-stay patients. *J Ment Health* **2**, 43–56.

Black, N. (1990). Quality assurance of medical care. *J Public Health Med* **12**, 97–104.

Bowling, A. (1991). *Measuring Health: A Review of Quality of Life Scales*. Open University Press, Milton Keynes.

Burgner, T. (1996). *The Regulation and Inspection of Social Services*. Department of Health, London/Cardiff.

Challis, D. (1992). Providing alternatives to long-stay hospital care for frail elderly patients: is it cost-effective? [Editorial] *Int J Geriatr Psychiatry* **7**, 773–781.

Dalley, G. (1997). A better home life: the components of quality in continuing care. In: *Achieving a Better Home Life: Establishing and Maintaining Quality in Continuing Care for Older People*. Centre for Policy on Ageing, London, pp. 5–11.

Darton, R. (1994) Review of recent research on elderly people in residential care and nursing homes, with specific reference to dependency. Discussion paper, 1082. Personal Social Services Research Unit, University of Kent at Canterbury.

Department of Health (1989). *Caring for people: community care in the next decade and beyond*, Cm849. HMSO, London.

Department of Health (1996). Local monitoring of continuing care: developing a framework for health and social care. Department of Health, Wetherby.

Donabedian, A. (1980). *Explorations in Quality Assessment and Monitoring*, Vol. 1: *The Definition of Quality and Approaches to its Assessment*. Health Administration Press, Ann Arbor, MI.

Gibbs, I. and Sinclair, I. (1992). Consistency: a pre-requisite for inspecting old people's homes? *Br J Soc Work* **22**, 541–549.

Higginson, I. (1994). Quality of care and evaluating services. *Int Rev Psychiatry* **6**, 5–14.

Hugman, R. (1994). *Ageing and the care of older people in Europe*. Macmillan Press, London.

Moos, R. and Lemke, S. (1984). *Multiphasic Environmental Assessment Procedure (MEAP) Manual*. Social Ecology Laboratory, Stanford University, Palo Alto, CA.

Netten, A. and Beecham, J. (Eds) (1993). *Costing Community Care: Theory and Practice*. Personal Social Services Research Unit, University of Kent, Canterbury.

Oliver, J., Huxley, P., Bridges, K. and Mohamad, H. (1995). *Quality of Life and Mental Health Services*. Routledge, London.

Schneider, J., Mann, A., Blizard, B. *et al.* (1997). Exploring quality in residential care for elderly people. *Care J Pract Dev* **6**, 7–20.

Schneider, J., Mann, A., Blizard, B. *et al.* (1998). Home truths. *Health Service J* 15 January, 30–31.

Watkins, T. and Pearson, N. (1996). *Residential Homes: Quality of Life and Quality of Service*. Welsh Consumer Council, Cardiff.

Youll, P. and McCourt-Perring, C. (1993). *Raising Voices: Ensuring Quality in Residential Care, An Evaluation of the Caring in Homes Initiative*. Brunel University and HMSO, London.

10

The Old Age Forensic Psychiatrist

ROBIN JACOBY

Professor of Old Age Psychiatry, University of Oxford, Oxford, UK

INTRODUCTION

There are always many strands to national life, but one of the most prominent in the lives of the British has been the mercantile tradition. For many
years we exported and imported goods, building at the same time an empire
which until recent times covered a great part of the world. One of our less
desirable mercantile traditions, however, has been the export of criminals.

In Georgian England there was a crisis of crime (Hughes, 1987). Among
the many causes were the increasing affluence of the relatively small middle
and upper classes, together with a much larger increase in the urban poor,
many of whom had arrived in towns from the countryside with no means of
earning a living. It is generally acknowledged that this indigent segment of
society was in many respects driven to crime simply to survive. Late
eighteenth century British governments were faced with an identical problem
to that which Tony Blair's faces today, namely what to do with such a large
number of offenders. Today's solutions are to build more prisons or to find
alternative means of punishment within the community. Both solutions are
employed and we currently send more people to prison than any other
country in Europe but fewer than in the United States. In the eighteenth
century there were other ways of resolving the problem. Many were hanged
for crimes as trivial as theft, but export presented itself as a golden opportunity of getting rid of a tiresome, troublesome and ever-increasing group of
individuals. The United States of America would have been an ideal spot
but, unfortunately for His Majesty's ministers, a tea party was held in Boston
on 16 December 1773 and the prospect of sending the undesirables across
the Atlantic evaporated. However, there had recently been an unsuccessful
attempt in the South Pacific to use Norfolk Island, just over one thousand
miles NE of Sydney, as a source of timber and flax for masts and sails for

Table 1. Age and gender distribution of the first convict fleet to Australia, 1787–88.

Age	Men	Women
under 15	3	2
16–25	68	58
26–35	51	50
36–45	11	6
46–55	4	3
over 56	3	3
Total	140	122

Source: Hughes, 1987.

the British Indian Ocean fleet, which was our main bulwark against our traditional foes, the French. This failure was turned to good account by the establishment of a penal settlement in Australia and the first fleet containing convicts under the command of Captain Arthur Philip arrived in Botany Bay on 20 January 1788.

Table 1 shows some interesting facts. First, man's inhumanity to man is matched by the heroic endurance of 272 people who were forced to spend eight months confined below decks *en route* to the other side of the world. Secondly, the age distribution shows a remarkable similarity to that of modern offender populations in the USA and Britain, the great majority of offences being committed by those between 16 and 35. Thirdly, however, the almost equal number of women is at variance with current trends, where men vastly outnumber women. Fourthly, and lastly, although they were very few, some old people had fallen foul of the law and were paying a high price for it. Among those three women was one Dorothy Handland, a dealer in rags and clothes, who was 82 years old when sentenced to seven years for perjury in 1787. Not only does poor Dorothy have the dubious distinction of being one the oldest convicts transported, but she was also Australia's first suicide victim, for she hanged herself from a eucalyptus tree at Sydney Cove in 1789. As she was described as being in a state of 'befuddled despair' (Hughes, 1987), we might hazard a guess that not only was she depressed but perhaps even also in the early stages of dementia. If so, she highlights a number of issues relative to old age and crime which are as relevant today as they might have been 200 years ago. First, as a female offender she is a relatively rare creature – old women are very infrequent offenders. Secondly, she probably suffered from at least one and possibly two mental illnesses, depressive and dementing. Thirdly, her convict status put her at higher risk of committing suicide. And, finally, she exemplifies how with elderly offenders it is not always possible to distinguish a criminal from a victim.

STATISTICS

How much crime do elderly persons commit? Much less than younger people, that is for sure. Wilbanks (1984) pointed out that in Dade County, Florida, the highest rate of offending for any age, sex and ethnic group, which occurred in non-white 18–24-year-old men, was 3089 (three thousand and eighty nine!) times the lowest rate, which was in white women of 65 and over. An 18–24-year-old male was 389 times more likely to be charged with burglary than a male aged 65 to 74. In the elderly group as a whole, 81.5% of crimes were misdemeanours or minor offences and only 18.5% were felonies. The most frequent felony in Dade County was grand theft, which category includes shoplifting.

Statistics for indictable offences in England and Wales in 1995 (Home Office, 1994), for men at least, are not dissimilar to those from the first Australian convict fleet. Some 74% of indictable offences committed by men were committed by those under the age of 30, whereas those of 50 and over were responsible for only 4%, of which under 1% was perpetrated by those of 60 and over.

The author has not been able to obtain exactly the equivalent for the USA, but Table 2 might cautiously be taken as a reflection (US Department of Justice, Bureau of Statistics: data supplied on request). Of course the data are not the same as the British figures because a defendant has not been convicted, but presuming that an equal number from each age group were acquitted, it can be seen that 60% of felonies were committed by defendants under the age of 30. However, the problem with these data is that the oldest group is aged only 40 and above and, although it certainly must contain some old people, it also contains many who are not.

It is worth considering here the point that official statistics probably *underestimate* the number of crimes committed by older persons. Kercher (1987) has said that they 'substantially underestimate' it. He based this assertion on

Table 2. Felony defendants in 75 large urban counties in the USA by age group.

Age	%
<18	4
18–20	17
21–24	19
25–29	20
30–39	29
40+	11

Source: Reaves and Smith, 1995.

the fact that the number of crimes reported to the police overall is five times greater than the number of people arrested; and that only about half the crimes committed are reported to the police. He therefore estimated that people of 55 and over may have been responsible for some four million so called 'criminal violations' in the USA in 1979. Since the prison population and crime rates have risen considerably since 1979 without a concomitant increase in detection or reporting rates, the present estimate must be far greater; estimate, however, it remains.

In Britain the authorities try to avoid sending elderly offenders to prison at all. In Brixton Prison, London, Taylor and Parrott (1988) found only 1.9% of men remanded in custody before trial to be over 65, whereas older men represented 11.1% in the local population. For those between the ages of 15 and 24 the situation was reversed since they formed a greater proportion (22.8%) of the remanded sample than they did in the local population (17.4%). Only five out of 23 of the men over 65 had a home to go to, so that the remaining 18 probably ended up in prison only because they were homeless.

The proportion of convicted men (i.e. after trial) over 59 in prison establishments in England and Wales actually rose between 1983 and 1993 (Home Office, 1995), whereas the proportion of young men aged 15–24 fell over the corresponding period. The raw totals of older men were, of course, much lower than for the young males – 259 and 17 097 respectively in 1983 compared with 442 and 11 074 in 1993 – but the near doubling of older men within the system over 10 years has important implications for the provision of services in the UK. The number of women over the age of 59 in prison in England and Wales is tiny – eight in 1993, as it was in 1983 – and proportions did not change.

This is to be contrasted with the fact that over the same period (1983/93) the numbers of men received into prison declined in all age groups except 25–29 where it rose, but only slightly. Of those of 60 and over, 539 were admitted in 1983 whereas it was 323 in 1993. The apparently paradoxical trends among the older men of a rising prison population but falling admission rate can be explained by the fact that those who committed less serious offences were diverted away from custody, but those who committed more serious offences attracted lengthier sentences.

As regards America, it is not very easy to know what the incarcerated population is because there are jails and prisons (not the same thing) and state and federal institutions, but the state prison population rose from 450 416 to 711 643 between 1986 and 1991. The proportions by age group, however, remained remarkably constant.

It is not known how many of the older men serving sentences in prison are suffering from mental disorders. If their group characteristics reflect those on remand in Brixton Prison in London (Taylor and Parrott, 1988), it is likely to be a considerable number, since a much greater proportion of the older men were showing signs of mental disorder than the younger groups. It is reasonable to assume that several would have received alternative noncustodial disposal or acquittal at their trials. In Oxford the author's team is about to embark on a two-year study funded by the Wellcome Trust of the epidemiology of mental disorders in elderly *convicted* prisoners in England. It can be predicted that a significant number will be suffering from mental illness and that alternative placement would be more appropriate.

There has been some interest in the American literature in the elderly prison population from the standpoints of gerontology and sociology (Flynn, 1992; Rubenstein, 1982) but little, if any, from psychiatry. What is published seems to have been based as much on speculation and theory on the back of crime statistics as it has on experimental data. Older inmates are described as showing a deterioration of their mental and physical condition on entry to prison, becoming depressed and anxious and depending on the warden and staff for protection (Rubenstein, 1982). Wooden and Parker, quoted by Rubinstein (1982), stated that older prisoners cope better as 'they cause less trouble because they are more mature and less sexually involved'. But, as this newspaper snippet shows, one may not make watertight generalizations about older people.

> **Crime of Passion**
> A man aged 83 who stabbed his 73-year-old wife to
> death with scissors after she refused sex gave himself
> up in Salonica, northern Greece ...
> *Sunday Telegraph*, 31 August 1997

SEXUAL OFFENCES

Although they commit fewer crimes than younger persons, the elderly by and large commit the same types as younger ones, except illegal drug offences. However, proportions vary greatly at different ages. In all age groups theft and handling stolen goods make up the largest proportion of offences. A cursory glance at official statistics, however, might lead one to assume that elderly men commit more sexual offences, and the data therefore provide some evidence to support the commonly held concept of the 'dirty old man'. But, in fact, all the figures say about the matter is that sexual offences constitute a greater proportion of all offences committed by older men or that they commit a lesser proportion of other offences.

Figure 1 (Home Office, 1994) shows that younger age groups of 10–20 and 21–29 consume respectively twice and three times more of the sexual offences pie than do those of 60 and over. It thus seems a little strange to

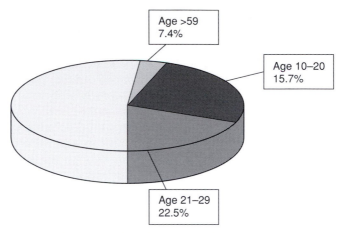

Figure 1. Proportion of all convictions for sexual offences in oldest and two youngest age groups (source: Home Office, 1994).

discover that 43% of all elderly offenders who go to prison are convicted of sexual offences, whereas of young offenders in the age groups 21–24, 25–29 and 30–39 the proportions are 1.4, 2.2 and 5.7%, respectively. Taking these data together with what appears in the papers or on television, one may conclude only that the concept of the dirty old man is less of a reality than the notion that English judges take a more punitive stance towards crimes against property in younger defendants than older ones, but compensate by taking a more severe approach to sexual offences committed by older men.

Hucker (1984) suggested that one possible explanation (for sex crimes apparently being more common in the elderly) is that elderly offenders are less likely to be charged with 'minor offences'. In Britain, there is some evidence to support this contention. Of 367 elderly arrestees referred to the Community Services Branch of the Essex Police, only 36, or 9.8% were actually prosecuted. Of the remainder, those who admitted to the offence were cautioned or subject to no further action (Needham-Bennett *et al.*, 1996).

One should also bear in mind that the term 'sexual offences' covers a multitude of sins in older offenders. On the one hand there are those who have committed such offences at various times throughout their lives and whose activities in old age are merely a continuation of a lifelong pattern. On the other hand there are those whose first sexual offence occurs in old age, which might be for one of a number of reasons, for example isolation due to loss of a parent, or as a consequence of organic brain disorder, sometimes of frontal lobe type.

Farragher (Farragher and O'Connor, 1995) conducted a retrospective review of elderly cases referred to a forensic psychiatry clinic in Dublin over a 20-year period. Only 42 patients in all were referred, i.e. a very small number averaging about two a year. The precise number of those charged with sexual offences is not easily determined from the paper but of that number 66% suffered from organic brain disorder. This compares with the findings of another Dublin study (O'Connor and O'Neill, 1990) where the predominant psychiatric diagnosis was that of personality disorder when sex offenders of all ages were taken into account. When looked at from the perspective of an ordinary old age psychiatry service in Dublin, McAleer and Wrigley (1999) found 13 patients referred for sexual offences between 1989 and 1997. About half were essentially trivial, such as making lewd remarks in public, and the other half were more serious, such as indecent assault, including three cases of incest. Of more interest, however, was the finding that only two of the 13 sex offenders did *not* have a psychiatric diagnosis assigned to them. Of those who did, one suffered from a depressive and another from a schizophrenic illness. The remaining nine had some form of organic brain disease. Sexual offences can certainly vary from the serious to the trivial where elderly offenders are concerned but as Hucker (1984) has pointed out, sexual offences committed by younger men are much more likely to be violent and aggressive, whereas with older men they are more frequently of a passive nature.

SHOP THEFT

The elderly shoplifter has attracted quite a lot of attention, more in the USA than in Britain. There are differing views as to whether this is an increasing or decreasing problem. The reason for this is that the statistics wrap up shop theft along with other categories of larceny or theft. As with so much in the criminological literature pertaining to the elderly, there is a good deal of speculation and very little by way of hard fact. For example, Feinberg (1984) in concluding a chapter on the elderly shoplifter states, 'The elderly are ... set adrift and society has provided them with neither map, itinerary, or friendly shore. They are on their own, captain and mate, actor and agent of their own destiny ...', a view more touchingly romantic than substantial. Admittedly, there is not much research evidence on shoplifting available. Some authors suggest that the reason why older people steal from shops is because it does not require some of the physical and motor skills which are demanded by some of the more dashing crimes committed by younger people. As Feinberg, again, puts it, '... it does not require an apprenticeship or the acquisition of new skills, ...it can be integrated with one's normal daily activities ...' Curran (1984) does base some of her conclusions on elderly shoplifters on a now rather old study in Palm Beach County, Florida. She states that, contrary to public perception, 'the picture emerges that the phenomenon of elderly shoplifting is not a major problem'. Overwhelmingly, she reports, shoplifting by older persons proves to be a first and last offence.

The most modern study which touches on this topic was by Needham-Bennett and colleagues based on persons referred to the Community Services Branch (CSB) of the Essex Police, now disbanded for budgetary reasons, to which the elderly arrestee was referred to see if alternatives to prosecution were appropriate (Needham-Bennett *et al.*, 1996). They found that shoplifting constituted 63.4% of all CSB cases, most involving trivial amounts of money, usually theft of groceries not exceeding £15 in value. Eleven out of the 14 cases who were identified as suffering from a mental disorder were shoplifters. Of all the shoplifters, only one was eventually prosecuted in court, even though 38% of them had a previous conviction. This study does provide some evidence for the hypothesis that many elderly people are probably diverted away from the criminal justice system if at all possible.

HOMICIDE

Although homicide is the crime which attracts much, if not the most, interest among the public at large, the elderly are responsible for very few such crimes. In 1993 in England and Wales 548 persons (men and women) were charged with either of the two categories of homicide, murder and manslaughter, but of these only eight, or 1.46%, were older than 59. Although the raw number of older people is very small, half of those (two out of four) convicted of manslaughter received hospital orders, whereas only 3% (seven out of 217 of those younger than 60) were sent to special hospitals. There were a further 10 younger arrestees who were found unfit to plead, presumably because of insanity. But, even if it is assumed that most or all were sent to hospital, the *proportion* of older people sent there was still higher.

It has not been possible to obtain the equivalent figures for the USA but a report from 75 urban USA counties (Dawson and Boland, 1988) showed that a similarly very small proportion of murder defendants were 55 and over. Of the total of 3005 under sentence of death in the USA in 1995 only 119, or 4%, were over 54.

Domestic homicides are the commonest type in the UK. Some data on spouse murder defendants in the same 75 large urban USA counties for the year 1988 revealed that there were 540 spouse murder defendants, of whom 431, or 81%, were ultimately convicted (Langan and Dawson, 1995). Their ages ranged from 18 to 87, with a mean of 39. Eleven per cent were over 59 years old. Of the 22 in the latter category, 12 were husbands and 10 were wives. It is not always easy to unpack the human tragedies from inside the framework of statistics, but Langan and Dawson (1995) do give some useful little sample vignettes. In younger people infidelity is often, if not mostly, the underlying cause. With the elderly it is usually quite different. Those heady days of affairs are over and done with. Here it is sometimes illness and dependency which are the provoking factor. For example, there was the case of a 68-year-old Philadelphia man whose 65-year-old wife's 'health and state of mind deteriorated rapidly and she had become mentally disturbed. He feels he can no longer meet her health demands and decides to put her out of her misery. He shoots her with a rifle'. Apart from the firearm dimension the scenario is not dissimilar from a desperately tragic British case reported in *The Guardian* (19 November 1997). The story was that a woman had severe Parkinson's disease and presumably also dementia. Her husband clearly became depressed and decreasingly able to cope. Eventually he snapped and smothered her with a blanket. He told the police that as he was killing her, he was shouting to her that he loved her. Neither the American nor the British man was sent to prison. Both were sentenced to probation. Another case from Philadelphia is similar to one reported by Dankwarth and Püschel (1991) from a German survey of elderly homicides. Here it is the killer who was demented. In Philadelphia it was a 73-year-old man with Alzheimer's disease who beat his wife of the same age to death with a crowbar. No motive is given in the vignette and he entered a plea of negligent manslaughter with the same result: probation. In the German case a 90-year-old man suffering from dementia after a stroke killed his 79-year-old wife and then hanged himself. No motivation could be established for the crime.

MENTAL DISORDER AND CRIME

Is there an association between mental disorder in old age and crime? As far as crime and *old age* schizophrenia are concerned, there is virtually no evidence of any association. Robert Howard (personal communication, 1996), who collected one of the largest series ever of patients with late-onset schizophrenia, found that not one of the 101 cases had acted upon their delusions so far as to commit a crime, although one is said to have tried to kidnap the son of his alleged persecutor. Nor is there any evidence that so-called 'graduates', most of whom suffer from schizophrenia, are prone to commit crime, although this is a group who require to be watched carefully, not for major headline-catching crime but for minor, almost unnoticed, offending. Having spent much of their lives in large Victorian asylums where all their basic needs were catered for without their having to do anything to be clothed and fed, they have been released into the community, often with minimal supervision. It is not surprising that a number have taken to life on the streets. Deluded and hallucinating some of them undoubtedly are, but most are in no position or state of volition to commit bizarre delusion-driven crimes. On the other hand, who knows how many are driven to steal food and drink to survive?

What about affective disorder? Here again there are relative few data. Taylor and Parrott (1988) in the study of prisoners on pre-trial remand in Brixton Prison, found 11% of elderly individuals with what they termed endogenous psychotic affective disorder, although we do not know if the illness had anything directly to do with their offences. One situation where affective disorder might well be directly implicated is in shoplifting, although the author knows of no study which has conclusively linked shop theft to old age affective disorder. The study by Needham-Bennett *et al.* (1996), already referred to above, found one subject with depressive psychosis and three with depressive neurosis reaching case level on the Geriatric Mental State Schedule. But the most dramatic association between crime and affective disorder in old age, as with younger people, concerns depression and homicide. One of Taylor and Parrott's (1988) illustrative cases was that of a 68-year-old man with severe depression who had suffered two previous depressive episodes. He killed his wife and tried unsuccessfully to commit suicide at the same time. The Englishman mentioned in the case vignettes above, who killed his wife who was suffering from Parkinson's disease and dementia, was depressed and spent six months in a mental hospital after he had done the deed.

Dementia has been implicated in case-reports of sexual offending, homicide and shoplifting. In a sample of violent offenders and nonviolent sex offenders seen at the Clark Institute in Toronto, Hucker and Ben-Aron (1984) found a raised prevalence of organic brain syndrome in older offenders, but not significantly so when compared with young ones. Rosner *et al.* (1991), in a case-note study of elderly defendants from New York, found a high prevalence of organic brain syndromes (10/52), but sampling bias does not permit one to draw valid conclusions from this study about any clear association between crime and dementia. Taylor and Parrott (1988) in their Brixton Prison study found 'two or three cases of dementia within the older age groups ...' but give no further details. Hucker (1984) gives a detailed reference list of authors for and against an association between crime and senile dementia. Several of the papers are anecdotal and not data-based. In summary, there is no conclusive evidence that dementia predisposes to offending, although in individual cases there may clearly be a direct link. In everyday old age psychiatric practice aggression by demented patients is common, but it is mostly trivial verbal abuse or perhaps minor aggression to nurses or other carers. However, some patients are more seriously physically aggressive to spouses and other informal carers, usually during intimate care, but seldom with serious consequences.

ALCOHOL ABUSE

Alcohol abuse is one area in which some elderly people do fall foul of the law, but most alcohol-related offences in older men are relatively minor, as data from Dade County, Florida show (Wilbanks, 1984) (Figure 2). Most misdemeanours (column C) outnumber the more serious category of felonies (column A) by roughly four to one, but some 34% of the misdemeanours are alcohol-related. It is perhaps for this reason that there have been moves in some American states to decriminalize alcoholism.

In England and Wales in 1993 (Home Office, 1994) only 35 men and one woman in the over-60 age group were convicted of indictable motoring offences, of which some were presumably alcohol-related, but the total is tiny and highlights a clear difference between the UK and the USA in this area of offending. Although alcohol abuse can lead to serious consequences, notably in motor cars, the authorities tend to view most alcohol abusers in a different light to robbers, rapists and other sorts of criminals. One rather old study from California (Epstein *et al.*, 1970) revealed that cops and jailers regarded themselves more as social workers when dealing with drunken old men and thought they should not be prosecuted. On the other hand the

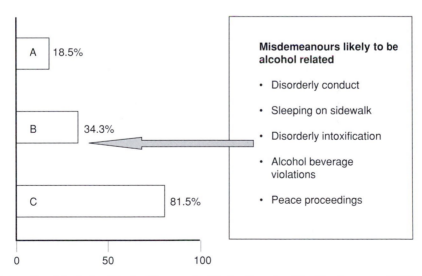

Figure 2. Alcohol-related offences in Dade County, Florida (source: Wilbanks, 1984), (A, total felonies; B, alcohol related misdemeanours; C, total misdemeanours.)

importance of alcohol as a factor in crime committed by older men should not be ignored. In the Brixton remand prisoners study (Taylor and Parrott, 1988) alcoholism rates in the 55–64-year-olds and the over-64-year-olds were 24% and 33% respectively, whereas the rate was less than 1% in the group aged 15–24 which is responsible for about half of all indictable offences.

CONCLUSION

The old age forensic psychiatrist does not, of course, exist (yet). At the moment he/she is a conceit in the Editor's mind, for elderly offenders are too few to warrant such special attention. Nevertheless, elderly criminals are a minority whose characteristics have plenty of interest for the journeyman old age psychiatrist and who are worthy of his/her attention. In Britain we have not always treated them well and, although we no longer transport 82-year-old women to Australia, who knows what generations 200 years hence will think of us for how we deal with them now. One way in which we might improve our care of the elderly offender is to take more notice of his or her mental health needs and then greater care of the offender within the criminal justice system.

REFERENCES

Curran, D. (1984). In: Wilbanks, W. and Kim, P.K.H.) (Eds), *Elderly Criminals*. Lanham, New York, pp. 123–141.

Dankwarth, G. and Püschel, K. (1991). Crimes against life – the elderly as victims and as perpetrators. *Z Gerontol* **24**, 266–270.

Dawson, J.M. and Boland, B. (1988). *Murder in Large Urban Countries*. United States Department of Justice Bureau of Statistics, Washington, DC.

Epstein, L.J., Mills, C. and Simon, A. (1970). Antisocial behavior of the elderly. *Compr Psychiatry* **11**, 36–42.

Farragher, B. and O'Connor, A. (1995). Forensic psychiatry and elderly people – a retrospective review. *Med Sci Law* **35**, 269–273.

Feinberg, G. (1984). In: Newman, E.S., Newman, D.J. and Gewirtz, M.L. (Eds), *Elderly Criminals*. Oelgeschlager, Gunn & Hain, Cambridge, MA, pp. 35–50.

Flynn, E.E. (1992). The graying of America's prison population. *Prison J* **72**, 77–98.

Home Office (1994). *Vol. CM2680. Criminal Statistics in England & Wales 1993*. HMSO, London.

Home Office (1995). *Vol. CM2893. Prison Statistics England & Wales 1993*. HMSO, London.

Hucker, S.J. (1984) In: Newman, E.S., Newman, D.J. and Gewirtz, M.L. (Eds), *Elderly Criminals*. Oelgeschlager, Gunn & Hain, Cambridge, MA, pp. 67–77.

Hucker, S.J. and Ben-Aron, M.H. (1984). In: Wilbanks, W. and Kim, P.K.H. (Eds), *Elderly Criminals*. Lanham, New York, pp. 69–81.

Hughes, R. (1987). *The Fatal Shore*. Collins Harvill, London.

Kercher, K. (1987). The causes and correlates of crime committed by the elderly. *Res Aging* **9**, 256–280.

Langan, P.A. and Dawson, J.M. (1995). *Spouse Murder Defendants in Large Urban Counties*. US Department of Justice Bureau of Justice Statistics, Washington, DC.

McAleer, A. and Wrigley, M. (1999). A study of sex offending in elderly people referred to a specialised psychiatry of old age service. *Ir J Psychol Med*, in press.

Needham-Bennett, H., Parrott, J. and Macdonald, A.J.D. (1996). Psychiatric disorder and policing the elderly offender. *Crim Behav Ment Health* **6**, 241–252.

O'Connor, A. and O'Neill, H. (1990). Male prison transfers to the Central Mental Hospital, a special hospital (1983–1988). *Ir J Psychol Med* **7**, 118–120.

Reaves, B.A. and Smith, P.Z. (1995). *Felony Defendants in Large Urban Counties*. US Department of Justice Bureau of Statistics, Washington, DC.

Rosner, R., Wiederlight, M., Harmon, R.B. and Cahn, D.J. (1991). Geriatric offenders examined at a forensic psychiatry clinic. *J Forens Sci* **36**, 1722–1731.

Rubenstein, D. (1982). The older person in prison. *Arch Gerontol Geriatr* **1**, 287–296.

Taylor, P.J. and Parrott, J.M. (1988). Elderly offenders. A study of age-related factors among custodially remanded prisoners. *Br J Psychiatry* **152**, 340–346.

Wilbanks, W. (1984). The elderly offender: relative frequency and pattern of offenses. *Int J Aging Hum Dev* **20**, 269–281.

Everything You Need to Know About Old Age Psychiatry . . .
Edited by Robert Howard
©1999 Wrightson Biomedical Publishing Ltd

11

Assisted Death in Dementia: The Case for Accelerated Deaths

SIR LUDOVIC KENNEDY

President of the Voluntary Euthanasia Society, London, UK

There can be little doubt that, as we approach the third millennium, the most important issue in the field of medical ethics is that concerning the rights and/or wrongs of requests for, and the granting of, accelerated deaths. Voluntary euthanasia, or physician-assisted suicide (PAS) is one means to this, though it is unfortunate that to different people the word 'euthanasia' seems to mean different things. It comes from the Greek, *eu*, meaning well or good, and *thanatos*, death – the good death, so that Dr Nick Maurice, who practises in a Marlborough surgery, was able to write in a recent surgery newsletter, 'We doctors are practising euthanasia all the time and should be proud of it', by which he meant that by giving suffering patients in terminal decline enough diamorphine to ease their pain, he was also ensuring for them a comfortable, though accelerated, death. This practice is known as 'doubt effect' and is routinely practised by most doctors in Western countries, though the law being what it is, few are courageous enough to admit to it.

Dr Maurice's interpretation of euthanasia is unfortunately not that of everybody. Certainly not that of the Pope, who said in 1980 that suffering in the last stages of life was part of God's saving plan for humanity – a notion which seems medieval in its conception and cruel in its lack of compassion. Nor of the Roman Catholic faith as a whole, which takes an unequivocal view of the sanctity of life which throughout history has been honoured more in the breach than the observance. This is an illogical attitude, for the Catholic Church has no objection to capital punishment and traditionally its priests have always been ready to bless the colours of soldiers preparing to kill in battle. In any case, as the Age Concern paper of 1998a, *Values and Attitudes in a Changing Society*, makes clear,

'Few people in liberal democratic societies would think it legitimate for a particular religious perspective to dominate the wider policy-making process.'

The British Medical Association (BMA) was once the most strident opponent of accelerated death, as it had been of contraception and abortion, but has since modified its attitude considerably, stating that in some cases voluntary euthanasia may be the only alternative and admitting that recent polls show that there are now marginally more doctors in favour of voluntary euthanasia or PAS than against (BMA, 1996). For instance, a System Three poll prepared for Professor Sheila McLean of Glasgow University's Medical Law Unit in 1996 showed that 54% of general practitioners (GPs) in Scotland supported voluntary euthanasia and would be prepared to practise it were it legalized, with 46% against.

The real stumbling block to making voluntary euthanasia legal is Members of Parliament. To them the word has overtones of Hitler's extermination programme of Jews, gypsies, the handicapped and other so-called 'undesirables', and signifies the putting to death of people against their will; the qualification, the vital qualification, 'voluntary' tends to be forgotten. They think, mistakenly, that their constituents share their fears, but paradoxically this is not so. Polls conducted by British Social Attitudes have shown an increase in those favouring voluntary euthanasia from 75% of those canvassed in 1984 (and 24% against) to 82% in 1994 (and only 15% against). The same pattern is to be found in other Western countries, in some of which (Holland, Switzerland, Germany, the American State of Oregon) physician-assisted suicide is now permitted, while in others, such as the American State of Maine, and also South Australia, it is hoped it soon will be. The Voluntary Euthanasia Society is fully aware of the pejorative connotations of the word 'euthanasia' and at present is considering changing the name to one no less truthful but less threatening to political susceptibilities. The Society is already affiliated to the World Federation of Right to Die Societies.

The other pathway to the legalization of accelerated death is to be found in the movement favouring 'advance directives', sometimes called living wills, whereby a person in good health signs a declaration that if at any time he or she becomes permanently noncompetent they do not wish to be kept alive artificially.

Like most other advance directives, the one sponsored by the Voluntary Euthanasia Society is addressed to 'my family, my doctor and all other persons concerned' and made 'at a time when I am of sound mind and after consideration'. It continues:

I DECLARE that if at any time the following circumstances exist, namely:

1. I suffer from one or more of the conditions mentioned in the schedule; and
2. I have become unable to participate effectively in decisions about my medical care; and
3. two independent doctors (one a consultant) are of the opinion that I am unlikely to recover from illness or impairment involving severe distress or incapacity for rational existence,

THEN AND IN THOSE CIRCUMSTANCES my directions are as follows:

1. that I am not to be subjected to any medical intervention or treatment aimed at prolonging or sustaining my life;
2. that any distressing symptoms (including any caused by lack of food or fluid) are to be fully controlled by appropriate analgesic or other treatment, even though that treatment may shorten my life.

After absolving medical attendants from any civil liability arising from anything they have done or omitted to do in carrying out his or her directions, the petitioner declares, 'I wish it to be understood that I fear degeneration and indignity far more than I fear death. I ask my medical attendants and any person consulted by them to bear this statement in mind when considering what my intentions would be in any uncertain situation.' And finally,

'I reserve the right to revoke this directive at any time, but unless I do so, it should be taken to represent my continuing directions.'

There follows the schedule of conditions for which the patient forbids any treatment directed towards prolonging his or life:

1. Advanced disseminated malignant disease (e.g. widespread lung cancer)
2. Severe immune deficiency (e.g. AIDS)
3. Advanced degenerative disease of the nervous system (e.g. motor neurone disease)
4. Severe and lasting brain damage due to injury, stroke, disease or other cause
5. Senile or presenile dementia (e.g. Alzheimer's disease)
6. Any other condition of comparable gravity

Attached to the declaration is a form in which petitioners can nominate others to speak on their behalf if they are no longer able to do so themselves. Finally, the declaration must be witnessed by two persons.

WE TESTIFY that the maker of this Directive signed it in our presence, and made it clear to us that he/she understood what it meant. We do not know of any pressure being brought to bear on him/her to make such a directive, and we believe it was made by his/her own wish. So far as we are aware, we do not stand to gain from his/her death.

One copy of the Directive should be handed to the petitioner's GP, another to his or her solicitor and a third to the next of kin.

Advance directives were confirmed as common law in December 1992 when the Appeal Court was considering the case of the youth Tony Bland, who had been in a persistent vegetative state (PVS) for several years after having been crushed and starved of oxygen during the Hillsborough football ground tragedy. In his judgement the then Master of the Rolls, Sir Thomas Bingham ruled as follows:

> If ... Mr Bland had given instructions that he should not be artificially fed or treated with antibiotics if he should become a PVS patient, his doctors would not act unlawfully in complying with those instructions but would act unlawfully if they did not comply, even though the patient's death would inevitably follow (NHS Airedale Trust v. Bland 1993).

This judgement was in keeping with the doctrine of patient autonomy, then fully recognized by our courts, whereby any treatment of a patient which he or she has not sanctioned is an invasion of their person and therefore unlawful. The House of Lords concurred, and permission was given for the nourishment and hydration that was keeping Tony Bland alive to be withdrawn, and three weeks later he died. Ending his life by a lethal injection, as would be given to a loved pet in similar circumstances, would have spared his family the agony of sitting by his bedside and watching him die, but it was deemed that public opinion and the medical profession were not yet ready for so positive and euthanasia-like an act, though as the judge, Lord Mustill, stated in his judgement in the Lords, 'However much the terminologies may differ, the ethical status of the two courses of action is for relevant purposes indistinguishable', i.e. the end result of accelerated death was the same.

From then on there was growing public support for the statutory confirmation of advance directives, and in March 1998 a MORI poll for the Parents Association found that from a sample of 1960 people canvassed, 65% were in favour of legislation and only 21% against (MORI, 1998). Meanwhile, and acting on the recommendations of the Law Commission, the Lord Chancellor (1997) issued his Green Paper, *Who Decides?* The introduction of the all-important section, 'Advance Statements about Health Care' referred to a misconception that the Law Commission's proposals were advocating euthanasia, which was not so. Like most politicians who want to instil fear in people's minds on the subject, the Lord Chancellor could not bring himself to include the word 'voluntary', the only kind of euthanasia that might be, and, in the author's view, some day soon will be, acceptable.

The Green Paper was a consultative document and in it the Lord Chancellor (1997) called for responses to more than 100 questions relating to the treatment of those who had become noncompetent, or, as he put it, 'without capacity'. The response of the Voluntary Euthanasia Society was to approve of 'advance refusals' being recognized in law, i.e. that if a patient degenerated into a permanent and irreversible state of noncompetence, either through injury or dementia, their wish not to be kept artificially alive would be respected. Asked if an advance refusal should include the right to refuse basic care, the Society said that it should not, but in answer to a further question as to how basic care should be defined, it included bodily hygiene and the alleviation of severe pain but not the giving of nutrition and hydration (which the Green Paper had posited) if it was against the patient's expressed wishes. Asked what should be done were any doubts to arise about the execution of the advance refusal, the Society proposed that a forum similar to a mental health tribunal be set up (rather than the courts) to resolve them.

With two outstanding exceptions the Green Paper was well received by press and public. The press exception was an editorial in the *Daily Telegraph* of 1 April 1998 which falsely claimed that it 'would raise the question whether a doctor was obliged to carry out the killing of patients in order to comply with the terms of a living will'. On the contrary, the Green Paper specifically condemned any such action, declaring it to be, as it is now, illegal and therefore murder. 'The right to die,' the editorial went on, 'is the start of a slippery slope towards the killing of anybody who is helpless.' Such is the contempt with which the *Daily Telegraph* leader writer regards this country's doctors. Nor could the leader writer resist the opportunity offered to take a swipe at voluntary euthanasia, claiming that if it was accepted it would 'inevitably be extended to new categories of people through psychological coercion'. Elderly patients, the leader asserted, 'would feel obliged to do "the honourable thing" to relieve pressure on their families and ultimately perhaps on the state itself'. This is pure fantasy, conjuring up a situation where elderly patients who wanted to live offered themselves up to their doctor for voluntary euthanasia on the assumption that all doctors in this country would be prepared to dispense voluntary euthanasia for purely social reasons.

The other critic of the Green Paper was the Roman Catholic Church, Cardinals Basil Hume, Archbishop of Westminster, Thomas Winning, Archbishop of Scotland and Archbishop Sean Brady, Primate of All Ireland wrote a joint letter to the *Daily Telegraph* on 1 April 1998 claiming, as they put it, 'Legislation of Advance Directives would result in grave injustice being perpetrated on some of the country's most vulnerable people'.

So far as those in PVS are concerned, this criticism was misjudged. Where is the injustice in people in good health declaring that, if ever they were reduced to a state of noncompetence and had become no more than oxygenated vegetables, without personality and the capacity to think and act and maintain relationships, they did not wish to be kept artificially alive?

The Lord Chancellor's Green Paper was published in December 1997. Six months later the British Medical Association's Medical Ethics Committee issued a consultative paper of its own on the ethics of withdrawing or withholding treatment from patients who have no prospect of recovery, particularly those who are mentally incapacitated and whose wishes are not known.

Recognizing, yet without saying so explicitly, that these patients are a burden on the community, either on their relatives or on the National Health Service (NHS), the BMA seeks advice on how to deal with them. Here are some of the questions they pose.

1. When patients lack the ability to make decisions for themselves, and there is no clear indication of their wishes, should withdrawing or withholding treatment be an issue to be decided by health professionals and families alone?
2. Is there a role for ethics committees to be involved in making decisions about withdrawing or withholding treatment from patients who cannot express their own views?
3. How should 'best interests' be defined for incapacitated people? What criteria should be taken into account?
4. If a patient has left no indication of who should be consulted on his or her behalf, how widely should views be sought from people caring for an incapacitated adult? Should the views of blood relatives take precedence over others?

The unspoken assumption is that, when a person is noncompetent and his or her wishes as to treatment or disposal are unknown, it is up to other people, perhaps professional medical people, perhaps the courts, perhaps a mental health tribunal, perhaps the relatives, perhaps a combination of all of them, to take the decision by proxy. This seems unsatisfactory because no suggestions are put forward as to how the patient's unknown wishes are to be made known; and it seems imperative that they should be made known. And when they are, the questions raised by the BMA become irrelevant. But how are the patient's wishes to be made known? The answer is the advance directive. These are now to be found in many doctors' surgeries in the country and, as the Lord Chancellor's Green Paper explains, will before long have the force of statute law.

But that is not enough. The author would like to see the Government mounting a campaign to encourage people to make out advance directives while still of sound mind, so that, should a time come when the person becomes noncompetent, those caring for him or her will know exactly what to do. In the last resort the preparation of advance directives should be compulsory, so that it becomes as routine a task as filling in an application for a driving licence or making out one's tax returns. This would not only be in the patient's best interests, but also in the best interests of the medical people, the legal people, the relatives and so on, who would have been left clear instructions as to what to do in any situation because the patient, and only the patient, had willed it. And thus the voluntary principle would be preserved. These are the author's personal views and not those of the Voluntary Euthanasia Society, though in time they may be.

And now a word – or rather two words – of warning; the first about patients in PVS, and the second about patients with dementia. In the BMA's consultative document, a PVS is defined as 'the loss of specific and definable neurological pathways leading to permanent loss of sensitivity to external stimuli, and difficulty in swallowing, so that the patient feels no pain or distress at the withdrawal of nutrition and hydration'. It would seem to follow from this, the document goes on, that life is a value to be preserved only in so far as it contains some potentiality of human relationships. It then adds this warning: that there are some areas where it is not always possible to distinguish between a patient who is in a PVS and another – perhaps suffering from the effects of a severe stroke – who is not. 'Patients,' the document says, 'who previously indicated an advance decision to decline feeding may show enjoyment of life and an acceptance of nutrition after their competence has been lost.' Such patients should not, in the BMA's view, be candidates, at least at that moment, for the withdrawal of nutrition and hydration. The old adage, 'When in doubt, don't!' still, and particularly in these cases, forcibly applies.

Dementia, of course, is different from PVS in a number of ways. First, the number of cases of PVS at any one time is comparatively small, between 1000 and 2000 at most, whereas cases of dementia multiply every year. Secondly, dementia is a progressive illness, and it may take months or even years for a patient to reach a point where doctors can truthfully declare that he or she is no longer competent. Thirdly, dementia is a terminal condition whereas a PVS patient, if fed and watered, can survive for years.

Assume for a moment that a patient with dementia has reached the stage when he or she is no longer competent, and assume too that he or she, when they were competent, completed and signed an advance directive, stipulating that if ever they did become noncompetent, they did not wish to be kept artificially alive. By common law, as it exists today, to be confirmed by statute law in the near future, the patient's doctors would be breaking the law if they did not accede to their instructions – though, of course, much depends on how one defines the word 'artificially'.

How to resolve this dilemma is what is of concern today. The express wish of the patient, made in good health and updated from time to time, is paramount. It should, in the author's view override all other objections, particularly because it has the backing of the law. For the partner who is left behind this may be – almost certainly will be – distressing but only temporarily so. The affection that the healthy partner feels for the demented one is not based on the person they have become but on the person they once were, on the memories which they once shared; and when the decision has been taken to execute the advance directive and it has been executed, the surviving partner may well feel after a period of grieving, a sense of relief, even of exhilaration (so paradoxical is human nature) that the burden of caring he or she so willingly assumed has been lifted from them. They were sustained by memories before; and they will be sustained by memories in no less degree after.

If society is not yet ready for such a proposal then there is still much that the medical profession can do. Because dementia is both a progressive and a terminal condition, a time will come when the mental deterioration of the patient is matched by physical deterioration. And when, say, pneumonia sets in, as it is apt to, the wise doctor will refrain from prescribing antibiotics and allow nature to take its course.

The demand for accelerated death is going to grow, not diminish, because we are living at a time of increasingly ageing populations. By the year 2030, it has been estimated (Age Concern, 1998b) more than half the population of Europe will be over 60, sustained by an ever-diminishing workforce. The author's great and abiding fear is that unless our political leaders can be persuaded to make provision soon for permitting accelerated deaths with adequate safeguards, but only for those who have requested it (both now and as an insurance for the future), then thousands of old people are going to suffer neglect, and possibly abuse, because there will not be enough carers to look after them. Indeed, if some of the stories of the deficiencies emanating at present from residential homes are only half true, then neglect and abuse are already with us.

Death is not the worst thing that can happen to us; for many who are suffering it is the best. As Robert Louis Stevenson put it:

> It is not so much that death approaches as life withdraws and withers up round about him. He has outlived his own usefulness and almost his own enjoyment; and if there is to be no recovery, if never again will he

be young and strong and passionate ... if in fact this be veritably night-fall, he will not wish for a continuance of a twilight that only strains and disappoints the eyes, but steadfastly await the perfect darkness.

Other poets – Shelley's unacknowledged legislators of the world – have said the same. Keats's wish was to 'cease upon the midnight with no pain'; Hamlet saw death as 'a consummation devoutly to be wished'. And, said another Shakespeare character, Claudio in *Measure for Measure*,

If I must die,
I will encounter darkness as a bride,
And hug it in my arms.

But if for most of us death has lost its sting, as I believe it has, the same cannot be said of dying. Modern medicine has lengthened the span of life but not its quality; and this has led to many patients enduring prolonged and miserable days – if not weeks and months – of dying, often accompanied by the discomfort of such indignities as double incontinence, vomiting or nausea, oedema, breathlessness, insomnia, bed sores and so on, leading cumulatively to the gradual disintegration of mind, body and personality. When will our politicians come to accept that all this suffering continues because of their lack of courage to end it by legalizing physician-assisted death and providing the necessary safeguards. Dr Pieter Admiraal, the pioneer of voluntary euthanasia in Holland described this sort of death as 'a last act of love and compassion'. People talk about the alternative of palliative care, but while one has the greatest admiration for the living care given to patients in the few hospices that exist, they are not for everybody; the idea of palliative care at the other end of the spectrum, keeping alive those who are to all intents and purposes already dead, seems not only pointless but an abuse of medical resources.

We must be grateful to the Lord Chancellor for at least, and at last, making a start in the matter of accelerated deaths with the proposals contained in his Green Paper. Patient autonomy is now recognized to the degree that a patient can refuse any treatment recommended, even if such a refusal is likely to lead to death: the Green Paper quoted the case of a man with a gangrenous leg which he refused to have amputated, though warned that the consequences could be fatal; in the event he survived and from that common-law decision all else has followed. The only autonomy the patient is still forbidden is requesting and being granted, subject to specific safeguards, the means to an accelerated death. The author believes and hopes that, for the sake of those still living but no longer wishing to do so, and equally for those who have reached a stage where they no longer know what they wish, we are on the threshold of seeing that final veto lifted.

REFERENCES

Age Concern (1998a). *The Millenium Papers: Values and Attitudes in a Changing Society*. Age Concern, London, April.

Age Concern (1998b) *Guide to the Millenium Debate*. Age Concern, London, April, p.3.

BMA (1996). News Review, Press Release, 30 August. British Medical Association, London.

Lord Chancellor (1997). Green Paper: *Who Decides? Making Decisions on Behalf of Mentally Incapicitated Adults*. December, Commissioned 3803. HMSO, London.

MORI (1998). MORI Poll for the Parents Association. *Times Educational Supplement*, 27 March.

Everything You Need to Know About Old Age Psychiatry . . .
Edited by Robert Howard
©1999 Wrightson Biomedical Publishing Ltd

12

Assisted Death in Dementia and the Old Age Psychiatrist

JOHN WATTIS

Medical Director, Leeds Community & Mental Health Services, Leeds, UK

INTRODUCTION

Defining terms

The euthanasia debate has been going on for years. The literal meaning of euthanasia is 'easy' or 'good death'. The popular press writes of 'mercy killing' and this captures the idea that death can be a welcome relief from suffering and that the death described involves an outside agent. Most commonly, in modern times, this is a physician and so we come to the term used today, 'assisted death', or, often, 'physician-assisted death'. In the present chapter it is assumed that 'assisted death' is appropriate only for somebody who is suffering from a severe terminal illness from which he or she is unlikely to recover. One could argue that the principle of autonomy is so pre-eminent that a physician should assist any mentally competent adult who chooses to die; but this argument will not be developed since the topic of this chapter is specifically that of a person suffering from dementia. The issue of euthanasia is bound up with the issue of suicide. In what is called voluntary euthanasia the person who is to die is the one who makes the decision and the person who assists is acting as their agent. In involuntary euthanasia the person who is to die is not involved in the decision. This second seems very close to the crime of murder and reminds us of the worst excesses of the Nazi regime with respect to mentally ill and learning disabled people and will not be discussed in detail here.

Different dimensions

Moral

Morality is rooted in history and in religious or philosophical convictions. In broad terms it is to do with right and wrong. Some hold the view that moral principles are unchanging, perhaps 'God-given'; others believe that morality is situational and constantly changing. In ancient times Seneca, the Greek philosopher, argued that it was as proper for a man to choose the means and time of his death as for him to choose the house he lived in. At the same time the Jewish tradition held that, in normal circumstances, only God should decide when a person should die. To take one's own life virtually amounted to murder by making a decision that only God was allowed to make. An exception was allowed when suicide was to protect the Jewish faith and the 'glory of God'. Traditional Christian theology and morality followed the Jewish view about not 'playing God' by taking one's own life. Indeed, Augustine argued that suicide was a worse transgression of the commandment 'Thou shalt not kill' than was straightforward murder. He believed this was the case because it left no room for repentance. He was writing at a time when martyrdom was a common consequence of Christian belief and was opposing the views of some who deliberately sought martyrdom 'to the glory of God', thus departing a little from the traditional Jewish view and at the same time setting the scene for a fierce Christian condemnation of suicide (and consequently of euthanasia) that has held until very recent times (See Wennberg, 1989.) This book is particularly recommended for a detailed consideration of some of the issues that can only be touched on in a brief account such as this. The period of the enlightenment brought with it the humanistic tradition and a secular moral view which in the West, at least, has elevated the principles of self-determination and autonomy to a position of pre-eminence amongst other moral and ethical principles. This view of each individual as 'master of his own destiny' has brought about a twentieth-century campaign for a revision of social views on the morality of suicide and euthanasia. On the other hand, a profound respect for human life is another aspect of most modern morality.

Ethical

Ethics are closely related to morality. In the sense used in medicine ethics relates to a set of moral principles by which doctors govern their relationship with their patients (and sometimes other aspects of their lives, too). Another ancient Greek, Hippocrates, incorporated in his famous oath the phrase, 'I will neither give a deadly drug to anybody if asked for it nor will I make a suggestion to this effect'. The same oath incorporated a ban on procuring abortion. It was congruent with traditional Christianity and was widely adopted as the basis for medical ethics certainly to the middle of this century and possibly beyond. However, in recent times it has been replaced by more modern statements such as the General Medical Council's (1997) statement on 'Good Medical Practice' (expounded on in more detail later). Ethical duties include respecting the autonomy of the patient but also doing good and doing no harm.

Legal

Suicide is no longer against the law in this country. Euthanasia is still illegal and a review of medical ethics by the House of Lords in 1994 suggested it should remain so. In Holland, whilst euthanasia is not strictly legalized, there is an understanding that if performed according to an agreed code, prosecution is unlikely to follow. This is leading to a body of information about what happens when euthanasia is permitted (Olde Scheper and Duursma, 1994; Van der Wal and Dillman, 1994). Experience suggests that some involuntary euthanasia is creeping in but that active euthanasia is much less common than decisions not to treat life-threatening conditions in terminally ill people. The Northern Territories of Australia attempted to legalize euthanasia several years ago (Zinn, 1995) but no information is available on the outcome.

Theological

Theological considerations interweave with discussions of morality. Even secular humanists, who do not have a theology, nevertheless find that their thoughts are influenced by the religious past, and we should not forget that many people in modern secular societies still have a belief in God which helps shape their consideration of moral issues. Perhaps the most famous theological contribution to the debate in recent times comes from the Roman Catholic tradition in the shape of the 'doctrine of double effect'. According to this principle it is permissible to give, for example, a high dose of morphine with the intention of relieving pain even where it is reasonably foreseen that this may hasten death.

The structure of this chapter

The remainder of this chapter will focus on the dangerous tendency of the euthanasia debate to polarize opinion and cause proponents of one side of the debate to be deaf to contrary arguments. The author will then revisit the ethical basis of practice and rehearse some of the arguments for and against 'assisted death' in the context of the particular problems posed for people suffering from dementia whose decision-making capacity may be eroded by illness.

POLARIZATION

There are few issues so likely to polarize argument as the issue of euthanasia. Proponents of both sides of the debate often take extreme views about the 'rightness' of their own position and the 'wrongness' of the contrary view.

A 'spectrum of beliefs'

In fact there is a spectrum of beliefs in society about when it is right to breach the taboo on taking human life, and medical opinion is equally divided (Ward and Tate, 1994). Most people hold that taking life in war, even on a large scale, can be morally justified, though, the author holds the minority view that war and killing in war is wrong. As Gandhi put it: 'I can think of many causes in which I would be prepared to lay down my life but none for which I would be willing to take the life of another.' The majority of public opinion is in favour of capital punishment for murder but Parliament refuses to bow to popular pressure, whereas in the USA capital punishment has been reinstated and there is now pressure to extend it to children. It was only relatively recently that 'therapeutic abortion' was legalized and popular opinion is still divided about the 'rightness' of abortion on demand. Nor do views 'segregate' in what might be the expected clusters. Opponents of abortion may be vociferous campaigners for capital punishment and vice versa. Specifically in the context of dementia, Helme (1995) discusses three models of care characterized as follows: 'warehousing', where preservation of life is the dominant value, 'horticultural' where respect for autonomy is the dominant value and 'euthanasia' where easing suffering dominates. The present author does not agree with his analysis, believing, for example, that good long-term care for people with dementia can be far more than just 'warehousing', as expounded by Kitwood and Bredin (1992a).

Projection, paranoia and demonization

Unfortunately in the euthanasia debate the tendency is for each side to demonize the other. A proponent of legalizing euthanasia has discussed some of the psychodynamic 'mental mechanisms' involved (Helme, 1993). The anti-euthanasia group doubt the moral principles of the pro-euthanasia group and mumble darkly about Hitler's extermination programme which started with people suffering from mental illness and learning difficulty before spreading to Jewish people and other dissidents. The pro-euthanasia group regard those who oppose them as 'old-fashioned' religious bigots; there is not much room for a meeting of minds. Part of this is no doubt due to the adversarial nature of our democracy and legal system. If I hold that euthanasia is wrong, in an adversarial situation I tend to overstate my case to ensure that any compromise reached is nearer to my point of view than that of my adversary. It is likely that he or she may do the same. Thus much heat is generated but not a great deal of light or understanding.

The need to listen and find a middle way

If we are to find a consensus we must learn to listen to each other and respect one another's hopes and fears. It is no good simply rejecting the arguments of one side or the other and perhaps also rejecting the people expressing contrary views.

ETHICAL BASIS OF PRACTICE

Universal principles?

It has been argued that there are certain fundamental principles of good human behaviour that are accepted in virtually all societies. These have been characterized as follows:

- A belief in *fairness* – treating others as we would want them to treat us
- A belief that *honesty and integrity* are better than dishonesty and corruption
- A belief in the importance of *human dignity*
- A belief in the value of *service* in the sense of working for the common good
- A belief that *quality and excellence* are to be preferred to shoddiness and mediocrity
- A belief in the *potential for growth* of people
- A belief in the virtue of *patience, forbearance and a nurturing attitude* (Covey, 1989)

Of course, this list can be criticized, but it does show how much people from different social, religious and philosophical backgrounds can share a great many core beliefs. The problem comes when we try to translate these values and principles into ethical actions in the real world. For example, a belief in the importance of human dignity can be used as an argument for or against euthanasia.

'Good medical practice'

The Hippocratic tradition has already been mentioned. The General Medical Council has recently produced a much more modern statement of the 'duties of a doctor registered with the General Medical Council' (General Medical Council, 1997) part of which is as follows: 'Patients must be able to trust doctors with their lives and well being. To justify that trust, we as a profession have a duty to maintain a good standard of practice and care and *to show respect for human life* [author's italics].'

The statement then goes on to consider 14 specific duties covering areas as diverse as respect for patients' dignity and privacy, listening to patients and respecting their views, keeping up to date, and being honest and trustworthy. These principles are expanded in an 18-page detailed document, but nowhere are the issues of suicide, euthanasia (or abortion) specifically mentioned. Thus the modern physician is provided with very explicit guidance about issues such as note-taking and delegation of responsibility but no guidance on issues that were considered of paramount importance by Hippocrates and his successors up to the middle of this century. We are now in a 'moral maze' when it comes to these important issues. However, the law at least provides us with some clarity. Legally we are not permitted actively to assist patients to die. We are also always expected to act in the patient's best interest when dealing with someone incapable of making their own decisions and, in law, to respect the autonomous decisions of those who are mentally competent.

ARGUMENTS FOR AND AGAINST ASSISTED DEATH

Arguments for assisted death

Autonomy: substituted judgement and best interest

There is a tradition in modern ethics which gives individual autonomy great value. Provided the exercise of autonomy does not interfere with the rights of others it is held to be virtually the pre-eminent principle of ethics, though doing good and doing no harm are also accorded great importance. Those who argue for autonomy as the main determinant of appropriate behaviour echo the view of Seneca that a person should be able to choose his or her own death. As the law stands at the moment, however, it is not only potentially unethical for a physician to assist a patient to die, it is positively illegal. Thus it is argued that the law needs to be changed to enable the physician to support his or her patient's autonomous choice. Further, it is argued that for the mentally incompetent adult the principle of substituted judgement should supplant the present principle of acting in the patient's best interest. This means that the doctor should try to determine what the patient would have chosen had they been able to choose. Perhaps the best way of determining this is through the advance directive or 'living will'. Such documents are already respected when considering active medical treatment. For example, a patient who had clearly expressed the wish not to be subject to cardiopulmonary resuscitation whilst of sound mind and whilst in possession of relevant information could expect to have that wish respected, even if unconscious. However, advance directives cannot require a doctor to do something illegal and may be called into doubt if the mental competence and understanding of the patient when making the directive is not assured.

Economy/utility

This argument, based on the principle of 'the greatest good for the greatest number' is harder to sustain. According to this argument we should not be 'wasting money' looking after those who have untreatable chronic illness but investing that same money where it will 'do more good' – perhaps in children's health services. In its coarsest form this argument has been used to justify eugenics programmes such as those carried out in Nazi Germany. In a less virulent form it is the assumption which underlies some of the ageist attitudes found in modern health services. Even if the argument is accepted as morally defensible, it is hard to justify in such a rich and luxurious society as that in which we now live.

Duty to relieve suffering

This is an important duty for doctors, nurses and other members of the 'caring professions'. More than that it is often the main motivating factor for those working in terminal care settings. Yet it is also advanced as an argument in favour of euthanasia, crudely expressed as 'I wouldn't let a dog suffer like that' or 'If he was a horse, they'd shoot him'. That is to say that in some cases suffering can be so intractable and so beyond relief that death seems the kindest option. In extreme situations, for example a soldier shooting a comrade who is suffering in circumstances where his death is certain and where truly nothing else can be done to relieve his agony, some will allow this is permissible. Many in the hospice movement would argue that this kind of situation rarely, if ever, occurs in the terminal care setting. Assisted death is seen by such people as not only morally wrong but also as a denial of what can be done to relieve pain, distress and discomfort when the best medical care is available. The distress of depressive disorder in the context of terminal illness can be difficult to manage but early diagnosis and treatment can certainly help. Even here, there is room for debate about whether the medical description of depressive disorder is appropriate or whether we should use a term like 'existential despair'. Certainly the author has seen people with terminal illness who have appeared to want an early death in the context of a depressive illness improve with treatment and enjoy a more settled and comfortable last few weeks or months.

Another variation on this argument is more disturbing. According to this argument, people with dementia lose their humanity as their brains deteriorate. This is on the same scale as the argument about when a fetus acquires 'personhood', which is an important part of the debate on abortion. *If* a person loses their personhood in severe dementia, *then* it may be argued that their life no longer has a uniquely human value. Thus, ending that life, particularly to relieve distress or pain, may be seen as less morally serious than ending the life of someone who is still fully mentally competent and therefore 'fully human'. Pushing this argument to its logical conclusion would be an argument for *involuntary* as well as *voluntary* euthanasia.

Arguments against assisted death

The 'sanctity' of human life

Stated in this way this is a theological argument. It harks back to the Judaeo-Christian tradition that only God can give and take away human life. However, we have already seen that many Christian (and other) religions permit exceptions to this rule in wartime. At a secular level the same principle is reflected by a belief in the dignity of human life sometimes expressed as respect for the person of each human being (Kitwood and Bredin, 1992b; Kitwood, 1993). Human life is something of tremendous intrinsic value and therefore should be respected and not ended by a voluntary act. Killing a person is a very serious matter and army training recognizes that people have to be desensitized to killing others. Those who hold this principle strongly will probably be against all killing of people. Others will hold that exceptions to the principle occur in wartime, in judicial executions, in induced abortion and perhaps in other circumstances, including terminal illness.

The 'slippery slope'

This is a pragmatic argument. It holds that once the absolute taboo on taking human life is broken, voluntary euthanasia may or perhaps will lead on to involuntary or avolitional euthanasia of those who are seen as a burden on society and then, possibly, to the killing of other 'misfits' including minority ethnic groups. The pattern of euthanasia in the Third Reich, followed by mass extermination of Jewish people, and the way in which the liberalization of abortion law appears to have led to far more abortions on far less obvious grounds than originally envisaged are cited in support of this argument. On the other hand, society has for years managed to hold that murder is wrong whilst accepting large-scale killing in war. Further possible evidence for the validity of the slippery slope theory comes from the Dutch experience where at least one case of assisted euthanasia occurred in a patient who may have been suffering from a treatable depressive illness that (to use the quaint legal phrase) 'affected the balance of her mind' (Ogilvie and Potts, 1994). To some extent where one stands on this argument depends on how optimistic or pessimistic a view one takes about human nature.

Practicalities

When it comes to people with dementia there are a further group of pragmatic arguments which are predicated on the nature of the disease and its effect on human personality and decision-making capacity.

Who decides, and when?

For example, if we imagine somebody with severe dementia without the capacity to make a decision about ending his or her own life, who would make a decision for them and when, if one was considering active 'treatment' to end life? How would we even know when the capacity to make or reverse such a decision had occurred (Wattis, 1995). How could the decision-maker know what the patient wanted? How could he or she judge 'quality of life'? Perhaps more importantly, how should the decision be made if quality of life was poor because of inadequate care and the decision-maker knew that a few streets away, in another better-managed residential home, people with the same level of dementia were enjoying an altogether superior quality of life?

Problems with advance directives

Nor can these problems be solved completely by advance directives. To give consent to a medical procedure in the present a patient has a right to expect to be reasonably well informed. But in writing an advance directive in his or her fifties how can a person know what treatment may be available for dementia in 20 years' time or whether their acceptance of chronic disability might increase with increasing maturity. Again, if we are considering active euthanasia, how will the physician determine whether the patient has reached an appropriate stage of dementia? Will it be a question of 'Kill me if my mini-Mental State score falls below 10'? What if the patient wrote the advance directive whilst in a pessimistic frame of mind (or even when suffering from an undiagnosed depressive illness) and is now demented but cheerful? Of course, the purist could argue that these practicalities should not stand in the way of the principle of self-determination.

WHERE DO WE 'DRAW THE LINE'?

Medicine is an intensely practical occupation. Life and death decisions have to be made, often in the face of less than adequate information and understanding, so where do we 'draw the line'? Indeed, should we be thinking in terms of drawing lines at all except in so far as we are constrained by legislation?

An ethical perspective

The modern ethical principles stated by the General Medical Council (GMC) do not help a great deal here. We are to make the care of the patient our first concern. But which is more caring, to preserve life at all costs or to allow or even 'help' somebody to die with relative dignity? In the UK, in contrast to other countries where tube-feeding of patients with dementia is or has been relatively commonplace (e.g. parts of USA and Scandinavia), there is a long tradition of easing death by not indulging in heroic treatment for patients with severe dementia. Many of us would find moving a step further, by actively and intentionally causing the death of a patient, to be a step too far.

The legal position

So does the law help by prohibiting physicians from actively and intentionally causing the deaths of patients? Many of us feel it does help us to draw the line at an appropriate place, to seek to provide the best care possible but not to 'strive officiously' to keep alive. Some do not like the ambiguity of the present position where withholding treatment for a life-threatening chest infection is arguably acceptable but active intervention to cause death is not. They argue that there is not a true moral or ethical distinction between causing the death of a person by omission or by commission. They would like active intervention to cause death to be made legal in certain circumstances, arguing that this would be a more honest and open position. Others would argue that there is a difference in *intent* between 'letting nature take its course' and active killing and that the law should preserve its ban on active killing.

A personal view

In the end this is an intensely personal issue for patient and doctor. The author would certainly like to see the law around consent and the incapacitated adult clarified along the lines suggested by the Law Commission and accepted by the Lord Chancellor (The Lord Chancellor's Department,

1997). A carefully drafted statute law should be enacted to set appropriate limits on advance directives while giving them formal recognition. These directives should not be allowed to require active intervention to end life. The day when active intentional killing becomes part of a doctor's role would be a black one, even were it requested by a patient who was of sound mind. The author would be even more reluctant to see the law changed to enable him to kill patients with dementia. If such a law were enacted he would have to register as a 'conscientious objector' or perhaps retire from medical practice.

CONCLUSION

The issue of euthanasia is an emotional one but this should not stop us from listening respectfully to those who hold different views from ourselves. The moral, ethical and legal basis of respect for human life and dignity is deep and widely shared in many different societies and by those who espouse different religions and philosophies. Nevertheless, most societies accept that the taboo on killing can be broken in exceptional circumstances, as in war. Introducing the possibility of active 'mercy killing' into the physician–patient relationship is, however, of dubious value. Particular practical problems surround the issue of assisted death in patients with dementia and make it even more unacceptable for this group of patients than for those who are mentally competent.

REFERENCES

Covey, S.R. (1989). *The Seven Habits of Highly Effective People*. Simon and Schuster, London.

General Medical Council (1997). *Good Medical Practice*. General Medical Council, London.

Helme, T. (1993). A 'special defence': a psychiatric approach to formalising euthanasia. *Br J Psychiatry* **163**, 456–466.

Helme, T. (1995). Editorial comment: on euthanasia and other medical decisions in the terminal care of dementia patients. *Int J Geriatr Psychiatry* **10**, 727–733.

Kitwood, T. (1993). Towards a theory of dementia care: the interpersonal process. *Ageing Soc* **13**, 51–67.

Kitwood, T. and Bredin, K. (1992a). *Person to Person: a Guide to the Care of Those with Failing Mental Powers*. Gale Centre Publications, Loughton.

Kitwood, T. and Bredin, K. (1992b). Towards a theory of dementia care: personhood and well-being. *Ageing Soc* **12**, 269–287.

Lord Chancellor's Department (1997). *Who Decides? Making Decisions on Behalf of Mentally Incapacitated Adults*, Cm3803. HMSO, London.

Ogilvie, A.D. and Potts, S.G. (1994). Assisted suicide for depression: the slippery slope in action? *BMJ* **309**, 492–493.

Olde Scheper, T.M. and Duursma, S.A. (1994). Euthanasia: the Dutch experience. *Age Ageing* **23**, 3–6.

Van der Wal, G. and Dillman, R.J. (1994). Euthanasia in the Netherlands. *BMJ* **308**, 1346–1349.

Ward, B.J. and Tate, P.A. (1994). Attitudes among NHS doctors to requests for euthanasia. *BMJ* **308**, 1332–1334.

Wattis, J. (1995). Incompetence develops gradually. *BMJ* **310**, 1605.

Wennberg, R.N. (1989). *Terminal Choices: Euthanasia, Suicide and the Right to Die.* Wm B. Eerdmans, Grand Rapids, MI.

Zinn, C. (1995). Australia passes first euthanasia law. *BMJ* **310**, 1427–1428.

III

Management of Functional Disorders

13

Making Sense of Antidepressants

JOHN T. O'BRIEN

Department of Psychiatry and Institute for the Health of the Elderly, University of Newcastle upon Tyne, Newcastle upon Tyne, UK

INTRODUCTION

This chapter will review the use of antidepressants in elderly depressed subjects. This topic has been the subject of some excellent previous reviews (e.g. Baldwin *et al.*, 1995; Katona, 1997) and rather than repeat information from elsewhere, the current discussion will concentrate on the mechanism of action, efficacy and tolerability of recently introduced antidepressant medications. These will include the combined serotonergic and noradrenergic reuptake inhibitors venlafaxine and milnacipran, the specific noradrenergic reuptake inhibitor reboxetine as well as nefazodone and mirtazapine, which are thought to have their own distinct modes of action. Some practical guidelines will be offered about the very difficult but crucial clinical question of what should inform rational choice of antidepressants in the elderly and issues such as cost-effectiveness, treatment of resistant depression and the treatment of those with particular problems (e.g. the physically ill and those with dementia) will be addressed.

It is inevitable that any discussion about antidepressant medication in the elderly should begin by highlighting the relative dearth of evidence regarding efficacy in such subjects, who are often excluded from standard antidepressant drug trials (Gerson *et al.*, 1988; Anstey and Brodaty, 1995). This not only applies to those aged over 65 but, in particular, to those who form the mainstay of everyday clinical practice of old age psychiatrists – that is, the physically frail, those with concurrent illnesses and those with associated cognitive impairment and dementia (Evans *et al.*, 1997). The consequence of this is that the evidence-based management of depression in the elderly is based on very few double-blind studies, often with small sample sizes of patients who may be largely unrepresentative of clinical practice. Inevitably, undue weight has then to be placed either on open, uncontrolled studies or on extrapolations from work in younger subjects, the latter being particularly inappropriate in view of pharmacokinetic and pharmacodynamic changes which occur with ageing, the particular problems of co-morbidity and polypharmacy in the elderly, and increasing evidence that depression in late life may be a distinct subtype of depression (O'Brien *et al.*, 1996; Baldwin, 1997; Lebowitz *et al.*, 1997).

There are currently 29 drugs listed as antidepressants in the British National Formulary (BNF) and these are shown in Table 1. Despite the relative paucity of antidepressant studies in the elderly the main result emerging from all studies, which does very much parallel work in younger subjects, is that no single antidepressant has demonstrable superiority over another (Gerson *et al.*, 1988; Anstey and Brodaty, 1995). In general terms, all antidepressants have been shown to be more effective than placebo and, usually, as effective as comparitor 'gold standard' drugs (usually tricyclics)

Table 1.   Antidepressants available in the UK as of March 1998.

Tricyclic antidepressants
Amitriptyline hydrochloride (Lentizol, Tryptizol)
Amoxapine (Asendis)
Clomipramine hydrochloride (Anafranil)
Dothiepin hydrochloride (Prothiaden)
Doxepin (Sinequan)
Imipramine hydrochloride (Tofranil)
Lofepramine (Gamanil)
Nortriptyline (Allegron)
Protriptyline hydrochloride (Concordin)
Trimipramine (Surmontil)
  Related antidepressants
  Maprotiline hydrochloride (Ludiomil)
  Mianserin hydrochloride (Mianserin)
  Mirtazapine (Zispin)
  Trazodone hydrochloride (Molipaxin)
  Viloxazine hydrochloride (Vivalan)

Monoamine-oxidase inhibitors
Phenelzine (Nardil)
Isocarboxazid
Tranylcypromine (Parnate)
  Reversible Monoamine-oxidase inhibitors
  Moclobemide (Manerix)

Selective serotonin reuptake inhibitors
Fluoxetine (Prozac)
Citalopram (Cipramil)
Fluvoxamine maleate (Faverin)
Paroxetine (Seroxat)
Sertraline (Lustral)
  Related antidepressants
  Nefazodone hydrochloride (Dutonin)

Selective noradrenergic and serotonergic reuptake inhibitors
Venlafaxine (Efexor)

Noradrenergic noradrenaline reuptake inhibitors
Reboxetine (Edronax)

Other antidepressant drugs
Flupenthixol (Fluanxol)
Tryptophan (Optimax)

but never more so. The issue of whether newer compounds are really as effective as older tricyclics, however, remains. For example, Perry (1996) argues that when considering melancholic depression, pooled study data do indicate evidence of the superiority of tricyclics over selective serotonin reuptake inhibitors (SSRIs). In addition, as Katona (1997) rightly points out, caution is necessary in interpreting results of studies showing no differences between newer drugs and tricyclics, as studies have almost always been underpowered to allow sufficient confidence to conclude that no real differences exist.

Pharmacokinetic changes with ageing

Several changes occur with ageing which may have relevance for the prescribing of antidepressants. In general, absorption in the elderly is slower and there is a reduction in renal and hepatic clearance with age. There is an increase in the proportion of water compared to fat in the body with age and a decrease in serum albumin, reducing the capacity for protein-binding. Most antidepressant drugs are highly protein-bound (80–90%), an exception being venlafaxine which is only 30% bound. Depending on the particular properties of the antidepressant, these effects can lead to either little change or a great increase in circulating drug levels following an equivalent dose regimen in older compared with younger patients. For example, with tricyclic antidepressants considerably higher steady state plasma levels are seen in older subjects. Of perhaps more importance, however, is an increase in inter-individual variability, making it extremely difficult to predict the likely therapeutic dose of drug for any particular subject. The SSRIs differ considerably in how they are influenced by age. For example, the plasma half-lives of fluvoxamine and fluoxetine are relatively unaffected by age. However, the half-lives of paroxetine and the major metabolites of sertraline and citalopram are prolonged in the elderly.

Side-effects

The multiple side-effects of tricyclic antidepressants in the elderly are well recognized. These include anticholinergic effects of dry mouth, gastrointestinal problems, blurred vision and urinary retention. Sedation is often a major difficulty as is the development of postural hypotension (α_1 blocking effect). Although such drugs can be used in the presence of stable heart conditions, tricyclics are cardiotoxic and are contraindicated in patients with certain arrhythmias or who have had a recent myocardial infarction. The findings of most reviews of antidepressant studies in the elderly concur with the experience of the majority of clinicians which is that, because of these side-effects, tricyclic antidepressants are less well tolerated in the elderly than other newer drugs (Anstey and Brodaty, 1995). However, there is no doubt that when they can be tolerated they are effective compounds and this is undoubtedly why some clinicians still feel they should be the drug of first choice, even in elderly patients. Other antidepressants have their own problems. Mianserin can cause agranulocytosis and monoamine-oxidase inhibitors such as moclobemide can cause nausea, dizziness and insomnia. Venlafaxine can cause hypertension. The SSRIs have major advantages in that they lack the cardiotoxicity and major cholinergic and adrenergic side-effects of tricyclics. They do, however, have their own typical side-effect profile of nausea, insomnia and headache, along with gastrointestinal problems, and it is important to remember that their side-effects are different from tricyclics, rather than fewer, though overall they do appear to be better tolerated. Withdrawal reactions with antidepressants, particularly SSRIs, have aroused much interest recently (Price *et al.*, 1996; Stahl *et al.*, 1997a; Rosenbaum *et al.*, 1998). Withdrawal reactions do seem higher with paroxetine than other SSRIs, though withdrawal reactions have been described with all antidepressants, and rather than simply avoiding drugs that may be particular offenders, a sensible approach is probably to always advise gradual and cautious dose-tailing in any subject stopping antidepressant medication.

Drug interactions

Elderly depressed patients, who often have associated co-morbid physical illnesses, are frequently on other medications, making the frequency and nature of drug interactions an important consideration. Particular attention has recently been paid to the potential of some SSRIs to inhibit hepatic enzyme oxidation (the cytochrome P450 system). By inhibiting this system, the pharmacokinetics of other hepatically oxidized drugs can be affected. For example, most SSRIs (especially paroxetine and fluoxetine) are potent inhibitors of the cytochrome P450 CYP 2D6 which can affect other drugs metabolized by this system, including tricyclic antidepressants and trazodone, neuroleptics, lipophilic beta-blockers, some antiarrhythmics, and other drugs such as codeine. Some drugs inhibit the P450 enzyme that is responsible for their own metabolism (e.g. fluoxetine and paroxetine and the 2D6 system) leading to nonlinear kinetics with increasing drug dose. Some 5–10% of the population genetically lack the CYP 2D6 enzyme. This means that they are poor metabolizers of drugs oxidized by this pathway, though equally they are unaffected by problems caused by compounds which inhibit this system. Fluvoxamine, fluoxetine and sertraline are inhibitors of the P450 CYP 2C19 and 2C9 isoenzymes which are important in the metabolism of warfarin, diazepam and some anticonvulsants (e.g. phenytoin). Because of the potential for such interactions, prescription of an antidepressant always requires careful consideration of what other medication the patient is on and, though such interactions do not necessarily preclude co-prescription, they do indicate the need for increased caution and more careful clinical monitoring. The practice of co-prescription of a tricyclic and an SSRI, something that was becoming fashionable before newer agents such as venlafaxine were available, is not recommended by the author because of the risk of toxic levels of tricyclics occurring (Westermeyer, 1991). For a fuller discussion of drug interactions of antidepressants in the elderly readers are referred to Pollock (1998).

SOME RECENTLY INTRODUCED ANTIDEPRESSANTS

Mirtazapine

Mirtazapine (Zispin, Organon) is a drug which has effects on both the noradrenergic and serotonergic systems. Its overall effect is to enhance central noradrenergic and $5HT_1$-receptor-mediated serotonergic neurotransmission. It is an antagonist at the α_2 adrenergic presynaptic autoreceptor and also blocks $5HT_2$ and $5HT_3$ receptors. The effects of α_2 blockade are to increase noradrenergic release (de Boer, 1996). Serotonergic activity is also increased, partly because noradrenergic release directly stimulates excitatory α_1 receptors located on serotonergic neurones and partly because α_2 receptors are also located on serotonergic nerve terminals where they exert an inhibitory effect on serotonin release. The direct blockade by mirtazapine of these receptors will, therefore, enhance serotonin release. Since mirtazapine directly blocks $5HT_2$ and $5HT_3$ receptors (de Boer, 1996), the net effect of the drug is enhanced noradrenergic and $5HT_1$-mediated serotonergic neurotransmission. The latter effect may be important as some argue that the final common pathway of all antidepressant therapies (including electroconvulsive therapy (ECT)) is of enhanced $5HT_1$ neurotransmission (Blier and de Montigny, 1994).

Differences in pharmacokinetics with age are considered minor (Timmer *et al.*, 1996) and no dose adjustment is needed in the elderly. Efficacy in younger subjects has been assessed in comparison with placebo, amitriptyline, clomipramine, doxepin, trazodone, imipramine and fluoxetine (Stahl *et al.*, 1997b). Two studies, involving a total of 265 subjects, have involved older patients (Halkas, 1995; Hoyberg *et al.*, 1996). Hoyberg *et al.* (1996) compared mirtazapine (15–45 mg, mean dose 37 mg) to amitriptyline (30–90 mg, mean dose 74 mg) in a six-week study of 115 in- and outpatients aged 60–85 (mean age 70) in centres in Norway and the UK. No significant differences were observed at any time-point and a similar proportion of patients improved in each group (amitriptyline 81%, mirtazapine 74%). Perhaps surprisingly, both drugs were well tolerated and side-effect profiles were remarkably similar (dry mouth, constipation, blurred vision, fatigue, dizziness, sedation). This fits with the main side-effects of mirtazapine reported in other studies (dry mouth, drowsiness and excessive sedation, increased appetite and weight gain) though, interestingly, the classic side-effects associated with the SSRIs such as nausea, vomiting, diarrhoea, insomnia and sexual dysfunction are not particularly associated with mirtazapine (Montgomery, 1995). The absence of such side-effects may be due to the drug's $5HT_2$- and $5HT_3$-blocking properties.

The second study (Halkas, 1995) was of the very 'young elderly' and included 150 outpatients aged over 55 (mean age 62) who were randomized to receive placebo, mirtazapine (5–35 mg, mean dose 28 mg) or trazodone (40–280 mg, mean dose 220 mg) for six weeks. Mirtazapine treatment was significantly more effective than placebo, with a difference being seen at two weeks, but was not significantly different from trazodone. The finding that trazodone was only significantly more effective than placebo at weeks 2 and 3, but not at the study end, probably reflects the lack of power in a study where group sizes before drop-outs were only 50.

Nefazodone

Nefazodone (Dutonin, Bristol-Myers Squibb) is an inhibitor of serotonin reuptake and also blocks postsynaptic $5HT_2$ receptors. Again, this dual action may lead to a relative potentiation of $5HT_1$ neurotransmission. Plasma levels of nefazodone do appear to be higher in older female subjects (Barbhaiya *et al.*, 1996) and the product information states that because of this the effects of starting dose and the rate of dose titration should be carefully assessed. There appear to be no published double-blind studies specifically regarding nefazodone in elderly subjects, though an open-label report (yet to be published) on 40 subjects over the age of 65 with major depression or dysthymia shows similar response rates to younger subjects, perhaps not surprisingly in view of the small sample size (Wilcox *et al.*, 1999). The most frequent adverse effects noted in the elderly were headache, somnolence, nausea, dizziness and diarrhoea. Nefazodone caused no significant orthostatic hypotension or electrocardiogram (ECG) changes in 12 elderly controls, though supine blood pressure was lowered (Breuel *et al.*, 1993) and postural hypotension has been reported as an infrequent side-effect in younger subjects.

Reboxetine

Reboxetine (Edronax, Pharmacia & Upjohn) is the first in a new class of drugs which are selective noradrenergic reuptake inhibitors. There are no placebo-controlled studies in the elderly and, at the time of writing, use in the elderly is not recommended because of this. Plasma concentrations appear higher in older subjects and dose reduction may be advised (Dostert *et al.*, 1997). There is one eight-week study in elderly subjects which compares reboxetine (4–6 mg) with imipramine (75–100 mg) in the treatment of 218 patients (aged 56–94, mean 74) with major depressive disorder or dysthymia (Montgomery, 1997). An identical response rate (52%) was seen in both groups and the frequency of adverse events was very similar in the two treatment groups, though hypotension was more common in imipramine-treated subjects. Adverse events led to treatment discontinuation in 11% of reboxetine- and 16% of imipramine-treated subjects (Mucci, 1997). Full details of this trial, however, have not yet been published. However, increases in heart rate values to 100 beats per minute or higher occurred in a higher proportion of patients (12%) in the reboxetine group than in imipramine-treated subjects (6%). Similarly, rhythm disorders (which included tachycardia and occasional atrial and ventricular ectopic beats) were found in 13% of the reboxetine group and 6% of the imipramine group. Further details of efficacy and side-effect profile in elderly subjects are awaited, though the suggestion that some cardiac side-effects may be more common with reboxetine than imipramine is worrying.

Venlafaxine

Venlafaxine (Efexor, Wyeth) was the first combined noradrenergic and serotonergic reuptake inhibitor to be licensed in the UK. Pharmacokinetic changes with ageing appear to be minor and no dose reduction is necessary. Khan et al. (1995) conducted a 12-month open-label study of venlafaxine (75–225 mg) in 58 depressed outpatients aged over 65. Most common side-effects were headache, nausea, dry mouth and sweating. Significant improvements were seen, though only 24 completed 12 months of treatment. A double-blind study comparing venlafaxine and dothiepin (maximum dose 150 mg for both drugs) in 92 elderly subjects (age 64–87) found no significant differences between response rates (60% in each) or withdrawal rates because of adverse events between groups (Mahapatra and Hackett, 1997). Changes in blood pressure were significantly more common with dothiepin. Dierick (1996) reported an open-label study of 116 elderly depressed subjects treated for one year. Clinical response was seen in 64% of subjects by three months and the majority (81%) felt they had no side-effects. A randomized study of 170 elderly depressed subjects of six weeks' treatment with venlafaxine, trazodone or clomipramine has been reported in abstract form (Smeraldi *et al.*, 1997). Response rates were 80% for clomipramine, 67% for venlafaxine and 50% for trazodone. Both venlafaxine and clomipramine were significantly superior to trazodone at week 6 but not significantly different from each other.

Milnacipran

This drug, like venlafaxine, is a combined inhibitor of both serotonin and noradrenalin reuptake. At the time of writing, it is not yet licensed for prescription in the UK but may become available towards the end of 1999. It lacks anticholinergic and monoamine oxidase inhibitory activities and several studies have confirmed efficacy in younger subjects against tricyclics and SSRIs with, as expected, a low level of anticholinergic side-effects. Plasma levels appear only 20% higher in elderly subjects and no specific dose adjustment is needed, except in those with moderate and severe renal impairment (Puozzo and Leonard, 1996). Only one study (Tignol *et al.*, 1998) has compared milnacipran (50 mg twice daily) to imipramine (50 mg twice daily) in 219 patients (aged 65–93, mean age 74) with major depressive disorder over an eight-week period. No significant differences were found between milnacipran and imipramine in antidepressant efficacy, though a significantly greater number of side-effects were observed in the imipramine group. Sixteen per cent of imipramine patients dropped out of treatment because of adverse events compared with only 6% of those treated with milnacipran. However, figures were reversed (14% of milnacipran patients compared with 7.5% of imipramine patients) regarding drop-outs because of treatment failure. The only side-effect which was more common in milnacipran patients than imipramine subjects was nausea (though not a significant difference) and the only significant difference in side-effects between groups was in terms of dry mouth, seen in just over 35% of imipramine-treated subjects but 17% of those treated with milnacipran. Both imipramine and milnacipran had similar effects on cardiovascular parameters including tachycardia and lengthening of the QRS interval on the electrocardiogram.

Summary

As with more established drugs, there are few double-blind placebo-controlled studies of these newer compounds in the elderly, particularly with regard to nefazodone. Mirtazapine has been compared with placebo and active comparators and results support its efficacy as an antidepressant with a side-effect profile appearing to resemble that of the tricyclics rather than SSRIs, though seemingly with fewer cardiac effects than tricyclics. Other compounds (reboxetine, venlafaxine, milnacipran) have been compared with active comparators and generally found to be as effective, though never more so, than tricyclics. The small size of most of the studies makes it difficult to draw any firm conclusions about their current role in the management of elderly depressed subjects and while there are theoretical attractions about newer, better tolerated drugs that have a similar pharmacological profile to tricyclics, the evidence-base to support their use in the elderly in preference to drugs such as the SSRIs is lacking. There have been no controlled studies involving comparisons with SSRIs in the elderly and experience of use in the frail elderly and those with concurrent cognitive impairment is severely limited.

COST-EFFECTIVENESS

That the newer antidepressants are more expensive than older drugs such as tricyclics is self-evident from basic drug costs taken from the BNF and illustrated in Table 2, with the most expensive antidepressant being some 30 times the cost of the cheapest. This has, inevitably, caused some to advocate widespread prescription of cheaper antidepressant drugs as first-line agents. However, the notion that newer drugs are more expensive overall has been challenged by several economic analyses which, when taking account of *all* costs of treating depression rather than simply drug costs, often show similar costs or even an economic advantage of newer compounds over older drugs (Jonsson and Bebbington, 1994; Montgomery *et al.*, 1996; D'Mello *et al.*, 1995; Crott and Gilis, 1998; Hylan *et al.*, 1998). For example, Jonsson and Bebbington (1994) found costs per successfully treated patient to be lower for paroxetine (£824) than imipramine (£1024), while Montgomery *et al.* (1996) found overall annual costs lower for nefazodone (£219) than imipramine (£254). The main reason is that the greater costs of newer compounds are generally offset by higher costs of 'treatment failure' because of higher drop-out rates from older drugs. Costs of treatment failure include

Table 2.   Cost of treating depression for 30 days with selected antidepressants using a typical daily dose.

Drug name	Dose (mg)	Cost (%)
Amitriptyline	150	1.56
Dothiepin	150	6.46
Lofepramine	210	15.41
Mirtazapine	30	25.71
Moclobemide	300	21.00
Fluoxetine	20	20.77
Citalopram	20	22.80
Paroxetine	20	20.77
Sertraline	50	21.31
Sertraline	100	42.61
Nefazodone	400	18.00
Venlafaxine	75	25.68
Venlafaxine	150	51.36
Reboxetine	8	39.60

Costs listed are taken from the British National Formulary, March 1998.

not only the costs of switching to another antidepressant but also specialist referral, hospital admission for some patients, further expensive treatments (e.g. ECT) in some cases and the continued expense of remaining ill. The cost of overdose with older tricyclics has been shown to be up to four times greater than newer drugs (D'Mello *et al.*, 1995), largely because of longer hospital stay. Studies vary considerably in their levels of economic sophistication (Hylan *et al.*, 1998) and are usually based on assumptions from clinical research studies that may not always mirror clinical practice. The only prospective economic study found a nonsignificant trend for lower overall costs for fluoxetine compared with imipramine and desipramine (Simon *et al.*, 1996). All these studies have been in younger patients; cost-effectiveness has not been satisfactorily addressed in the elderly and reliance on such analyses may not be appropriate. For example, late-life depression is associated with increased mortality and, if successful treatment were to reduce mortality, it is possible that economic analyses would paradoxically show an increase in costs for a group who may then be well but reliant on the provision of social and nursing care for a longer period. However, despite various methodological problems, the general finding that current studies of cost-effectiveness do not demonstrate newer compounds to be more expensive when overall costs of treatment are considered (reviewed by Crott and Gilis, 1998) should suffice to firmly rebut any short-sighted economic pressure to prescribe antidepressants on the basis of cost alone.

WHICH ANTIDEPRESSANT DRUG IS THE DRUG OF FIRST CHOICE IN THE ELDERLY?

There is no universal consensus on this issue. If the principle is accepted that no single antidepressant has demonstrable superiority over another in terms of efficacy, then the choice of a first-line agent will always remain a difficult, controversial and often idiosyncratic one. Despite the cardiotoxicity of older tricyclic compounds and their high propensity to cause hypotension, confusion and other side-effects, many clinicians still feel they are the 'gold standard' and that, if the dosage is appropriately adjusted and monitored ('start low, go slow'), and side-effects are carefully explained to patients and families, then many older subjects can tolerate these. However, the experience of many other clinicians, including the author, is that there are major advantages in the greater tolerability of newer compounds, which leads to antidepressant treatment which is more effective (i.e. is more often delivered) rather than being more efficacious (i.e. has greater antidepressant effect).

Porter and O'Brien (1998) argued that rational choice of antidepressant can be made after consideration of several factors which are summarized in Table 3. If a patient has had a previous episode of depression which

Table 3. Factors to consider when selecting an antidepressant drug for an elderly subject (after Porter and O'Brien, 1998).

- History of response of previous episode to a particular agent
- History of tolerance (or intolerance) to particular drugs
- Type of depression (agitated/retarded)
- Concomitant drug treatment and possible drug interactions
- Compliance
- Concurrent physical illness
- Liability to particular side-effects such as hypotension, cognitive impairment and sedation

responded well to a particular agent, and which the patient could tolerate, there would seem to be no good reason not to prescribe the same drug again unless some clinical change had occurred to influence drug prescribing (e.g. the development of cardiac disease). Similarly, if a patient has been shown to be intolerant of a particular drug, there would seem little point in trying this again unless, for example, the intolerance could be shown to be for a clear reason (for example the injudicious use of a particularly high starting dose). Concurrent physical illness and associated cognitive impairment will be important factors in determining choice of compounds. There will be few clinicians who would want to give patients with compromised cognitive function, either because of dementia or some other cause, a drug that was a potent anticholinergic. Similarly, those with a history of urinary difficulties or a tendency to postural hypotension should not be prescribed drugs that will exacerbate this. Cardiac disease is common and the tendency of tricyclics to cause bradycardia and arrhythmias would make these unsuitable drugs for many elderly subjects. Concurrent drug treatment and possible drug interactions are also important considerations. For patients on warfarin, it may be sensible to avoid drugs such as fluvoxamine. Similarly, in patients who insist on continuing to drink large quantities of alcohol, drugs that have relatively few interactions (e.g. citalopram) may be preferable. Finally, compliance is a very important issue. The necessity for careful dosing of older tricyclic compounds (and some newer drugs) may make it inadvisable for them to be prescribed to patients who might not comply with frequent follow-up. Similarly, a once-daily dosage may be preferable to drugs that have to be taken more frequently and one advantage of some of the newer drugs, such as the SSRIs, is that they can be prescribed in a once-daily effective dose from day one. Associated features such as suicidal ideation may also influence prescribing. It does appear that older tricyclic drugs such as amitriptyline and dothiepin are particularly toxic in overdose (Power *et al.*, 1995; Henry *et al.*, 1995). However, it is most important for clinicians to remember that only the minority (perhaps only 4%) of all suicides are caused by overdose of prescribed antidepressant drugs. The majority are by other means and, if they involve overdoses, are more likely to involve other drugs such as analgesics. A patient at high risk of suicide requires management for this in its own right, be it careful clinical monitoring or admission to hospital, rather than just prescribing a drug that is safer in overdose (Jick *et al.*, 1995). The cost of different antidepressants is increasingly becoming a factor that is influencing choice of antidepressant, with newer drugs in many regions limited to prescription by specialists in psychiatry. The arguments over cost-effectiveness are complex and, until a consensus emerges on whether newer, more expensive drugs are more or less cost-effective overall than tricyclics, cost should be one of the least important factors in determining rational choice of an antidepressant drug.

ANTIDEPRESSANT USE IN PARTICULAR PATIENT GROUPS

There are enormous logistical problems with antidepressant studies involving particular patient groups such as elderly subjects with concurrent severe physical illness and those with dementia. A Cochrane review regarding the efficacy of antidepressants in dementia is in preparation. One difficulty with research in this area is that patients with dementia and depression appear to have a high rate of spontaneous recovery and high placebo response rate, making the study of large numbers of patients necessary. Some positive studies, however, have been reported. For example, citalopram was found to improve a variety of emotional symptoms, including depressed mood, in dementia (Nyth and Gottfries, 1990) while moclobemide significantly improved depressive symptoms in those with concurrent dementia (Roth *et al.*, 1996). Evans *et al.* (1997) have recently reported one of the few attempts at a placebo-controlled study in depressed subjects with severe physical illness. The study was underpowered as only 21 subjects in each group completed eight weeks of treatment with fluoxetine or placebo. Overall, no significant differences were seen, though those with severe illness did significantly better with fluoxetine treatment, suggesting that antidepressant therapy was still appropriate in this group. The logistic problems inherent in such studies (Koenig *et al.*, 1989) mean that large controlled studies of such patients are unlikely to be feasible.

TREATMENT OF RESISTANT DEPRESSION

Several strategies have been suggested for the management of depressed subjects who do not respond to full dose treatment of a single antidepressant for an adequate length of time. These include: augmentation with lithium, T3 or anticonvulsants; changing to another antidepressant; the addition of an SSRI to a tricyclic; the use of ECT; and augmentation with other agents including pindolol, buspirone and amphetamine. A recent comprehensive review of evidence in younger patients (Schweitzer *et al.*, 1997) concluded that solid evidence in the form of well conducted double-blind studies was only available for augmentation with lithium and T3. Evidence in the elderly is, not surprisingly, even more limited, though open studies have reported similar response rates to lithium augmentation in the treatment-resistant elderly (20–60%) as are seen in younger subjects (van Marwijk *et al.*, 1990; Zimmer *et al.*, 1991; Flint and Rifat, 1994; Reynolds *et al.*, 1996). Other strategies, such as combining SSRI and tricyclic drugs are not advocated for pharmacokinetic reasons (see above). Further data are needed regarding the use of augmentation strategies in the elderly, including the important question regarding the duration that adjunctive medication should be prescribed. Reynolds et al (1996) found that elderly subjects requiring augmentation (which was then stopped) had higher relapse rates during continuation therapy than those not requiring augmentation (52% versus 6%), suggesting that, as has been shown for antidepressants (OADIG, 1993; Reynolds *et al.*, 1998), long-term prescription of adjunctive medication may be needed to prevent relapse into depression once remission and recovery have occurred. However, only future prospective studies can address the issue of for how long such treatments should continue.

REFERENCES

Anstey, K. and Brodaty, H. (1995). Antidepressants and the elderly: double-blind trials 1987–1989. *Intl J Geriatr Psychiatry* **10**, 265–279.

Baldwin, R.C. (1997). Depressive illness. In: Jacoby, R. and Oppenheimer, C. (Eds), *Psychiatry in the Elderly*. Oxford University Press, Oxford, pp. 536–573.

Baldwin, R.C., Simpson, S. and Leitch, D.S. (1995). Antidepressants in the elderly. In: Levy, R. and Howard, E. (Eds), *Developments in Dementia and Functional Disorders in the Elderly*. Wrightson Biomedical, Petersfield, pp. 127–150.

Barbhaiya, R.H., Buch, A.B. and Greene, D.S. (1996). A study of the effect of age and gender on the pharmacokinetics of nefazodone after single and multiple doses. *J Clin Psychopharmacol* **16**, 19–25.

Blier, P. and de Montigny, C. (1994). Current advances and trends in the treatment of depression. *Trends Pharmacol Sci* **15**(7), 220–226.

Breuel, H.P., DeLeenheer, I., Coninx, L. *et al.* (1993). Comparison of the cardiovascular effects of nefazodone, imipramine and placebo in healthy elderly volunteers. *Europ Neuropsychopharmacol* Sept, 423.

Crott, R. and Gilis, P. (1998). Economic comparisons of the pharmacotherapy of depression: an overview. *Acta Psychiatr Scand* **97**, 241–252.

De Boer, T. (1996). The pharmacological profile of mirtazapine. *J Clin Psychiatry* **57** (suppl. 4), 19–25.

D'Mello, D.A., Finkbeiner, D.S. and Kocher, K.N. (1995). The cost of antidepressant overdose. *Gen Hosp Psychiatry* **17**, 454–455.

Dierick, M. (1996). An open-label evaluation of the long-term safety or oral venlafaxine in depressed elderly patients. *Ann Clin Psychiatry* **8**, 169–178.

Dostert, P., Benedetti, M.S. and Poggesi, I. (1997). Review of the pharmacokinetics and metabolism of reboxetine, a selective noradrenaline reuptake inhibitor. *Eur Neuropsychopharmacol* **7**(suppl), 23–35.

Evans, M., Hammond, M., Wilson, K., Lye, M. and Copeland, J. (1997). Placebo-controlled treatment trial of depression in elderly physically ill patients. *Int J Geriatr Psychiatry* **12**, 817–824.

Flint, A.J. and Rifat, S.L. (1994). A prospective study of lithium augmentation in antidepressant-resistant geriatric depression. *J Clin Psychopharmacol* **14**, 353–356.

Gerson, S.C., Plotkin, D.A. and Jarvik, L.F. (1988). Antidepressant drug studies 1946 to 1986: empirical evidence of aging patients. *J Clin Psychopharmacol* **8**, 311–322.

Halkas, J.A. (1995). Org. 3770 (mirtazapine) versus trazadone: a placebo controlled trial in depressed elderly patients. *Hum Psychopharmacol* **10** (suppl 2), S125–S133.

Henry, J.A., Alexander, C.A. and Sener, E.K. (1995). Relative mortality from overdose of antidepressants. *BMJ* **310**, 215–219.

Hoyberg, O.J., Maragakis, B., Mullin, J. *et al.*, (1996). A double-blind multi-centre comparison of mirtazapine and amitriptyline in elderly depressed patients. *Acta Psychiatr Scand* **93**, 184–190.

Hylan, T.R., Buesching, D.P. and Tollefson, G.D. (1998). Health economic evaluations of antidepressants: a review. *Depress Anxiety* **7**, 53–64.

Jick, S.S., Dean, A.D. and Jick, H. (1995). Antidepressants and suicide. *BMJ* **310**, 215–218.

Jonsson, B. and Bebbington, P.E. (1994). What price depression? The cost of depression and the cost-effectiveness of pharmacological treatment. *Br J Psychiatry* **164**, 665–673.

Katona, C.L.E. (1997). New antidepressants in the elderly. In: Homes, C. and Howard, R. (Eds), *Advances in Old Age Psychiatry*. Wrightson Biomedical, Petersfield, pp. 143–160.

Khan, A., Rudolph, R., Baumel, B., Ferguson, J., Ryan, P. and Shrivastava, R. (1995). Venlafaxine in depressed geriatric outpatients: an open-label clinical study. *Psychopharmacol Bull* **31**, 753–758.

Koenig, H.G., Goli, V., Shelp, F. *et al.* (1989). Antidepressant use in elderly medical inpatients: lessons from an attempted clinical trial. *J Gen Int Med* **4**, 498–505.

Lebowitz, B.D., Pearson, J.L., Schneider, L.S. *et al.* (1997). Diagnosis and treatment of depression in late life. *JAMA* **278**, 1186–1190.

Mahapatra, S.N. and Hackett, D. (1997). A randomised, double-blind, parallel-group comparison of venlafaxine and dothiepin in geriatric patients with major depression. *Int J Clin Pract* **51**, 209–213.

Montgomery, S.A. (1995). Safety of mirtazapine: a review. *Int Clin Psychopharmacol* **10**(4), 37–45.

Montgomery, S.A. (1997). Reboxetine: additional benefits to the depressed patient. *J Psychopharmacol* **11**, S9–S15.

Montgomery, S.A., Brown, R.E. and Clarke, M. (1996). Economic analysis of treating depression with nefazodone v. imipramine. *Br J Psychiatry* **168**, 768–771.

Mucci, M. (1997). Reboxetine: a review of antidepressant tolerability. *J Psychopharmacol* **11**(4), S33–S37.

Nyth, A.L. and Gottfries, C.G. (1990). The clinical efficacy of citalopram in treatment of emotional disturbances in dementia disorders. *Br J Psychiatry* **157**, 894–901.

OADIG (Old Age Depression Interest Group) (1993). How long should the elderly take antidepressants? A double blind placebo-controlled study of continuation/prophylaxis therapy with dothiepin. *Br J Psychiatry* **162**, 175–182.

O'Brien, J., Desmond, P., Ames, D., Schweitzer, I., Harrigan, S. and Tress, B. (1996). A magnetic resonance imaging study of white matter lesions in depression and Alzheimer's disease. *Br J Psychiatry* **168**, 477–485.

Perry, P.J. (1996). Pharmacotherapy for major depression with melancholic features: relative efficacy of tricyclic versus selective serotonin reuptake inhibitor antidepressants. *J Affect Disord* **39**, 1–6.

Pollock, B.G. (1998). Drug interactions. In: Craig Nelson, J. (Ed.), *Geriatric Psychopharmacology*. Marcel Dekker, New York, pp. 43–60.

Porter, R.J. and O'Brien, J.T. (1998). SSRIs may well be best treatment for elderly depressed subjects. *BMJ* **316**, 631.

Power, B.M., Hackett, P.L., Dusci, L.J. and Ilett, K.F. (1995). Antidepressant toxicity and the need for identification and concentration monitoring in overdose. *Clin Pharmacol* **29**, 154–171.

Price, J.S., Waller, P.C., Wood, S.M. and Mackay, A.V.P. (1996). A comparison of the post-marketing safety of four selective serotonin re-uptake inhibitors including the investigation of symptoms occurring on withdrawal. *Br J Clin Pharmacol* **42**, 757–763.

Puozzo, C. and Leonard, B.E. (1996). Pharmacokinetics of milnacipran in comparison with other antidepressants. *Int Clin Psychopharmacol* **11** (suppl 4), 15–27.

Reynolds, C.F., Frank, E., Perel, J.M. *et al.* (1996). High relapse rate after discontinuation of adjunctive medication for elderly patients with recurrent major depression. *Am J Psychiatry* **153**, 1418–1422.

Reynolds, C.F., Frank, E., Perel, J.M. and Kupfer, D.J. (1998). Maintenance therapies for late-life recurrent major depression: research and review circa 1996. In: Craig Nelson, J. (Ed.), *Geriatric Psychopharmacology*. Marcel Dekker, New York, pp. 127–139.

Rosenbaum, J.F., Fava, M., Hoog, S.L., Ascroft, R.C. and Krebs, W.B. (1998). Selective serotonin reuptake inhibitor discontinuation syndrome: a randomised clinical trial. *Biol Psychiatry* **44**, 77–87.

Roth, M., Mountjoy, R., Amrein and the International Collaborative Study Group. (1996). Moclobemide in elderly patients with cognitive decline and depression. An international double-blind, placebo-controlled trial. *Br J Psychiatry* **168**, 149–157.

Schweitzer, I., Tuckwell, V. and Johnson, G. (1997). A review of the use of augmentation therapy for the treatment of resistant depression: implications for the clinician. *Aust N Z J Psychiatry* **31**, 340–352.

Simon, G.E., Von Korff, M., Heiligenstein, J.H. *et al.* (1996). Initial antidepressant choice in primary care. Effectiveness and cost of fluoxetine vs. tricyclic antidepressants. *JAMA* **275**, 1897–1902.

Smeraldi, E., Aguglia, A., Cattaneo, M. *et al.* (1997). Double-blind, randomised study of venlafaxine, clomipramine and trazodone in geriatric patients with major depression. Abstract presented at the 10th European College of Neuropsychopharmacology meeting, Vienna, September, 1997.

Stahl, S., Lindquist, M., Pettersson, M. *et al.* (1997a). Withdrawal reactions with selective serotonin re-uptake inhibitors as reported to the WHO system. *Eur J Clin Pharmacol* **53**, 163–169.

Stahl, S., Zivkov, M., Reimitz, P.E., Panagides, J. and Hoff, W. (1997b). Meta-analysis of randomized, double blind, placebo-controlled, efficacy and safety studies of mirtazapine versus amitriptyline in major depression. *Acta Psychiatr Scand* **96** (suppl 39), 22–30.

Tignol, J., Pujol, D.J., Chartres, J.P. *et al.* (1998). Double-blind study of the efficacy and safety of milnacipran and imipramine in elderly patients with major depressive episode. *Acta Psychiatr Scand* **97**, 157–165.

Timmer, C.J., Paanakker, J.E., and van Hal, H.J.M. (1996). Pharmacokinetics of mirtazpine from orally adminstered tablets: influence of age, gender and treatment regimen. *Hum Psychopharmacol* **11**, 497–509.

van Marwijk, H.W.J., Bekker, F.M., Nolen, W.A., Jansen, P.A., Nieuwkerk, J.F. and Hop, W.C. (1990). Lithium augmentation in geriatric depression. *J Affect Disord* **20**, 217–223.

Westermeyer, J. (1991). Fluoxetine-induced tricylic toxicity: extent and duration. *J Clin Pharmacol* **31**, 388–392.

Wilcox, C.S., Linden, R.D., D'Amica, M.F. *et al.* (1999). Nefazodone in the treatment of elderly patients with depression. *Arch Fam Med* (in press).

Zimmer, B., Rosen, J., Thornton, J.E., Perel, J.M. and Reynold, C.F. (1991). Adjunctive lithium carbonate in nortriptyline-resistant elderly depressed patients. *J Clin Psychopharmacol* **11**, 254–256.

Everything You Need to Know About Old Age Psychiatry . . .
Edited by Robert Howard
©1999 Wrightson Biomedical Publishing Ltd

14

Approaches to Treatment-Resistant Depression in the Elderly

ROBERT C. BALDWIN

Department of Psychiatry for the Elderly, Central Manchester Healthcare Trust, Manchester, UK

INTRODUCTION

About one-third of patients, young (Katona *et al.*, 1995) and old (Flint, 1995), do not respond to first-line antidepressant therapy. The human cost of chronic depression is highlighted by the Medical Outcomes Study where it was found that functional impairment and interference with quality of life associated with depression was comparable to or worse than that of eight major chronic medical conditions. These included diabetes, arthritis and severe coronary artery disease (Wells *et al.*, 1989). The ultimate cost of untreated depression may be suicide.

This chapter will discuss the difficulties in defining what is meant by 'resistant' or 'refractory' depression, its management and the pharmacological strategies available, with whatever evidence there is to support their use in older patients. It is important from the outset to address common terms which cause confusion such as 'double depression' and 'chronic depression'. The former refers to depression superimposed upon dysthymia (chronic subsyndromal depression); the definition of the latter is persistence of symptoms for two or more years (Scott, 1988). Likewise, one must not confuse depressive disorders which are hard to treat, perhaps because of problems with tolerability of antidepressants or medical co-morbidity, with patients who have genuinely failed to respond to adequate treatment. These issues, of course, overlap and will be discussed.

REFRACTORY DEPRESSION: DEFINITIONS AND CONCEPTUALIZATION

Patients who do not recover with a course of an antidepressant are often termed refractory. Literally this means 'obstinate' or 'unmanageable'. As such, 'refractory depression' is merely descriptive – the patient has not responded to treatment. 'Treatment-resistant depression' is not much better a term unless the precise treatments offered, along with duration and dosages, are clarified.

Attempts to define resistance/refractoriness in operational terms have not been particularly successful. For example, 'relative' and 'absolute' resistance, originally proposed by the 1974 World Psychiatric Association (Lehman, 1974), have no agreed meaning. Other definitions seem sensible but are nevertheless arbitrary. For example, Renwick (1985) suggested '... an ongoing and unremitting depressed state in a patient as defined by his/her physician and who has been unsuccessfully treated with at least two different antidepressants or an antidepressant and/or course of ECT'. A widely used definition is that of Nierenberg and Amsterdam (1990), namely a failure to cause a decrease in the Hamilton Rating Scale for Depression (HAM-D) by 50% and a post-treatment residual score of >7. However, this is perhaps more relevant to clinical pharmaceutical trials.

An interesting approach proposed by Thase and Rush (1995) is to stage the depression based on prior treatment response (see Table 1). This has the advantage of being applicable across a range of treatment types. In their view, treatment-refractory depression is present when stage 2 has been completed; that is, failure to respond to two trials of different antidepressants from different classes in sufficient dose for an adequate period of time.

Table 1. Proposed staging of depression based on prior treatment response (after Thase and Rush, 1995).

0	No adequate trial of medication
1	Non-response to antidepressant monotherapy
2	Non-response to two trials of monotherapy from drugs of different classes
3	Stage 2 plus failure to respond to one augmentation strategy
4	Stage 3 plus failure of a second augmentation strategy
5	Stage 4 plus failure to respond to course of electroconvulsive therapy (ECT)

The clinical utility of terms such as 'resistance' or 'refractory depression' could be improved if there was a clearer conceptualization of the process of depression management. An advance is the approach proposed by Guscott and Grof (1993) (Table 2). They suggest that the clinician ask six questions when faced with a 'refractory' patient:

Table 2. A stepped-care approach to depression management (after Guscott and Groff, 1991).

1) Is the diagnosis correct (for example, organic mood disorder overlooked)?
2) Has the patient received adequate treatment?
3) Has a stepped-care pharmacological approach been used?
4) Has outcome been measured appropriately?
5) Has medical and/or psychiatric co-morbidity been addressed?
6) Are there factors in the treatment setting that have been overlooked?

1) Is the diagnosis correct? For example, some patients with resistant depressive symptoms do not have a primary affective disorder. Rather, their symptoms are secondary to another psychiatric illness, or an organic mood disorder. The prognosis for 'secondary' depression is poor (Keller et al., 1984). Patients with psychotic depression may conceal psychotic symptoms which also confer a poorer overall prognosis.

2) Has the patient received adequate treatment? Adequacy must be evaluated along the axes of duration, dosage and compliance (including the use of serum monitoring where available), and tolerability (discussed later).

3) Was a stepped-care approach used (see below)?

4) How was outcome measured? For example, antidepressants generally improve depressive symptomatology but improvement in social function may be less dramatic.

5) Is there a co-existing medical or psychiatric disorder that interferes with response to treatment?

6) Are there factors in the clinical setting that interfere with treatment? External factors to consider are poor social circumstances, chronic adversity and an investment in invalidism, perhaps to secure continuing attention from carers.

Lastly, Guscott and Grof point to clinician-related factors. These include the balance struck in a particular treatment facility between psychological and physical treatment modes and the frustration and anger which patients with resistant depression engender in the treating clinician, sometimes leading to avoidance or erroneous reassignment of the case as primarily due to 'personality'.

To expand slightly point number 5, there has recently been interest in what has been termed 'vascular depression' (Alexopoulos et al., 1997). This proposes that late-onset depression is associated with a high rate of cerebrovascular disease which influences the clinical presentation. 'Vascular depression' is suggested by the presence of psychomotor retardation, limited depressive ideation such as guilt, poor insight, apathy and greater disability and the finding on magnetic resonance imaging (MRI) of white matter hyperintensities and other brain changes (Krishnan *et al.*, 1995; Alexopoulos *et al.*, 1997). In the work of the author's team (Simpson *et al.*, 1997; Simpson *et al.*, 1998), it has been shown that white matter hyperintensities and basal ganglia lesions are also associated with poorer response to antidepressant therapy, but that it is not merely the presence of such lesions but their location which is important in this respect. In particular, lesions in the deep frontal white matter, basal ganglia and pons are associated with refractoriness in the acute phase of treatment to antidepressant drugs but not to ECT. Clearly it would be helpful if there were clinical markers at onset, rather than those seen only on MRI scans, which could identify which patients were least likely to recover with antidepressant therapy and who therefore might move on quite swiftly to second-line treatments such as ECT. These observations (Simpson *et al.*, in press) indicate that there may be some neurological markers such as the presence of mild parkinsonism and poor performance on a simple motor sequencing task which may help in this respect, although of course these findings need to be replicated.

Addressing questions 1, 2, 4, 5 and 6 of Guscott and Grof's approach will result in the recovery of a substantial number of patients. The precise figure is undetermined as most experience is in highly specialized tertiary referral centres, but a rough estimate is 50% (Bridges, 1995; Smith and Singh, 1995). Guscott and Grof (1991) go as far as to state: 'The evidence clearly points to undertreatment as the primary cause of so-called refractory depression.' Bridges *et al.* (1995), dealing with patients under the age of 65 in the main, suggest that dosages of 300–400 mg of amitriptyline equivalents, plus or minus substantial doses of thioridazine, may be required to overcome resistance to treatment. Elderly patients are unlikely to tolerate such high doses of tricyclics so that so-called refractoriness in an older patient may represent intolerance of the chosen drug as much as genuine non-response. Alternative strategies become even more important with older patients.

It is at this point that Guscott and Grof's question 3, a rational, stepped-care approach to treatment becomes relevant. By this they mean that treatment decisions (the 'steps') are based on scientifically grounded principles, but they concede that, unlike a number of general medical conditions, such principles in psychiatry are based on shaky, often untested or contentious grounds.

TREATMENT STRATEGIES FOR THE REFRACTORY PATIENT

What then are the steps which in practice clinicians may adopt? They may be summarized as follows (see Table 3).

Table 3.   Strategies for treatment-resistant depression.

1) Increase dose
2) Increase length of treatment
3) Switch class – intraclass or between classes
4) Augmentation – tricyclic antidepressant (TCA) or selective serotonin reuptake inhibitor (SSRI); thyroid; lithium; neuroleptic; anticonvulsants
5) Monoamine-oxidase inhibitor
6) ECT
7) Psychotherapy

Increase dose

First, the dose of the antidepressant can be increased. This may be beneficial with tricyclic drugs but there is little evidence that increasing the dose significantly alters outcome for patients treated with the selective serotonin reuptake inhibitors (SSRIs) (Thase and Rush, 1995). As discussed, the high dosages recommended for younger resistant patients are unlikely to be tolerated by older patients.

Increase length of treatment

A second strategy is to continue a therapeutic trial beyond what would usually be considered an 'adequate' period of time. In the past a four-week therapeutic trial was considered long enough. Quitkin *et al.* (1984) have suggested at least six weeks as a minimum adequate trial. Many psychiatrists would accept this, but would change to ECT before this if the patient's suffering was intolerable or his/her condition grave. Although the strategy of continuing beyond six weeks has never been properly tested there is evidence from studies of geriatric patients that an extension to nine weeks or even longer may result in further recovery (Georgotas and McCue, 1989). In a small open study of 23 patients almost 50% responded with this approach (Georgotas *et al.*, 1989). If therapy is given beyond 12 weeks a natural remission becomes more probable. This may artificially inflate the supposed drug response rate.

Class-switching

Switching between drugs of the same class has little logic to it. Although some success has been reported this may be due to better tolerability of the second drug rather than better efficacy (Bridges *et al.*, 1995). The most popular strategy clinically is a change from one antidepressant to another from a different class; for example, from a tricyclic antidepressant (TCA) to an SSRI, or vice versa (Shaw, 1977; Akiskal, 1985). The basis of this strategy is that there may be noradrenergic and serotonergic types of depression. It is remarkable how little real evidence there is for this. Nolen *et al.* (1988), in a double-blind partial crossover study, studied 71 patients, all under 65 years, and crossed them over either from oxaprotiline (a TCA) to fluvoxamine (an SSRI) or vice versa. Only 13% overall responded, 27% to oxaprotiline and none to fluvoxamine. The authors conclude that '... non-responders to "noradrenergic" antidepressants do not appear to have much chance of responding to "serotonergic" antidepressants and vice versa'. Criticisms of this study include the length of treatment phase, which at four weeks is shorter than the recommendation of Quitkin *et al.* (1984). Also, the side-effects of fluvoxamine, principally nausea, might have resulted in subtherapeutic dosages being used. Despite the theoretical appeal of this approach, there is limited evidence to date that this strategy is effective in mixed-aged and younger adult patients, and no evidence at all of efficacy in elderly patients. The only available data have have to be extrapolated from mixed-aged or younger subjects. Summarizing such data, Thase and Rush (1995) have suggested that between 30 and 70% of resistant patients may respond to a change from a tricyclic to an SSRI. The wide range is probably due to many of the studies being uncontrolled, with a tendency to report only positive results.

Even less is known about the other type of switch, from an SSRI to a tricyclic. As Thase and Rush (1995) highlight, North American psychiatrists, and increasingly European ones, routinely prescribe SSRIs as drugs of first choice in mixed-aged patients so that this is an important strategy to study. Evans and co-workers reported good results when they treated elderly physically ill patients with fluoxetine (Evans, 1992; Evans *et al.*, 1997). Tolerability was good, the rate of serious adverse effects low and, against expectations, outcome was best in those with the most grave physical illnesses. In contrast to this, Roose *et al.* (1994) found that 22 depressed patients with heart disease with a mean age of 73 years responded less well to fluoxetine than 42 comparable patients treated with nortriptyline (mean age 70). Only five of the 22 fluoxetine-treated patients responded; those with melancholic subtype of major depression (the majority) had a particularly poor outcome. The number of drop-outs in each group was similar. So although the newer antidepressants appear to have a role here, the evidence for their efficacy over established antidepressants is far from convincing, perhaps especially in the more severe forms of depressive disorder.

There are several newer antidepressants which either act in novel ways or constitute a new class of drug. Nefazodone has similarities to trazodone but differs from the latter in lacking H_1 antagonism, thereby causing less sedation. Its place in resistant therapy is unclear, although possibly it may benefit patients who are trazodone responders but cannot tolerate its side-effects. Mirtazepine is an analogue of mianserin. It antagonizes presynaptic alpha-2 receptors and, less strongly, alpha-1 receptors, as well as 5-HT receptors but it does not inhibit monoamine reuptake. It is termed a noradrenaline and specific serotonergic antidepressant (NaSSA). In resistant depression it may have a place in patients who fail to respond to a reuptake inhibitor (tricyclics, SSRIs and venlafaxine). A rational, but unproven, strategy would be to use it as adjunctive treatment in resistant cases. The first nontricyclic selective noradrenaline reuptake inhibitor (NARI), reboxetine, has been introduced. Currently, European regulatory authorities have not recommended its use in the elderly until placebo-controlled trials have been conducted.

Venlafaxine, a serotonin and noradrenaline reuptake inhibitor (SNRI) shows some promise in resistant patients, but evaluation is confined to clinical experience (Bowskill and Bridges, 1997) or open trials (Nierenberg et al., 1994). As with established antidepressants, some resistant patients may require doses above the recommended maximum in specialist settings.

Augmentation

Traditionally, the combination of a tricyclic antidepressant with an older MAOI was thought to be a potent treatment for resistant cases. However, the regimen is potentially dangerous and has never been tested in an elderly patient group. Furthermore, O'Brien et al. (1993) have cast doubt on the efficacy of this combination. They allocated 80 patients (none elderly) to either tranylcypramine and amitriptyline or either drug alone. The combination was only marginally more effective than the single drug and was associated with significantly more side-effects.

Another fashionable strategy is of combining a TCA with an SSRI. Seth et al. (1992) reported a small series of mainly elderly patients who responded to the combination of nortriptyline and fluoxetine. Most had not responded to ECT. However, there is a risk of elevating TCA levels into the toxic range with this combination. Preskorn et al. (1990) described a 69-year-old patient given desipramine and fluoxetine, with the development of delirium within 10 days which resolved on discontinuation of both drugs. The strategy has not been subjected to proper controlled evaluation.

An approach for which there is a larger literature is that of augmenting antidepressants with lithium (LA). De Montigny et al. (1981) were the first to report a series of patients who responded to the addition of lithium to a tricyclic antidepressant, pointing out that improvement was sometimes not only dramatic but occurred within days. Austin et al. (1991) conducted a meta-analysis of five small double-blind trials and found that 18/50 of patients augmented with lithium responded compared with 6/49 of those who were given a placebo. While this difference is statistically significant, the response rate of 36% in the augmented group is not as impressive as earlier open studies and clearly the response rate of 12% in the placebo group is not negligible. In contrast, Schou (1990) grouped all studies of LA in the literature into those of fewer than 10 subjects, those with more than this but uncontrolled, and those studies with controls. He concluded that the enthusiastic positive reports in uncontrolled settings were not matched by those from controlled studies. In a more recent placebo-controlled trial of LA with fluoxetine compared with LA and lofepramine (Katona *et al.*, 1995), 15/29 responded to augmentation, which was significantly more than the placebo group (8/32), but again this latter rate is surprising and suggests that merely prolonging any antidepressant trial, in this case to 12 weeks in all, will result in some further improvement.

De Montigny *et al.* (1981) originally suggested that LA works within days but this has not been substantiated by more recent research. Three weeks of treatment is the suggested minimum time for a trial but longer may be required (Katona *et al.*, 1995; Schou, 1990).

Unfortunately there has been very little evaluation of LA in older patients. Flint (1995) reviewed 25 cases from several reports. He found that 76% of patients had a complete response and 16% a partial one. However, there was a lack of standardization regarding what was meant by resistant depression and what was regarded as a successful outcome and why. Also, one could not guarantee that the prior antidepressant trial had been adequate.

Three retrospective case series (Lafferman *et al.*, 1988; Finch and Katona, 1989; van Marwijk *et al.*, 1990) have involved 74 patients with less striking results, only 40% showing a complete response and 26% a partial one. Seymour and Wattis (1992) described three cases of refractory depression in the elderly which improved with lithium and lofepramine where a previous trial of lithium plus fluoxetine had failed. Lastly, the combination of lithium with an SSRI can potentially cause a serotonin syndrome.

There have been four prospective studies of LA in elderly patients to date. Zimmer *et al.* (1988) and Flint and Rifat (1994) found response rates of 20% and 23% respectively, much lower than open studies of younger adults. Parker *et al.* (1994) compared a group treated with a single antidepressant ($n = 23$) with a lithium-augmented group ($n = 21$) in a prospective study. The latter group was found to have significantly lower depression severity scores on the Montgomery Asberg Depression Scale at follow-up and a trend for lower scores on the Geriatric Depression Scale (two well-known depression scales which have been used in elderly patients). Although all but one patient in the LA group experienced side-effects, the total burden of them was greater in the group on an antidepressant alone, probably because the latter had residual depressive symptoms, and depressed patients are known to report more side-effects. However, this study did not utilize random allocation or blinded measures, so the results can only be viewed as encouraging. There have been no double-blind placebo-controlled trials of augmentation therapy in elderly patients.

The issue of side-effects and compliance with LA is addressed by Katona *et al.* (1995), who reported that despite careful monitoring only 16 of 29 LA patients achieved adequate lithium levels. Flint and Rifat (1994) found in their study that half their elderly patients on lithium developed dose-limiting side-effects.

The issue of the optimum dose of lithium in LA has not been settled. For example, Zusky *et al.* (1988) studied 18 patients aged 18–80 using lithium in dosages of between 100 and 500 mg (serum levels 0.1–0.8 mmol/l) and found poor results. Kushnir (1986) reported a series of five physically ill depressed elderly patients and found that low-dose lithium (150–300 mg; serum levels 0.15–0.25 mmol/l) was effective.

Foster (1992) reviewed the use of lithium in elderly patients and found that nontoxic side-effects are common. For example, polydipsia occurred in 50–74%, polyuria in 25–58%, tremor in 33–58%, dry mouth in 53%, nausea in 33% and memory impairment in 33%. Of concern was Foster's finding that the frequency of acute lithium toxicity appears to be in the range of 11–23% for elderly patients. This is not dissimilar to Stone's study of mania (Stone, 1989), where a quarter of 45 patients developed lithium toxic symptoms and five required admission. A quarter of Stone's patients had some evidence of cerebral organic impairment, which might help explain this finding. However, late life depression, especially late-onset, is also associated with subtle structural brain damage which might predispose to lithium neurotoxicity. Not only, then, is the issue of efficacy of LA in elderly patients unresolved but elderly patients may be considerably more prone to adverse effects than younger adults.

Neuroleptics, such as thioridazine, can be a useful augmentor of antidepressants. The main effects are anxiolytic and sedative. Additionally, thioridazine increases plasma tricyclic antidepressant levels by inhibiting their metabolism, which might be how it acts in resistant depression.

Other approaches include thyroid augmentation and antiepileptic drugs. However, in Flint's (1995) review reports in the elderly were almost entirely based on case studies; there has been no controlled evaluation of them among elderly patients, and hence their routine use cannot be justified in elderly patients.

Monoamine-oxidase inhibitors (MAOIs)

With regard to a trial of an MAOI, Georgotas *et al.* (1983) gave phenelzine (15–75 mg/day) to 20 elderly patients with refractory depression with a 65% recovery rate. However, this was an unusually chronically ill group and many older patients are intolerant of MAOIs. Few old age psychiatrists nowadays would use them as drugs of first choice. Whether the newer reversible inhibitors of monoamine oxidase A, represented by moclobemide in the UK, have anything to offer elderly patients with refractory depression is perhaps too early to say. Bowskill and Bridges (1997) have reported good clinical results with moclobemide in refractory cases, although they comment that some patients require more than the maximum recommended dose of 600 mg.

Electroconvulsive therapy (ECT)

Another step to be included in a 'stepped-care' approach is ECT which is effective in around 50% of 'refractory' cases (Prudec *et al.*, 1994). ECT is safe and effective in older patients and improves a wider range of symptoms arising as part of a depressive disorder, for example anxiety (Benbow, 1989). Whilst it seems reasonable to extrapolate research evidence from younger patients with resistant depression, more is needed of ECT use in older refractory patients.

There is no consensus as to the time of introduction of ECT. Should it be before augmentation strategies have been tried, or after? The use of ECT has decreased in recent years, probably because of increased acknowledgement of undertreatment with antidepressants and the wide variety of antidepressants available today, so that almost all patients can be given a drug which they can tolerate. The adverse publicity which surrounds ECT and the fact that often it is difficult to give to older people as an outpatient may discourage clinicians, but it remains the most effective remedy for patients with depressive disorder of all ages.

CONCLUSIONS

Extrapolating from studies of younger patients, a typical 'stepped-care' approach for a patient who has not responded to a course of an antidepressant correctly complied with over at least six weeks is as follows. The simplest strategy, of increasing the dose and prolonging the original antidepressant course beyond six weeks, has some merit. There is some evidence that this is effective in elderly patients. For older patients dose-limiting side-effects may make a substantial dose increase difficult. An alternative is that the original antidepressant can be changed to one of another class, given, if feasible for at least six weeks. Although the evidence for this is mixed, it is an attractive option for older depressed patients, given the dose-limiting side-effects of the older tricyclics, which often means they are never given at full therapeutic dosage.

If these measures are ineffective, the next two strategies for which there is reasonable evidence of efficacy are lithium augmentation and ECT. The former may be preferred as it can be given as an outpatient but there is no doubt that ECT remains the most effective of all physical treatments for depression. Such evidence as there is suggests lower response rates for LA compared with younger patients, and a higher risk of both dose-limiting side-effects and toxicity. There are difficulties with lithium compliance at all ages. In the absence of any sound evidence, it seems wise to adhere to the current recommended serum levels for use in older patients (0.35–0.70 mmol/l) and to give a trial for at least three to four weeks.

None of these strategies has been subjected to prospective double-blind evaluation in elderly depressed patients. A study which would clarify which is the best option would be to compare three groups in a parallel study lasting 12 weeks. In group 1, patients would be maintained on the same antidepressant, at maximum tolerated dose in the case of tricyclics, for a total of 12 weeks. In group 2, the drug would be changed to one of another class after six weeks if there had not been an adequate response. In the third group, patients would be given LA after six weeks if full recovery had not occurred. No such study has been conducted.

REFERENCES

Akiskal, H.S. (1985). A proposed approach to chronic and 'resistant' depressions: evaluation and treatment. *J Clin Psychiatry* **46**, 32–36.

Alexopoulos, G.S., Meyers, B.S., Young, R.C., Campbell, S., Silbersweig, D. and Charlson, M. (1997). 'Vascular depression' hypothesis. *Arch Gen Psychiatry* **54**, 915–922.

Austin, M.P.V., Souza, F.G.M. and Goodwin, G.M. (1991). Lithium augmentation in antidepressant-resistant patients: a quantitative analysis. *Br J Psychiatry* **159**, 510–514.

Benbow, S.B. (1989). The role of electroconvulsive therapy in the treatment of depressive illness in old age. *Br J Psychiatry* **155**, 147–152.

Bowskill, R.J. and Bridges, P.K. (1997). Treatment-resistant affective disorders. *Br J Hosp Med* **57**, 171–172.

Bridges, P.K., Hodgkiss, A.D. and Malizia, A.L. (1995). Practical management of treatment-resistant affective disorders. *Br J Hosp Med* **54**, 501–506.

De Montigny, C., Grunberg, F., Mayer, A. and Deschenes, J.P. (1981). Lithium induces rapid relief of depression in tricyclic antidepressant drug non-responders. *Br J Psychiatry* **138**, 252–256.

Evans, M.E. (1992). Depression in elderly physically ill inpatients: a 12 month prospective study. *Int J Geriatr Psychiatry* **8**, 587–592.

Evans, M.E., Hammond, M., Wilson, K., Lye, M. and Copeland, J. (1997). Placebo-controlled treatment trial of depression in elderly physically ill patients. *Int J Geriatr Psychiatry* **12**, 817–824.

Finch, E.J.L. and Katona, C.L.E. (1989). Lithium augmentation in the treatment of refractory depression in old age. *Int J Geriatr Depress* **4**, 41–46.

Flint, A.J. (1995). Augmentation strategies in geriatric depression. *Int J Geriatr Psychiatry* **10**, 137–146.

Flint, A.J. and Rifat, S.L. (1994). A prospective study of lithium augmentation in antidepressant-resistant geriatric depression. *J Clin Psychopharmacol* **14**, 353–356.

Foster, J.R. (1992). Use of lithium in elderly psychiatric patients: a review of the literature. *Lithium* **3**, 77–93.

Georgotas, A. and McCue, R. (1989). The additional benefit of extending an antidepressant trial past seven weeks in the depressed elderly. *Int J Geriatr Psychiatry* **4**, 191–195.

Georgotas, A., Friedman, E., McCarthy, M. *et al.* (1983). Resistant geriatric depressions and therapeutic response to monoamine oxidase inhibitors. *Biol Psychiatry* **18**, 195–205.

Georgotas, A., McCue, R.E. and Cooper, T.B. (1989). A placebo-controlled comparison of nortriptyline and phenelzine in maintenance therapy of elderly depressed patients. *Arch Gen Psychiatry* **46**, 783–786.

Guscott, R. and Grof, P. (1991). The clinical meaning of refractory depression: a review for the clinician. *Am J Psychiatry* **148**, 695–704.

Katona, C.L.E., Abou-Saleh, M.T., Harrison, D.H. *et al.* (1995). Placebo-controlled trial of lithium augmentation of fluoxetine and lofepramine. *Br J Psychiatry* **166**, 80–86.

Keller, M.B., Klerman, G.L. and Lavori, P.W. (1984). Long-term outcome of episodes of major depression. *JAMA* **252**, 788–792.

Krishnan, K.R.R., Hays, J.C., Tupler, L.A., George, L.K. and Blazer, D.G. (1995). Clinical and phenomenological comparisons of late-onset and early-onset depression. *Am J Psychiatry* **152**, 785–788.

Kushnir, S.L. (1986). Lithium-antidepressant combinations in the treatment of depressed, physically ill geriatric patients. *Am J Psychiatry* **143**, 378–379.

Lafferman, J., Soloman, K. and Ruskin, P. (1988). Lithium augmentation for treatment-resistant depression. *J Geriatr Psychiatry Neurol*, **1**, 49–52.

Lehman, H.E. (1974). Therapy-resistant depressions: a clinical classification. *Pharmacopsychiatr Neuropsychopharmakol* **7**, 156–163.

Nierenberg, A.A. and Amsterdam, J.D. (1990). Treatment resistant depression: definitions and treatment approaches. *J Clin Psychiatry* **51** (suppl 6): 39–47.

Nierenberg, A.A., Feighner, J.P., Rudolph, R., Cole, J.O. and Sullivan, J. (1994). Venlafaxine for treatment-resistant unipolar depression. *J Clin Psychopharmacol* **14**, 419–423.

Nolen, W.A., van de Putte, Dijken, W.A. *et al.* (1988). Treatment strategy in depression 1. Non-tricyclic and selective reuptake inhibitors in resistant depression: a double-blind partial crossover study on the effects of oxaprotiline and fluvoxamine. *Acta Psychiatr Scand* **78**, 668–675.

O'Brien, S., McKeon, P. and O'Ryan, M. (1993). The efficacy and tolerability of combined antidepressant treatment in different depressive subgroups. *Br J Psychiatry* **162**, 363–368.

Parker, K.L., Mittmann, N., Shear, N.H. *et al.* (1994). Lithium augmentation in geriatric depressed outpatients: a clinical report. *Int J Geriatr Depress* **9**, 995–1002.

Preskhorn, S.H., Beber, J.H. and Faul, J.C. (1990). Serious adverse effects of combining fluoxetine and TCAs. *Am J Psychiatry* **147**, 532.

Prudec, J.M., Sackeim, H.A. and Rifas, S. (1994). Medication resistance, response to ECT, and prevention of relapse. *Psychiatr Ann* **24**, 228–231.

Quitkin, F.M., Rabkin, J.G., Ross, D. and McGrath, P.J. (1984). Duration of antidepressant treatment: what is an adequate trial? *Arch Gen Psychiatry* **41**, 238–245.

Renwick, R.A. (1985). Treatment resistant depression. *Psychiatr J Univ Ottawa* **46**, 576–584.

Roose, S.P., Glassman, A.H., Attia, E. and Woodring, S. (1994). Comparative efficacy of selective serotonin reuptake inhibitors and tricyclics in the treatment of melancholia. *Am J Psychiatry* **151**, 1735–1739.

Schou, M. (1990). Lithium and treatment-resistant depression: a review. *Lithium* **1**, 3–8.

Scott, J. (1988). Chronic depression. *Br J Psychiatry* **153**, 287–297.

Seth, R., Jennings, A.L., Bindman, J., Phillips, J. and Bergmann, K. (1992). Combination treatment with noradrenalin and serotonin reuptake inhibitors in resistant depression. *Br J Psychiatry* **161**, 562–565.

Seymour, J. and Wattis, J.P. (1992). Treatment resistant depression in the elderly: three cases. *Int Clin Psychopharmacol*, **7**, 55–57.

Shaw, D.M. (1977). The practical management of affective disorders. *Br J Psychiatry* **130**, 432–451.

Simpson, S.W., Jackson, A., Baldwin, R.C. and Burns, A. (1997). Subcortical hyperintensities in late-life depression: acute response to treatment and neuropsychological impairment. *Int Psychogeriatrics* **9**, 257–275.

Simpson, S., Baldwin, R.C., Jackson, A. and Burns, A. (1998). Neurological, neuropsychological and neuroradiological correlates of treatment response in depression in late life. *Psychol Med* **28**, 1015–1026.

Smith, A. and Singh, S. (1995). Treatment resistant depression: causes and consequences. *Psychiatr Bull* **19**, 676–680.

Stone, K. (1989). Mania in the elderly. *Br J Psychiatry* **155**, 220–224.

Thase, M.E. and Rush, A.J. (1995). Treatment-resistant depression. In: Bloom, F.E. and Kupfer, D. (Eds), *Psychopharmacology: The Fourth Generation of Progress*. Raven Press, New York, pp. 1081–1215.

Van Marwijk, D.W.J., Bekker, F.M., Nolen, W.A., Jansen, P.A.F., van Nieuwkerk, J.F. and Hop, W.C.J. (1990). Lithium augmentation in geriatric depression. *J Affect Disord* **20**, 217–223.

Wells, K.B., Stewart, A., Hays, R.D. *et al.* (1989). The functioning and well-being of depressed patients: results from the Medical Outcomes Study. *JAMA* **262**, 914–919.

Zimmer, B., Rosen, J., Thornton, J.E., Peral, J.M. and Reynolds, C.F. (1988). Adjunctive low dose lithium carbonate in treatment resistant depression: a placebo-controlled study. *J Clin Psychopharmacol* **8**, 120–124.

Zusky, P.M., Biederman, J., Rosenbaum, J.F. *et al.* (1988). Adjunct low dose lithium carbonate in treatment-resistant depression: a placebo-controlled study. *J Clin Psychopharmacol* **8**, 120–124.

Everything You Need to Know About Old Age Psychiatry . . .
Edited by Robert Howard
©1999 Wrightson Biomedical Publishing Ltd

15

Advances in Electroconvulsive Therapy in the Elderly

MICHAEL PHILPOT

Old Age Psychiatry Directorate, Maudsley Hospital, London, UK

The use of electroconvulsive therapy (ECT) in psychiatry has had a chequered history. Its credibility in the early years was damaged by its indiscriminate use in a wide range of psychiatric disorders. During the last 20 years the indications for its use have narrowed such that most patients receiving the treatment nowadays suffer from severe depressive disorder. In addition, the majority of patients given ECT are middle-aged or elderly, a feature which is probably associated with the relative age of onset of depression with psychotic features or melancholia. What follows is a review of some of the areas of recent research interest selected from the literature pertaining to the treatment of depression in older people. For a general introduction to ECT the reader should consult The ECT Handbook (Royal College of Psychiatrists, 1995).

IMMEDIATE OUTCOME AND EFFECTIVENESS

Mulsant *et al.* (1991) reviewed a group of studies carried out in depressed elderly patients until 1989 (Table 1). The response rate was quite varied and was not consistently related to type of treatment, the age of the patient or other clinical factors. However, these studies were case series, mostly retrospective and not to be confused with randomized controlled trials. Inclusion criteria varied: some only included patients resistant to medication, others included patients receiving ECT as a first-line treatment and most included a small number of patients with dementia and depression. Unquestionably, these studies were written up by advocates of the treatment who emphasize the benefits. But, like the pessimist who says the bottle is half empty, one

Table 1.   ECT for depression in older people: immediate outcome in studies pre-1990
(after Mulsant *et al.*, 1991).

Authors	Year of publication	n	Mean age/range	Outcome (%)		
				Good	Fair	Poor
Fraser and Glass	1980	29*	73	100		0
Gaspar and Samarasinghe	1982	33*	74	79	9	12
Meikle *et al.*	1984	24*	60–80	75	25	0
Karlinsky and Shulman	1984	73	73	42	36	21
Burke *et al.*	1985	30	72	60	23	17
Kramer	1987	50	74	92		8
Benbow	1987	122*	55–89	52	28	20
Godber *et al.*	1987	163*	65+	51	23	21
Magni *et al.*	1988	30	73	63		37
Coffey *et al.*	1988	44*	60–86	54	44	2
Figiel *et al.*	1989	51*	60+	82		18

*Sample includes patients with dementia and depression.

could highlight the proportion of patients who do not do so well, up to 37%
in one study.

Since 1989, a number of other studies have examined immediate outcome
in older depressed patients (Table 2). The samples here are a little different
in that they exclude patients with dementia but do include younger patients.
However, the outcome is as varied as before. Wilkinson *et al.* (1993) found
a significant correlation between the fall in depression scores and age: greater
improvement was found in older patients. The study by Prudic *et al.* (1996)
introduces another area of recent interest: whether the rigorousness of
antidepressant treatments given prior to ECT has a bearing on the outcome.
Patients were subdivided into two groups on the basis of a quantitative
assessment of their pre-ECT drug treatment: 65% were deemed to have been
medication-resistant and the remaining 35% to have received inadequate
medication for a variety of reasons. The inadequate group were significantly
older than the resistant group, as might be expected. A good response to
ECT was found in only 64% of the resistant group but in 94% of the inadequate group. ECT response was worse in those who had been resistant to
tricyclic antidepressants whereas serotonergic and other antidepressant
classes had no predictive effects on response rate. The authors felt that this
had particular implications for the drugs which might best be used as continuation treatments and this point will be dealt with later. Lastly, it was alarm-
ing to see that, in this well conducted study, improvement in some patients
was transient. The number of treatments was titrated against mood state, as
is usual, and each group received a mean of approximately nine treatments,
but even then 21% of the immediate responders had become depressed again

Table 2. ECT for depression in older people: immediate outcome in studies post-1990.

Authors	Year of publication	n	Mean age/range	Outcome (%)		
				Good	Fair	Poor
Fraser and Glass	1980	29*	73	100		0
Mulsant et al.	1991	42	74	55	14	26
Wilkinson et al.	1993	43	65–88	73		27
Sackeim et al.	1993	96	56	70		30
Philibert et al.	1995	108	72	40	55	5
Prudic et al.	1996	100	62	73		23
Lauritzen et al.	1996	87	65	95		5
Folkerts et al.	1997	21	50	71		29
Flint and Rifat	1998a	15	74	88		12

*Sample includes patients with dementia and depression.

after one week. Slipping back was more likely in the medication-resistant group.

Folkerts et al. (1997) compared outcome in depressed patients randomly allocated to acute treatment with either six sessions of ECT followed by two weeks of paroxetine or four weeks of paroxetine alone. The mean dose was relatively high at 44 mg/day. Of the ECT group 71% responded compared with 28% of the paroxetine group. Again, those resistant to medication prior to ECT did worse. Lastly, O'Leary et al. (1994) described the effects of ECT in the elderly participants of the Nottingham trial. There was a better immediate response to real ECT but real and simulated ECT groups were rated as having similar mood at one, three and six months after treatment. This finding should remind us that while ECT may be useful for 'jump-starting' recovery in treatment-resistant patients and thereby providing short-term gains, the advantages over medication are short-lived.

RELAPSE/RECURRENCE RATE

One problem with ECT in the treatment of depression (or perhaps it is a problem with the patients to whom ECT is given) is the relatively high relapse rate. Table 3 shows studies which report either recurrence or readmission rates in older people, usually without a comparison group. Even so, from our knowledge of the classic outcome studies (see Baldwin, 1997, for review), these recurrence rates do seem rather high. The general trend is that most patients who will relapse do so during the first six months; the rate flattens out after about a year. Frederiksen et al. (1993) compared data from the 1940s with 1974–83 data to determine historical trends before and after the introduction of effective continuation treatments such as antidepressants and

Table 3. ECT for depression in older people: relapse rate.

Authors	Year of publication	Relapse/recurrence rate (%)			
		Six months	One year	Two years	Three years
Godber *et al.*	1987	28			67
Benbow	1987	26*			
Sackeim *et al.*	1993	50	60		
Frederiksen *et al.*	1993	45			70
Lauritzen *et al.*	1996	65			
Wesson *et al.*	1997			——58——	
Flint and Rifat	1998(b)	53			

*Readmission rate.

lithium. The six-month relapse rate was 14% in the 1940s but rose to 45% in the later period. Similarly, three-year recurrence rate increased from 41% to 70%. Women under the age of 50 had the worst prognosis while older men, over 50 years, had the best. Explanations provided by the authors include the possibility that ECT was reserved for the more treatment-resistant patients during the later period, *or* that the use of anticonvulsant anaesthetics, which were not available in the 1940s, actually reduced the antidepressant properties of ECT.

PREVENTION OF RELAPSE/RECURRENCE OF DEPRESSION

What can be done to reduce the high tendency to relapse? Continuation or maintenance ECT is an option and although compliance can be a problem this may be the only effective alternative in some patients. More usually, however, patients are maintained on antidepressants. Are some medications more suitable for this purpose than others?

A Danish study from Lauritzen *et al.* (1996) compared recurrence rates in patients treated with ECT and given either imipramine or paroxetine in the acute and continuation phase. Patients were allocated to one of two groups depending on their cardiac status. Group A – with cardiovascular abnormalities – were then randomly allocated to paroxetine or placebo. The healthier group B were randomly allocated to receive either paroxetine or imipramine. As would be expected, group A were older than group B. Those receiving imipramine during ECT did better in the acute phase but those receiving paroxetine fared better during the six-month follow-up period. However, the difference in relapse rate between the paroxetine group and the placebo group became nonsignificant by the six-month point. The additional implication was that older patients did worse than the younger patients when paroxetine was used as the continuation therapy. The authors suggest that serotonergic antidepressants are better at controlling the early signs of depressive relapse – symptoms such as lack of interest, impaired concentration, depressed mood, and anxiety.

There is some evidence that lithium may be more effective than antidepressants as continuation therapy following ECT (Shapira *et al.*, 1995) but no studies have yet been carried out in older patients. As yet there have been no trials of the newer antidepressants such as venlafaxine or nefazodone.

COGNITIVE EFFECTS OF ECT

Some patients complain bitterly about these problems and it is essential that we prepare them in an honest way. However, the literature on cognitive effects in the elderly is rather confusing and inconsistent. In the studies reviewed by Mulsant *et al.* (1991) between 10 and 30% of elderly patients developed severe disorientation and transient cognitive impairment, particularly with bilateral ECT. On the other hand, Fraser and Glass (1980) found patients improved on tests of memory and attention after ECT. Russ *et al.* (1990) found no differences in objective cognitive performance before and after treatment. However, both these studies reassessed patients at two to three weeks after the last treatment and probably failed to pick up the immediate cognitive problems. Rosen *et al.* (1992) tracked cognitive performance during treatment in a small group of elderly patients. Even though unilateral ECT was being used there was a progressive fall in Mini-Mental State Examination (MMSE) score and a modified version of the Digit Symbol Substitution test which assessed cognitive processing time. The extent of the fall was affected by the number of treatments and the cumulative seizure duration.

The study by Sackeim *et al.* (1993) examined the cognitive effects of ECT in great detail before and after treatment. The following impairments were significantly more common in those receiving bilateral ECT: immediate effects (after 90 minutes) included an increased rate of prolonged disorientation and greater impairment of word recall; short-term effects (in the week following ECT) included reduced performance on MMSE, and greater impairment of new learning for words and memory of personal events. However, subjective ratings of memory performance increased in all patients. Two months later, performance on most tests was unchanged in comparison to that before treatment, but performance on the MMSE, word and face learning and subjective memory had all improved significantly.

A number of strategies have been identified which help reduce the likelihood of post-ECT cognitive impairment. These measures are not specific to the treatment of older patients but may have more impact in them. Reports of severe and long-standing memory impairment largely date from the days before the use of machines which generated brief pulse stimuli. Twice-weekly administration is associated with less severe cognitive effects than thrice-weekly administration (Shapira *et al.*, 1998) and there is now plenty of evidence that unilateral ECT is associated with fewer cognitive effects (see Sackeim *et al.*, (1993) for review). Choosing the lowest optimal dose of electrical charge for each patient requires the use of a stimulus-dosing method to determine the seizure threshold. This in turn requires an ECT machine capable of delivering a wide range of electrical charge. The recent audit on behalf of the Royal College of Psychiatrists (Duffett and Lelliott, 1998) found that 41% of the machines in use in the UK were unable to do this and were no longer recommended. Effective oxygenation before and after treatment can reduce immediate confusion. Propofol, which is usually contraindicated in ECT because it raises the seizure threshold and shortens seizure duration, may actually have a role in patients prone to post-ictal confusion. The almost instant recovery from the anaesthetic can outweigh the other problems with its use if care is taken. Lastly, T_3 is thought to have a neuroprotective effect and has been shown to prevent the impairment in remote personal memory (Stern *et al.*, 1993).

ELECTROENCEPHALOGRAPHIC PREDICTORS OF CLINICAL RESPONSE

ECT machines which concurrently monitor the electroencephalographic status (EEG) are becoming increasingly fashionable. Some ECT/EEG machines automatically calculate a number of performance variables, but what is their significance? What measures have been shown to relate to effective treatment or 'quality' seizures? There is now general agreement that seizure duration is a poor indicator of therapeutic benefit even though seizures lasting less than 20 seconds are thought to be of little therapeutic value. Nobler *et al.* (1993) found that effective forms of ECT were associated with a shorter polyspike phase and a longer slow-wave phase. In contrast, Krystal *et al.* (1995) found that such forms of ECT were associated with a shorter time to slow-wave onset, greater interhemispheric coherence and greater spectral amplitude. Both studies found a positive relationship between effective ECT and post-ictal suppression, i.e. the degree to which the EEG becomes 'silent' after the seizure has terminated. Suppes *et al.* (1996) found this same measure correlated with the fall in depression score. Folkerts (1996) found that rapid clinical response was associated with a higher maximum frequency of complexes and greater frequency slowing during the spike and wave phase.

With the exception of post-ictal suppression none of these measures is automatically generated by the new machines and, in addition, there is little consistency about which measures are of importance. We need further studies in older patients to determine whether these measures have any real clinical significance. Recently, software packages which assist storage and analysis of EEG output have become available. It is hoped that these will act as a catalyst for further research in this area which, up to now, has necessitated laborious and time-consuming measurement of the printed output.

NATIONAL VARIATION IN THE USE OF ECT

It goes without saying that ECT is still a controversial treatment and some sections of the public continue to express concern. Enthusiasm for ECT varies considerably among psychiatrists themselves and surveys carried out by John Pippard in the UK showed a wide variation of use. For example, there was a 10-fold difference in ECT use between City and Hackney district and East Suffolk (Pippard, 1992). Old age psychiatrists are more generally in favour of ECT and Susan Benbow's survey in the late 1980s (Benbow, 1991) revealed that 98% would consider using ECT for appropriate patients.

There are even more extreme geographical and clinical variations in the use of ECT in the USA. A recent study by Olfson et al. (1998), limited to the use of ECT in recurrent depression, showed that ECT was more likely to be used in older, white patients, those with private insurance and those living in more affluent areas. Although ECT patients tended to have longer admissions, those who were given ECT within five days of admission spent a much shorter time in hospital and had less costly inpatient care. Similar effects of the early use of ECT on admission length were found by Ball et al. (1995), examining elderly patients at Guy's Hospital, London. The introduction of managed care protocols in the USA has complicated the prescription of ECT. Some protocols restrict access to the treatment, while others insist that ECT be considered very soon after admission, to save costs. Should we in the UK follow this path or retain clinical freedom based on individual cases?

The author's team recently carried out a survey among members of the European Association of Geriatric Psychiatrists (EAGP) with the intention of finding out what barriers prevented easy access to ECT at the national and regional level in Europe (Philpot et al., 1999). A postal questionnaire was sent to selected members of the EAGP in all 28 countries within the wider Europe; members from 23 countries responded. ECT was widely available in only 13 out of 23 countries.

The main restrictions could be grouped as follows: lack of resources; excessive legal requirements generated by public and political concern; and in some countries ECT was restricted to academic centres. Although it was clear from the responses that there was a consensus among old age psychiatrists within each country that ECT was indicated for severe depressive illness, many reserved this treatment for life-threatening conditions. Only Slovenia has specifically outlawed the use of ECT in the elderly but concern about its use in older people was expressed by respondents from Belgium, France, Italy, The Netherlands, Portugal and Spain.

CONCLUSIONS

ECT can still be regarded as an effective treatment for medication-resistant depressed patients. Some studies suggest that older patients may respond better than younger patients. 'Real' ECT has a temporary advantage over simulated ECT (O'Leary et al., 1994) and medication (Folkerts et al., 1997). Some medications may have advantages over others when given as continuation therapy. In any event there is little sense in keeping the patient on the same class of antidepressant to which they were resistant prior to the ECT course. Cognitive impairment following ECT is a problem for some patients and must be acknowledged. However, longer-term studies suggest that the impairment to retrograde and personal memory are temporary. So far, the only EEG variable which consistently seems to be associated with good outcome is the degree of post-ictal suppression induced in brain activity following the seizure. More research is needed in this area, particularly with reference to older patients.

Lastly, there are major national and regional variations in the use of ECT caused as much by the treatment preferences of individual psychiatrists prescribing ECT as by local legal and resource issues. All of which begs the question of what happens to patients not given ECT? Do they suffer unnecessarily or are other treatment approaches successful? It may be significant that some areas such as Germany, Spain, Israel, and parts of the USA where ECT is difficult to use, are in the forefront of research into rapid transcranial magnetic stimulation which has been heralded as becoming the replacement for ECT in the new millenium (Kirkaldie et al., 1997).

REFERENCES

Baldwin, R. (1997). The prognosis of depression in later life. In: Holmes, C. and Howard, R. (Eds), *Advanes in Old Age Psychiatry: Chromosomes to Community Care*. Wrightson Biomedical Publishing, Petersfield, pp. 194–224.

Ball, C.J., Fashola, Y. and Herzberg, J.L. (1995). Length of stay and the timing of ECT. *Int J Geriatr Psychiatry* **10**, 783–786.

Benbow, S.M. (1987). The use of electroconvulsive therapy in old age psychiatry. *Int J Geriatr Psychiatry* **2**, 25–30.

Benbow, S.M. (1991). Old age psychiatrists' views on the use of ECT. *Int J Geriatr Psychiatry* **6**, 317–322.

Burke, W.J., Rutherford, J.L., Zorumski, C.F. and Reich, T. (1985). Electroconvulsive therapy and the elderly. *Comp Psychiatry* **26**, 480–486.

Coffey, C.E., Figiel, G.S., Djang, W.T. *et al.* (1988). Leukoencephalopathy in elderly depressed patients referred for ECT. *Biol Psychiatry* **24**, 143–161.

Duffett, R. and Lelliott, P. (1998). Auditing electroconvulsive therapy. The third cycle. *Br J Psychiatry* **172**, 401–405.

Figiel, G.S., Coffey, C.E. and Weiner, R.D. (1989). Brain magnetic resonance imaging in elderly depressed patients receiving electroconvulsive therapy. *Convuls Ther* **5**, 321–329.

Flint, A.J. and Rifat, S.L. (1998a). The treatment of psychotic depression in later life: a comparison of pharmacotherapy and ECT. *Int J Geriatr Psychiatry* **13**, 23–28.

Flint, A.J. and Rifat, S.L. (1998b). Two-year outcome of psychotic depression in late life. *Am J Psychiatry* **155**, 178–183.

Folkerts, H. (1996). The ictal electroencephalogram as a marker for the efficacy of electroconvulsive therapy. *Eur Arch Psychiatry Clin Neurosc* **246**, 155–164.

Folkerts, H.W., Tolle, M.N., Schonauer, K., Mucke, S. and Schulze-Monking, H. (1997). Electroconvulsive therapy vs. paroxetine in treatment-resistant depression – a randomized study. *Acta Psychiatr Scand* **96**, 334–342.

Fraser, R.M. and Glass, I.B. (1980). Recovery from ECT in elderly patients. *Br J Psychiatry* **133**, 524–528.

Frederiksen, S.O., D'Elia, G., Thorell, L.-H. and Nilsson, M. (1993). Recurrence of depressive episodes after electroconvulsive therapy. *Nord J Psychiatry* **47**, 361–368.

Gaspar, D. and Samarasinghe, L.A. (1982). ECT in psychogeriatric practice – A study of risk factors, indications and outcome. *Comp Psychiatry,* **23**, 170–175.

Godber, C., Rosenvinge, H., Wilkinson, D. and Smithies, J. (1987). Depression in old age: prognosis after ECT. *Int J Geriatr Psychiatry* **2**, 19–24.

Karlinsky, H. and Shulman, K. (1984). The clinical use of electroconvulsive therapy in old age. *J Am Geriatr Soc* **32**, 183–187.

Kirkaldie, M.T., Pridmore, S.A. and Pascual-Leone, A. (1997). Transcranial magnetic stimulation as therapy for depression and other disorders. *Austr N Z J Psychiatry* **31**, 264–272.

Kramer, B.A. (1987). Electroconvulsive therapy use in geriatric depression. *J Nerv Ment Dis* **175**, 233–235.

Krystal, A.D., Weiner, R.D. and Coffey, C.E. (1995). The ictal EEG as a marker of adequate stimulus intensity with unilateral ECT. *J Neuropsychiatry Clin Neurosc* **7**, 295–303.

Lauritzen, L., Odgaard, K., Clemmesen, L. *et al.* (1996). Relapse prevention by means of paroxetine in ECT-treated patients with major depression: a comparison with imipramine and placebo in medium-term continuation therapy. *Acta Psychiatr Scand* **94**, 241–251.

Magni, G., Fisman, M. and Holmes, E. (1988). Clinical correlates of ECT resistant depression in the elderly. *J Clin Psychiatry* **49**, 405–407.

Meikle, D.H., Winstead, D.K., Goether, J.W. and Schwartz, B.D. (1984). Multiple-monitored electroconvulsive therapy: safety and efficacy in elderly depressed patients. *J Am Geriatr Soc* **32**, 180–182.

Mulsant, B.H., Rosen, J., Thornton, J.E. and Zubenko, G.S. (1991). A prospective naturalistic study of electroconvulsive therapy in late-life depression. *J Geriatr Psychiatry Neurol* **4**, 3–13.

Nobler, M.S., Sackeim, H.A., Solomou, M., Luber, B., Devanand, D.P. and Prudic, J. (1993). EEG manifestations during ECT: effects of electrode placement and stimulus intensity. *Biol Psychiatry* **34**, 321–330.

O'Leary, D., Gill, D., Gregory, S. and Shawcross, C. (1994). The effectiveness of real versus simulated electroconvulsive therapy in depressed elderly patients. *Int J Geriatr Psychiatry* **9**, 567–571.

Olfson, M., Marcus, S., Sackeim, H.A., Thompson, J. and Pincus, H.A. (1998). Use of ECT for the inpatient treatment of recurrent major depression. *Am J Psychiatry* **155**, 22–29.

Philibert, R.A., Richards, L., Lynch, C.F. and Winokur, G. (1995). Effects of ECT on mortality and clinical outcome in geriatric unipolar depression. *J Clin Psychiatry* **56**, 390–394.

Philpot, M., Treloar, A., Gormley, N. and Gustafson, L. (1999). Barriers to the use of ECT in Europe, (in preparation).

Pippard, J. (1992). Audit of electroconvulsive therapy in two National Health Service regions. *Br J Psychiatry* **160**, 621–637.

Prudic, J., Haskett, R.F., Mulsant, B. *et al.* (1996). Resistance to antidepressant medications and short-term clinical response to ECT. *Am J Psychiatry* **153**, 985–992

Rosen, J., Mulsant, B. and Nebes, R.D. (1992). A pilot study of interictal cognitive changes in elderly patients during ECT. *Int J Geriatr Psychiatry* **7**, 407–410.

Royal College of Psychiatrists (1995). *The ECT Handbook*. Council Report CR39. Royal College of Psychiatrists, London.

Russ, M.J., Ackerman, S.H., Burton, L. and Shindledecker, R.D. (1990). Cognitive effects of ECT in the elderly: preliminary findings. *Int J Geriatr Psychiatry* **5**, 115–118.

Sackeim, H.A., Prudic, J., Devanand, D.P. *et al.* (1993). Effects of stimulus intensity and electrode placement on the efficacy and cognitive effects of electroconvulsive therapy. *N Engl J Med* **328**, 839–846.

Shapira, B., Gorfine, M.A. and Lerer, B. (1995). A prospective study of lithium continuation therapy in depressed patients who have responded to electroconvulsive therapy. *Convuls Ther* **11**, 80–85.

Shapira, B., Tubi, N., Drexler, H., Lidsky, D., Calev, A. and Lerer, B. (1998). Cost and benefit in the choice of ECT schedule. Twice versus three times weekly ECT. *Br J Psychiatry* **172**, 44–48.

Stern, R.A., Steketee, M.C., Durr, A.L., Prange, A.J. and Golden R.N. (1993). Combined use of thyroid hormone and ECT. *Convuls Ther* **9**, 285–292.

Suppes, T., Webb, A., Carmody T. *et al.* (1996). Is postictal electrical silence a predictor of response to electroconvulsive therapy? *J Affect Disord* **41**, 55–58.

Wesson, M.L., Wilkinson, A.M., Anderson, D.N. and McCracken, C. (1997). Does age predict the long-term outcome of depression treated with ECT? (A prospective study of the long-term outcome of ECT-treated depression with respect to age.) *Int J Geriatr Psychiatry* **12**, 45–51.

Wilkinson, A.M., Anderson, D.N. and Peters, S. (1993). Age and the effects of ECT. *Int J Geriatr Psychiatry* **8**, 401–406.

Everything You Need to Know About Old Age Psychiatry . . .
Edited by Robert Howard
©1999 Wrightson Biomedical Publishing Ltd

16

The Anxiety–Stress Model and its Implications for the Rational Treatment of Anxiety and Panic in Old Age

CHRISTOPHER G. KRASUCKI

Section of Old Age Psychiatry, Institute of Psychiatry, London, UK

THE THERAPEUTIC PARADOX OF ANXIETY – THE 'INVISIBLE MAN' OF PSYCHIATRY

It has been demonstrated in population (Krasucki *et al.*, 1998) and primary care (Oxman *et al.*, 1987) studies that the prevalence of anxiety disorders diminishes with increasing age. Indeed, conditions such as panic disorder and obsessive-compulsive disorder are very rare above the age of 65. Therefore anxiety, particularly in its more severe and debilitating forms, would not seem to pose a major therapeutic problem in the elderly. However, matters are complicated by the fact that as psychiatrists we attempt to assign patients to diagnostic categories, order these categories according to an arbitrary consensus hierarchy of importance, and apply the diagnosis that has the highest ranking within the hierarchy (WHO, 1992; APA, 1994). Anxiety has always been the lowest category in the hierarchy, and so is not diagnosed as a disorder in its own right unless organic brain syndromes, psychoses and clinically significant depression are absent. Although anxiety runs as a common thread through every psychiatric disorder, such a hierarchical approach effectively renders it diagnostically invisible. This problem is compounded by increasing age, as physical health problems and cognitive impairment make it even more difficult to regard anxiety as a primary disorder. After all, if the anxiety is 'understandable' in the light of the increasing physical frailty or diminishing mental faculties of an individual, is it really a pathological phenomenon? It is here that the paradox lies, for anxiety, which as a mental state is almost by definition unpleasant and unwanted, is extremely common in patients with organic brain syndrome, psychotic states, depression, and somatic illness, but is unlikely to be recognized and treated in its own right. One way of circumventing this problem is to adopt a dimensional approach to the diagnosis and classification of mental disorder in the elderly (Krasucki et al., 1998). Another way is to create a model for the way that anxiety influences and is influenced by other psychic and somatic disorders, and thus appreciate its central role in the illness process. Such a model has the potential for generating predictions and testable hypotheses about how anxiety controls and is controlled by other illness variables. It may also allow us to understand, classify and refine existing anxiety treatments, and perhaps develop novel others in a rational way.

PSYCHOLOGICAL HOMEOSTASIS, THE ANXIETY–STRESS MODEL, AND ANXIETY IN THE ELDERLY

Theoretical background

It is a fundamental characteristic of living organisms that perturbations in their internal environment initiate compensatory physiological processes with the aim of returning the organism to its original state of physiological equilibrium. If the cause of such a perturbation is described as a 'stressor', then 'stress' can be defined as anything that causes an alteration of physiological homeostatic processes, in other words, a 'stress response' (Selye, 1956; Burchfield, 1979). The powerful concept of homeostasis can be conceptually extended beyond that of simple physiological stressors eliciting a physiological stress response. Indeed, in human beings, many if not most physiological stressors are likely to be dealt with by automatic and subconscious homeostatic mechanisms and will either not be noticed or, if noticed, not subjectively regarded as 'stressful'. However, if one restricts the definition of a stressor to an event or state that influences psychological homeostasis (Engel, 1953), then the homeostatic response will consist of a subjective psychological component ('stress') and, usually, a physiological component also (Schachter and Singer, 1962). These two components together have been characterized as the 'fight-flight' response. The subjective experience of 'stress' is phenomenologically indistinguishable from 'fear' (when the stressor is well defined and recent) and 'anxiety' (when the stressor is poorly defined or multiple, and temporally more remote). From the physiological point of view 'stress' involves an activation of the sympathetic nervous system and hypothalamo-pituitary-adrenal axis, the former resulting in immediate psychological and physiological arousal, and the latter in metabolic changes which begin immediately but whose maximal effects are delayed and prolonged beyond the duration of the stressor. Thus initial 'fright' prepares the individual for 'fight' or 'flight'. Severe 'fright' can also precipitate a 'freeze' response, particularly in the elderly (Jarvik and Russell, 1979). When, or if, the psychological challenge is neutralized, psychological homeostasis is restored, and the 'fright-fight-flight-freeze' or 'stress' response is switched off.

The anxiety–stress model of anxiety in action

When an individual is in psychological equilibrium, he or she is, psychologically speaking, where he or she needs or wants to be (Figure 1). The effect of a stressor is to create a discrepancy between where an individual is, and where they need or want to be. This creates psychological disequilibrium and initiates the psychological homeostatic mechanism (Figure 2). The degree of

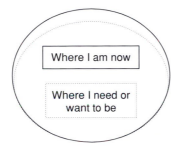

Figure 1. Psychological equilibrium.

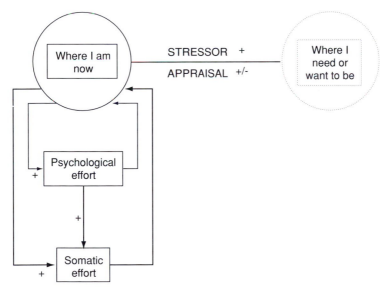

Figure 2. Psychological disequilibrium: the stress or fight-flight response.

psychological disequilibrium is likely to depend on the magnitude of the stressor, whether it is single or multiple, and how rapidly it is presented. Previous experience, with the same or similar stressors, and perceived coping resources, in other words appraisal of the potential stressor, will also modify the raw effects of the stressor. Modest degrees of disequilibrium will generate only modest amounts of psychological and physiological arousal and be perceived as 'challenge'. Greater disequilibrium will activate the fright-fight-flight-freeze response. This will be associated with the subjective experience of anxiety and the perception of 'threat'. The state of psychological disequilibrium and associated fright-fight-flight-freeze response will continue until

Table 1.   Stressors and desired states in the elderly.

Stressor	Desired state
Physical disability	Ability to carry out basic activities of daily living
Dependent state, e.g. heavy reliance on spouse or family, hospitalization, unwanted institutionalization	Independent adult existence
Isolated existence	No loneliness, adequate companionship, social support network
Cold or damp accommodation, difficult access (e.g. high location with no lifts), noise from neighbours or road traffic	Comfortable external (to body) environment
Chronic and poorly controlled sensations arising from the body, e.g. pain, nausea	Comfortable internal (to body) environment
High local levels of mugging, assault, burglary and fraud	Safety of self and belongings
Disputes and disagreements, e.g. about how often the family visits, the amount of help the family gives, finances, whether the elderly person lives with family or not, the status and authority of the elderly person	Good relations with spouse, family, friends and neighbours
No income additional to state pension, no one to offer financial support in a crisis	Financial security
Age-associated cognitive decline, dementia	Sufficient cognitive resources to deal with own problems
Inability to carry on with previously enjoyed activities, inability to find new ones to replace them	Meaningful occupation throughout the day
Insomnia, poor-quality sleep	Adequate restful sleep

and unless the process of psychological homeostasis, and the psychological and somatic effort that it entails, restores the individual to the resting state (Figure 1).

Stressors and desired states in relation to the anxiety–stress model

The conceptual framework of where an individual is, in contrast to where he or she needs or wants to be, can be used to classify the common stressors and corresponding desired states in the elderly (Table 1).

Translating the fright-fight-flight-freeze stress phenomenon into the wider phenomenology of acute anxiety

The fright-fight-flight-freeze stress response can be divided into psychological and physiological components (Figure 3). The psychological component can take the form of fright-flight, or fright-fight, or more usually a combination of these. The phenomenology of fright-flight is dominated by the subjective experience of anxiety, heightening of the senses, and mental arousal. The behaviours that are familiarly associated are escape from the stressor, and avoidance of it and similar situations. Very severe 'fright', which would otherwise result in 'flight' behaviour, may physically and psychologically immobilize an individual, causing 'freeze'. Seeking reassurance or nurturance is also recognized as an anxiety behaviour in children (WHO, 1992) and there is no reason why it should not also occur in adults at times of stress. Irritability and anger comprise the core phenomenology of fright-fight, and the associated behaviours encompass varying degrees of verbal and physical assault. The physiological component of the combined fight-flight response involves increased activity of the sympathetic nervous system on various end-organs, producing the so-called autonomic symptoms of anxiety, and increased motor activity leading to bodily tension and restlessness.

Patterns of stress response and their consequences

Time-limited stressor successfully overcome

If the stressor or stressors an individual is exposed to are overcome or dissipate spontaneously, the stress response should gradually subside and psychological equilibrium will be restored. The time required for this process may be prolonged in the elderly (Stokes *et al.*, 1996). The lesson learned by the individual is likely to be along the lines of 'I can do it.' The episode will be seen as a 'victory' over the stressor. Self-confidence and self-esteem will be boosted, and the individual may see himself or herself as self-sufficient rather

Psychological	
Fright-Flight	**Fright-Fight**
Mental phenomena	**Mental phenomena**
Preoccupation Concern Worry Anxiety Fear Arousal Sensory heightening Hypervigilance Insomnia	Irritability Easy loss of temper Hostility Anger Rage
Behaviours	**Behaviours**
Escape Avoidance Seeking nurturance or reassurance Freeze (inability to act)	Loud and/or rapid speech Swearing Shouting Physical assault
Physiological	
Autonomic	**Motor**
Heart – increased stroke volume and heart rate ('palpitations') Lungs – increased rate and depth of ventilation ('hyperventilation') Gut – increase in certain aspects of activity ('dyspepsia', 'irritable bowel') Bladder – lower threshold for emptying ('urgency', 'frequency') Skin – sweating, flushing	Muscle tension Inability to relax Tremor Fidgeting Restlessness Pacing

Figure 3. The acute anxiety phenomenology of the fright-fight-flight-freeze response.

than helpless. There are likely to be optimistic and hopeful views about the future. Appraisal of the same or similar stressor or stressors will tend to classify them as 'challenge' rather than 'threat', perhaps leading to a more limited stress response if they occur again.

Prolonged stressor, chronic stress and chronic anxiety

If the stressor is particularly severe, or prolonged, or there are multiple stressors, the fright-fight-flight-freeze stress response may continue to be active.

This may lead to perpetuation of what would normally be an acute, circum-scribed anxiety state. There is likely to be a chronic level of anxiety and irritability, with accompanying somatic phenomena.

The anxiety may, with or without provocation, reach a peak, resulting in intense fear, intense physiological arousal, and a powerful 'flight' drive to escape. This has been labelled panic disorder (WHO, 1992) and is best regarded as an acute exacerbation of an underlying chronic anxiety state (Tyrer, 1986). Full panic disorder is rare in the elderly (Krasucki et al., 1998). One possible reason for this is that the diagnosis relies heavily on the presence of multiple somatic symptoms of anxiety which tend to occur relatively infrequently in later life (Lindesay, 1991). Limited symptom attacks (APA, 1987) may therefore be a more accurate diagnostic representation of the panic phenomenon in the elderly. Another possible reason for the rarity of panic disorder in the elderly could be that increasing age makes it more likely that, in the face of overwhelming anxiety, the escape component will be supplanted by the 'freeze' response (Jarvik and Russell, 1979).

In a similar way, the irritability may, with or without provocation, reach a peak, resulting in intense anger or rage with an associated drive to attack, verbally or physically. The literature on anger and assault in cognitively intact elderly individuals appears to be very sparse. In this case, however, potential diagnostic labels tend to come under the rubric of personality disor-der. Elderly patients are therefore liable to be excluded because of the requirements for a presumed inborn rather than acquired origin and onset early in life.

When a stressor first occurs, the 'fright' component is directed precisely at it and is described as 'fear'. Perhaps over time the continued stress response modifies the cognitive element of the 'fright', such that the threshold for appraisal of other difficulties as stressors is lowered and there is consequently a 'generalization by association' of the originally circumscribed fear. This would be (free-floating) 'anxiety' and the condition generalized anxiety disorder (WHO, 1992). Anxious thoughts are characteristically unpleasant, unwelcome and repetitive. They can be consciously suppressed or minimized by distraction but tend to recur. If the generalization process that broadens 'fear' into 'anxiety' further generalizes and associates anxious thoughts with mental phenomena that could not be construed as stressors or potential stres-sors in their own right, then the distressing ideas, images and impulses of obsessional neurosis might result. Diagnostically this would be obsessive-compulsive disorder with predominant obsessional thoughts or ruminations (WHO, 1992).

The 'escape' aspect of 'flight' and the 'attack' aspect of 'fight' have been described above. However, 'flight' has two other behavioural components: 'avoidance' and 'nurture-seeking'. To avoid a feared stressor is a natural sequel to escaping it, and perhaps initially that avoidance is precisely targeted at the stressor. However, continuation of the stress response could, as with the cognitive elements, generalize to other situations resulting finally in widespread avoidance. Alternatively, or additionally, the instinct to 'hide' and retreat to a safe environment could be regarded as an integral behavioural component of fear and anxiety. In that case, one might expect that the more severe the anxiety, the more severe and widespread the avoidance, and this is what is found in the severe anxiety of panic disorder. The diagnostic category used for this phenomenon of avoidance in the face of 'fright' is agoraphobia (WHO, 1992). This is the phobia most frequently encountered in the elderly, and tends to start relatively late in life. The classical agoraphobic situations (crowds, public places, travelling away from home) can be seen as environments in which any individual might reasonably perceive their vulnerability to 'attack' as being greatest. Some include being at home alone, and being in a confined space, as agoraphobic fears (Lindesay et al., 1989). These additional fears are understandable in the 'fright-flight' context as being within places where there is vulnerability to 'entrapment'. Social phobia and specific phobia (WHO, 1992) represent more circumscribed types of avoidance. Social phobia in the elderly may have been acquired as a child or young adult. If social phobia occurs for the first time in old age it could be a partial variant of full agoraphobia, as the two conditions have as a unifying principle the fear of other people. Specific phobia is frequently a lifelong condition and probably represents heritable fear, early fearful exposure to the feared stimulus, or both. Support for the limited nature and chronicity of social and specific phobia is provided by the finding that neither is associated with much avoidance or somatic symptomatology in the elderly (Lindesay, 1991). In contrast to the 'passive' avoidance of potential harm that is seen in phobic behaviour, 'active' avoidance may also occur. Here individuals may carry out actions to avert potential danger to or caused by the individual, which could, again by a process of generalization, be transformed into the cleaning and checking rituals of obsessive-compulsive disorder with predominant compulsions (WHO, 1992).

The other behavioural element of 'fright-flight' is the 'nurture-seeking' phenomenon. This is recognized in children as a response to anxiety, and also in young animals on exposure to danger. In adults, and perhaps particularly in the elderly, 'nurture-seeking' could manifest as increased reliance and dependence on spouse, family and friends, or increased contact with health services. Doctors seeing the individual over time might consequently be tempted to diagnose them under one of the somatoform disorder categories (WHO, 1992).

Post-traumatic stress disorder (WHO, 1992) encapsulates all the major elements of the stress response. Exposure to a time-limited stressor that is extremely severe and unpleasant generates a powerful acute stress response that seems to 'engrave' its details on the mind, such that subsequently it is remembered so vividly that the memory constitutes a stressor in its own right. Repeated 'triggering' of the memory leads to repeated activation of the fright-fight-flight-freeze response, and effectively establishes the event and its memory as a chronic stressor in its own right, which the individual attempts to avoid. There is thus a 'fear of fear'. Post-traumatic stress symptoms can be reactivated as much as half a century after the original trauma (Krasucki et al., 1995). Less is known about the disorder when it arises in old age but there are indications that the prevalence of the disorder does not vary with age (Helzer et al., 1987); the elderly are just as vulnerable to its onset as the young, suffer more from symptoms, and are more resistant to therapy (Drozdek, 1997).

Whether the individual finally overcomes the stressor himself or herself, or the stressor continues to operate but perhaps in diminished or modified form, the stress response may shut down. If the stress response has been very severe or very prolonged, the individual might be left thinking 'I can't do it' or 'Nothing I do makes any difference'. The episode will be seen as a 'defeat'. Self-confidence and self-esteem are likely to be diminished, and the individual may see himself or herself as worthless or useless. As in our society adult humans are expected to overcome their own problems, the failure or delay in so doing may lead to self-blame and guilt. The individual may come to see himself or herself as dependent and possibly a burden. If those on whom the individual has depended, whether lay or professional, have not been able effectively to deal with the stressor either, a feeling of helplessness ('learned helplessness') may ensue. The loss of self-confidence, and helplessless if it is present, may lead to pessimism and ultimately hopelessness about the future. Appraisal of the same or similar stressors in the future will be more likely to classify them as 'threat' rather than 'challenge'. The appraisal process might in this way be 're-tuned' such that very minor stressors, or even circumstances where there is nothing that might reasonably be regarded as a stressor, could cause psychological disequilibrium and perpetuate or re-start the stress response. The individual would have thus become 'nervous', 'sensitive' or 'neurotic'.

Positive feedback loops (vicious circles) in the anxiety–stress model

Depression is strongly correlated with anxiety at the categorical, dimensional and phenomenological levels. This results in considerable confusion in the use of the terms in clinical practice, whether as diagnoses or as symptoms. As fear and anxiety are the subjective manifestations of the activation and arousal of an individual to deal with a stressor, it would seem natural to regard them as 'positive' phenomena, in the sense that they represent increased psychological (and physiological) activity. This increased activity may possibly lead sooner or later to underfunctioning, perhaps 'exhaustion',

of the central nervous system. Such a mechanism is supported by the observation that in those elderly people with chronic anxiety, depression is mostly
due to recent intercurrent, i.e. additional, stress (Bergmann, 1971). Two out
of the three core symptoms of depressive disorder – anergia and anhedonia
– seem to be plausibly 'negative' (in the sense that they represent underfunctioning) consequences of the central nervous system 'overdrive' that
occurs in the chronic anxiety-stress response. Combined, and in mild degree,
they seem to approximate to the concept of 'boredom'. The third core
symptom – depressed mood – may be less useful since in both clinical and

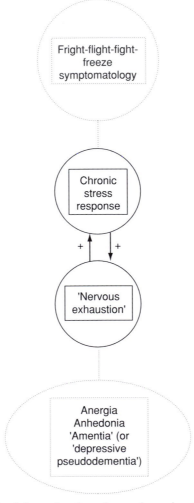

Figure 4. Positive feedback loop A: when depression arises in the context of anxiety.

lay usage it has a tendency to confound anxiety, depression and the various components of the two syndromes. The occurrence of anergia and anhedonia is liable to impair cognitive functioning in a reversible manner, causing 'depressive pseudodementia' (or 'amentia' if one wishes to describe the 'negative' syndrome anxiety as the three A's: anergia, anhedonia and amentia). It is also likely to diminish motivation, compound the social withdrawal that occurs with anxious avoidance, and limit the physical energy available for dealing with a stressor. This could effectively magnify the stressor, leading to exaggeration of the stress response and increased anxiety (positive feedback loop A; Figure 4). A vicious circle explanation of this kind could account for the ability of anxiety to generate depression and vice versa. It offers an explanation for the concept of the 'general neurotic syndrome' (Tyrer, 1987) and is supported by the observed tendency of anxiety and depression to change one into the other in elderly individuals (Larkin et al., 1992) as a 'bidirectional diagnostic interchange' (Krasucki et al., 1998). The anxiety–depression vicious circle is likely to compound the social difficulties of an individual.

The chronic stress response in general, and certain forms of anxiety in particular, have been implicated in end-organ changes. For example, phobic anxiety has been associated with fatal myocardial ischaemia (Haines et al., 1987) and panic disorder with increased likelihood of stroke and cardiovascular mortality (Flint et al., 1996). If the stress response and anxiety can lead to particular physical impairments, then each such impairment has the potential to become a direct (physiological) stressor in its own right as well as indirectly (psychologically) through a general debilitating effect on physical functioning. Such a multiplication of stressors is perhaps particularly likely to occur in elderly people where end-organ function is already compromised, and could effectively amplify the original stressor, leading to boosting of the stress response and increased anxiety (positive feedback loop B; Figure 5). The anxiety–physical impairment vicious circle has the effect of multiplying the medical problems of an individual.

The occurrence of anxiety in dementia, especially early in the course of the disorder, is recognized (Ballard et al., 1994) and predicted by the anxiety–stress model if one accepts that a significant reduction in cognitive functioning constitutes a stressor. It can also be argued that the various behaviours which increase with increasing severity of dementia and currently come under the umbrella term 'agitation' (Cohen-Mansfield and Billig, 1986; Cohen-Mansfield, 1986) are actually anxiety equivalents (Krasucki et al., 1998). Many can be interpreted in fright-flight-fight-freeze terms. If agitation is indeed the manifestation of fear and anxiety in patients with dementia, then the anxiety–stress model correctly predicts the increasing agitation that is found with increasing dementia severity. The reverse hypothesis is more challenging. Psychometric testing of the elderly does suggest that elevated

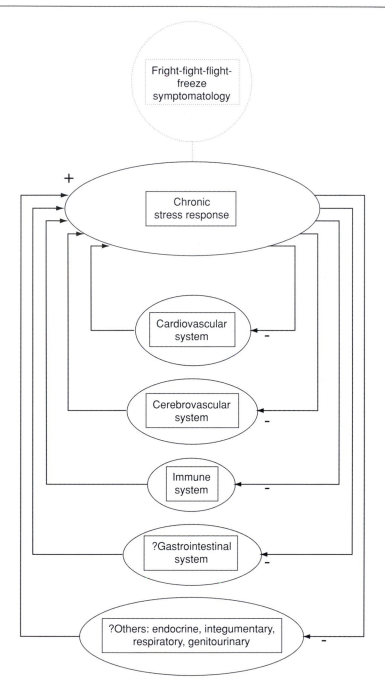

Figure 5. Positive feedback loop B: the psychosomatic link.

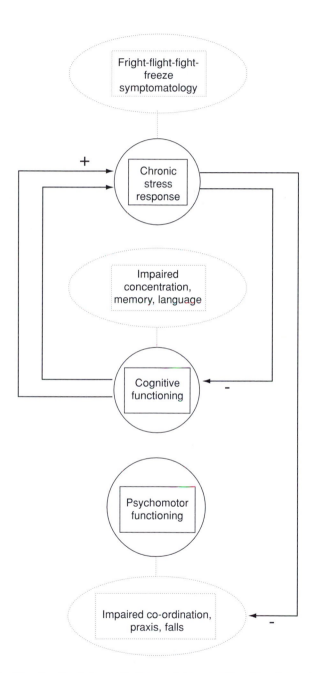

Figure 6. Positive feedback loop C: the anxiety–cognitive impairment interaction.

anxiety impairs test performance (Whitbourne, 1976; Cockburn and Smith, 1994) and this is what the Yerkes–Dodson Law (Yerkes and Dodson, 1908) would lead one to expect. However, there is accumulating evidence also that anxiety and the underlying stress response may have permanent neurotoxic effects (Figure 6). Animal experiments suggest that stress can exacerbate neuron loss and cytoskeletal pathology, in other words accelerate ageing, in the hippocampus (Stein-Behrens et al., 1994), and that this is mediated by the group of hormones that in humans are the prime movers of the chronic stress response, the glucocorticoids (McEwen et al., 1992; Seckl and Olsson, 1995). In humans, 'burn-out' into dementia could account numerically for the decline in anxiety and associated mental disorders with increasing age (Krasucki et al., 1998). Possibly psychomotor as well as purely cognitive function could be affected (Vetter and Ford, 1989). Such an anxiety–cognitive impairment vicious circle would not only hasten central nervous system decline, but also generate the 'excess disability' of established dementia and multiply the associated social difficulties.

Chronicity: of stressors, of the stress response and of anxiety

We are familiar with the idea of a discrete stressor such as a life-event precipitating a stress response and associated psychiatric disorder. Such an event would, it is hoped, resolve spontaneously or be overcome by the individual, allowing the corresponding reaction to it to gradually diminish and finally cease, leaving the individual in a unstressed and non-anxious state. However, the very fact of being elderly may modify this process. Many stressors that the elderly experience are not limited in time and can, at best, only be partially resolved. They may therefore continue to serve as chronic, active stressors, perpetuating the stress response and the anxiety that accompanies it. One could also predict that the greater the age of an individual the more stressors are likely to be experienced simultaneously. Therefore, even if all stressors could be removed or rendered inactive, an individual who was stressed to a sufficient degree and for a sufficient period of time might be left with the psychological and physiological elements of a stress response disengaged from or autonomous of the stressor or stressors that initiated it. This would represent a 'tuning-up' of the fright-fight-flight-freeze system leading to a greater likelihood of appraising future stressors as 'threat' rather than 'challenge', a greater vulnerability to such stressors, and a greater likelihood of suffering the adverse psychological and physiological consequences of a chronic stress response. Such a model receives support from evidence that the hypothalamo-pituitary-adrenal axis response to stressors is prolonged or disinhibited in the elderly (Stokes et al., 1996) and that stressors and the affective illness that accompanies them may leave residual traces leading to a greater vulnerability to similar illness in the future (Post, 1992).

THE ANXIETY–STRESS MODEL AND RATIONAL TREATMENT FOR ANXIETY

A rational approach to anxiety follows directly from this model. There are several logical points of attack, some of which are likely to owe at least part of their effect to the interruption of anxiety positive feedback loops A, B or C. The timing of therapeutic approaches is likely to be of importance. Anxiety symptoms when first detected may represent a 'window of opportunity' during which effective intervention may diminish or eliminate a subsequent chronic anxiety state. This is suggested by the impression in military psychiatry that prompt treatment of a psychologically traumatized individual with adequate doses of anxiolytic medication hastens the return to normal functioning and may prevent the later development of post-traumatic stress symptoms (O'Brien and Nutt, 1998). Perhaps the intense learning or 'engraving' mechanism triggered by the traumatic event is modified or disrupted by early pharmacological anxiolysis. This possibility awaits confirmation by clinical trials in both the young and the elderly.

Diminishing the effect by removing the cause: dealing with stressors

Ideally stressors should be neutralized or eliminated as soon as possible after they occur. This process can be passive or active from the point of view of the patient. Where stressors are severe, complex or multiple, outside help will probably be needed and this has been labelled 'environmental manipulation' (Pasnau and Bystritsky, 1990; McCullough, 1992). Clearly the range of potential stressors is very wide (Table 1) and made wider still by the individual appraisal process. With some, e.g. treating somatic illness, intervention on conventional medical lines is likely to be needed, while with others, social interventions will be appropriate. The advantage of a multidisciplinary approach with an associated range of skills is that a range and a mix of stressors can potentially be effectively addressed in a co-ordinated manner. Some individuals may be able to take an active role and receive counselling (Pasnau and Bystritsky, 1990) or problem-solving treatment (Gurian and Goisman, 1993; Mynors-Wallis and Gath, 1992), although neither appears to have been formally tested in the elderly. Theoretically 'helping the patient to help himself or herself' has the advantage of favourably altering appraisal. Future stressors are thus more likely to be viewed as challenging rather than threatening, and therefore diminished in their potential to generate a stress response.

Altering the threshold for a stress or anxiety response: appraisal

As the appraisal of stressors past and present modifies the likelihood of an event or situation being perceived as a stressor, altering appraisal has the potential to diminish current and future stress responses and therefore anxiety. Cognitive and dynamic psychotherapy (and perhaps religious observance also) attempt to link the meaning an individual attaches to certain events and circumstances with his or her mental state, and by altering the former benefit the latter. They could therefore be said to be modifying the appraisal process.

Cognitive therapy (Turnbull and Turnbull, 1985; Nakra and Grossberg, 1986; McCarthy *et al.*, 1991), either alone or as part of stress inoculation (Hussian, 1981; McCarthy *et al.*, 1991) or stress management (Turnbull and Turnbull, 1985; McCullough, 1992) approaches, has been recommended as an effective treatment for generalized anxiety disorder in the elderly but there is only sparse research evidence for this. In a randomized trial with 50 volunteers, mean age 75 years, cognitive-behavioural therapy produced a statistically significant reduction in state but not trait anxiety, but this was the same as that in the reminiscence therapy and recreational activity control groups (Harp Scates *et al.*, 1986). One possible explanation is that these three latter approaches do not alter appraisal as such but provide the 'nurturance' which is sought by anxious individuals. Various forms of dynamic psychotherapy have also been recommended for anxiety in the elderly (Barbee and McLaulin, 1990; Salzman, 1991; McCullough, 1992) but their efficacy has never been demonstrated in clinical trials. Psychotherapy is less frequently advocated for the obsessional element of obsessive-compulsive disorder (Turnbull and Turnbull, 1985). Indeed, the only supporting evidence appears to be a case report in which the treatment of an 84-year-old man suffering from self-harming obsessions and depression with a self-psychology approach for three years resulted in significant improvement by clinician rating (Weiner and White, 1985). Cognitive therapy has been described as the treatment of choice for panic disorder in the elderly (Hocking and Koenig, 1995) but there is no published evidence in support of this. In PTSD 'psychological debriefing' might be expected to alter *post hoc* appraisal of the traumatic stressor and therefore alter prognosis, but work with younger populations has shown it to be without effect (Deahl *et al.*, 1994) and it does not appear to have been tested in the elderly. However, case series data (Simpson *et al.*, 1996) suggest that elderly individuals with established PTSD may benefit from cognitive therapy. Psychodynamic working through of the traumatic experience in the elderly is, on the other hand, not recommended until symptoms have abated (Schreuder, 1996). In summary, there is currently insufficient evidence to decide whether it is possible to alter appraisal in the anxious elderly, and therefore whether altering appraisal can modify or protect against anxiety disorders.

Interfering with positive feedback loops: breaking the vicious circle of anxiety

The anxiety–stress model predicts that anxiety causes other impairments, which can both directly and indirectly act as stressors, thus maintaining and potentiating the anxiety. Breaking this circular process by diminishing the impairments should reduce anxiety levels.

Anxiety and depression

If positive feedback loop A (Figure 4) is correct, successfully treating anxiety should eliminate depression, but successful treatment of depression should improve but not necessarily eliminate anxiety. Writers have generally recommended antidepressant therapy (Pasnau and Bystritsky, 1990; Hocking and Koenig, 1995) for mixed anxiety–depression in the elderly, with or without adjunctive benzodiazepines. Suggested antidepressant compounds include the tricyclic antidepressants (Hershey and Kim, 1988; Richardson and Bell, 1989), especially imipramine and doxepin (Crook, 1985), and monoamine-oxidase inhibitors (Hershey and Kim, 1988; Richardson and Bell, 1989), especially tranylcypromine, phenelzine (Crook, 1985), trazodone and nefazodone (Weiss, 1996). When adjunctive benzodiazepines are used, short-acting compounds such as oxazepam or lorazepam are favoured (Crook, 1985). The use of the 5-HT_{1A} agonist, buspirone, is also advocated (Weiss, 1996). Unfortunately, none of these individual compounds has been formally tested in elderly individuals with mixed anxiety–depression. A study (Sinclair *et al.*, 1975) in which 72 elderly primary care attenders with mixed anxiety–depression were treated for 28 days with either fluphenazine/nortriptyline (Motival) or amitriptyline was flawed by the confounding effect of nitrazepam given in an uncontrolled manner as a hypnotic and a probable suboptimal dose (75 mg daily) and treatment duration of amitriptyline. In a more rigorously conducted mixed-age (range 18–82 years, mean 49 years) primary care study (Laws *et al.*, 1990) in which individuals with mixed anxiety–depression were treated with either fluvoxamine 50–300 mg daily or lorazepam 1–6 mg daily for six weeks, anxiety ratings improved significantly within the first week for both fluvoxamine and lorazepam and continued to improve over the course of the trial. Depression ratings improved in a parallel manner. There were no significant differences between fluvoxamine and lorazepam in terms of the magnitude or onset of anxiolytic or antidepressant effect, apart from in individuals aged 65 and over where anxiety improved much more rapidly with lorazepam. Elderly individuals treated with lorazepam also had significantly greater improvements in depression in the first two weeks of the study. This difference subsequently diminished but did not disappear. Both treatments were equally well tolerated. These findings support the concept of a positive feedback loop between anxiety and depression. Lorazepam, a prototypical anxiolytic with no intrinsic antidepressant action, had a primary effect on anxiety and a virtually simultaneous secondary effect on depression. Fluvoxamine, an antidepressant, was shown in the elderly group to have a lesser anxiolytic effect, as the model would predict, and an antidepressant effect that was delayed by about two weeks, as one would also predict for this class of agent. Although one cannot exclude the possibility that fluvoxamine, like lorazepam, exerts its antidepressant action through anxiolysis, together these findings support the prediction that anxiety is the dominant prognostic factor in mixed anxiety–depression. Further evidence for this is that elderly patients with a substantial anxiety component to their depression are less likely to respond to fluoxetine (Ackerman *et al.*, 1997), more likely to require augmentation of their antidepressant therapy (Reynolds *et al.*, 1996), and more likely to have a good outcome when electroconvulsive therapy (ECT) is given for depression (Fraser and Glass, 1980). Nearly one-third of elderly patients hospitalized for depressive illness will be left with chronic anxiety after resolution of the depression (Blazer *et al.*, 1989).

Anxiety and physical impairment

Positive feedback loop B (Figure 5) predicts that the anxiety–stress response can trigger or exacerbate physical impairment, and that physical impairment can initiate or maintain this response. Although anxiety in the elderly is associated with both particular physical disorders (Lindesay and Banerjee, 1994) and general physical ill-health (Himmelfarb and Murrel, 1984), whether the treatment of co-morbid anxiety in medical patients can substantially alter the overall prognoses of specific medical conditions remains a crucial research issue (Stoudemire, 1996). The reverse hypothesis in relation to anxiety similarly remains largely unexplored. However, there are early indications that in the elderly physical rehabilitation (Barbisoni *et al.*, 1996) and the provision of sensory aids (Appollonio *et al.*, 1996) can improve depressed mood, and therefore possibly anxiety as well.

Anxiety and cognitive impairment

Positive feedback loop C (Figure 6) predicts that the chronic stress response underlying chronic anxiety will exert a cumulative neurotoxic effect resulting eventually in an irreversible decrement in cognitive and psychomotor functioning, and that such a decrement will act itself as a stressor which is likely to maintain or exacerbate anxiety. Therefore although treatment of the anxiety would not be expected to produce a clinically significant improvement in cognitive or psychomotor functioning, one would expect interventions that reduce cognitive and psychomotor deficits to diminish anxiety. The literature on anxiety interventions in dementia has been dominated by the pharmacological approach. Evidence for the efficacy of psychological approaches to anxiety in dementia is currently very sparse and equivocal (Schneider and Sobin, 1991; Koder, 1998). On the other hand, a multitude of pharmacological agents have been recommended. These include potent and relatively non-sedating antipsychotics such as haloperidol, fluphenazine, trifluoperazine and thiothixene (Shader and Greenblatt, 1982); benzodi-azepines (Salzman, 1987; Salzman, 1988; Pomara *et al.*, 1991; Karlsson, 1996a) such as oxazepam 20–50 mg daily or diazepam 9–12 mg daily (Salzman, 1988); and selective serotonin reuptake inhibitors (Karlsson, 1996a) such as citalopram (Karlsson, 1996a; Karlsson, 1996b). Randomized controlled trials show that loxapine (Barnes *et al.*, 1982); the monoamine-oxidase-B inhibitor L-deprenyl (Tariot *et al.*, 1987); the 5-HT$_{1A}$ agonist buspirone (Cantillon *et al.*, 1994); and possibly the selective serotonin reuptake inhibitors citalopram (Nyth and Gottfries, 1990) and fluvoxamine (Olafsson *et al.*, 1992) can reduce anxiety in dementia. In addition, open studies suggest that trazodone is (Lebert *et al.*, 1994) but carbamazepine is not (Lemke, 1995) effective. No study lasted more than 10 weeks and so it is unclear whether these agents continue to be effective and acceptable in the longer term. Furthermore, none was shown to have any benefit on psychometric test results, which is in accordance with the predictions of the model. It is probably safe to conclude, however, that in the short term the above agents probably do have some effect in reducing anxiety and therefore 'excess disability' in dementia. Whether improvement of cognition can alleviate anxiety must await the development and testing of effective cognition-enhancing therapies with regard to their effect on mood as well as cognition.

Treating chronic anxiety directly

Treatments for chronic anxiety can be divided into psychological and pharmacological groupings. Psychological interventions tend either to use relaxation techniques that rely on physiological symptoms of anxiety or stress as a therapeutic target and measure of change, or to involve harnessing and turning to advantage 'nurture-seeking' behaviour.

Behavioural techniques (Carstensen, 1988; Barbee and McLaulin, 1990; Salzman, 1991; McCullough, 1992; Gurian and Goisman, 1993; Hocking and Koenig, 1995; Martin *et al.*, 1995) have been advocated, whether utilizing progressive muscle relaxation (Hussian, 1981; Handen, 1991; McCarthy *et al.*, 1991), autogenic training, hypnosis, meditation (Turnbull and Turnbull, 1985) or controlled breathing (McCarthy *et al.*, 1991). Research with the elderly supports the efficacy of progressive muscle relaxation in diminishing both the psychological and physiological components of chronic anxiety (Scogin *et al.*, 1992; Rankin *et al.*, 1993; Rickard *et al.*, 1994), but these improvements tend to be lost after the end of active treatment (Scogin *et al.*, 1992; Rankin *et al.*, 1993). In the only study to show continued improvement, one-third of subjects had dropped out at follow-up (Rickard *et al.*, 1994). Progressive muscle relax-ation is therefore palliative rather than curative, and continued practice is necessary for continued suppression of anxiety. Biofeedback using the amount of EEG alpha wave activity is also effective in reducing psychological and physiological anxiety over the treatment period (Brannon, 1976), but whether treatment effects persist is unknown. The effect of biofeedback is not additive to that of progressive muscle relaxation (West, 1978), suggesting the possibility that both work through a final common pathway. Whether psychological approaches can effectively deal with the severe anxiety of panic disorder is not known, although cognitive–behavioural therapy has been advocated (Hocking and Koenig, 1995). Behaviour therapy in conjunction with an antidepressant (dothiepin 100 mg daily) and cognitive therapy alone have been reported to be effective in PTSD (Simpson et al., 1996).

Some psychological therapies work by responding to and addressing the 'nurture-seeking' behaviour of anxious individuals. Supportive psychotherapies are often advocated (Turnbull and Turnbull, 1985; Nakra and Grossberg, 1986; Barbee and McLaulin, 1990) but are untested as interventions. One 'nurturing' treatment, 'therapeutic touch', was, however, shown to reduce anxiety in a single-blind randomized controlled trial (Simington and Laing, 1993). No follow-up data were provided and so whether the effects are maintained is unknown. 'Nurturing' treatments are neither recommended nor tested in panic disorder. In PTSD individuals may attend victim support groups but whether these are effective in reducing anxiety is unknown (Simpson et al., 1996). Nearly every doctor–patient or therapist–patient contact probably contains a 'nurturing' element, and therefore this may underlie both the appeal and outcome of many 'alternative' therapies and the substantial placebo response in anxious elderly individuals.

Virtually every conceivable psychotropic agent has at some point been recommended for generalized anxiety disorder in the elderly. The list includes sedative-hypnotics such as the benzodiazepines; antidepressants including the tricyclic, monamine-oxidase inhibitor and selective serotonin reuptake inhibitor classes; neuroleptics; and azapirones such as buspirone. Antihistamines have also been advocated but not subjected to trial (Jenike, 1983; Hershey and Kim, 1988; Salzman, 1990). Beta-blockers are said to reduce anxiety by acting on the physiological component of anxiety (Shader and Greenblatt, 1982; Jenike, 1983), but there is disagreement as to whether there is (Fernandez et al., 1995; Hocking and Koenig, 1995) or is not (Barbee and McLaulin, 1990) also a secondary effect on the psychological component. This breadth of potential treatment is matched by the finding that the noradrenergic, dopaminergic, serotonergic, and gamma-aminobutyric acid (GABA) neurotransmitter systems are are involved in the biochemistry of anxiety and panic states (Smith et al., 1995), each offering a potential pharmacological target for treatment.

If increased activity at central noradrenergic synapses is contributing to anxiety, then agents that further increase synaptic noradrenaline should, at least initially, increase anxiety. Indeed, tricyclic antidepressants, which inhibit noradrenaline reuptake, are initially anxiogenic but become anxiolytic on longer-term use, for reasons that are unclear (Nutt and Lawson, 1992) but could represent a densensitization process. Monoamine-oxidase inhibitors also increase synaptic noradrenaline but do not cause early exacerbation of anxiety symptoms because of their more gradual mode of action (Nutt, 1990). Neither class of agent appears to have been tested in elderly individuals with generalized anxiety or panic disorder although tranylcypramine produced complete resolution of obsessions of harm dating back to adolescence in a 69-year-old woman (Jenike *et al.*, 1987), trazodone improved bowel obsessions in a 66-year-old man (Ramchandi, 1990), and dothiepin in combination with behaviour therapy was found helpful in a PTSD case study (Simpson *et al.*, 1996). In individuals with dementia an open study found that trazodone could reduce anxiety (Lebert *et al.*, 1994) and a small double-blind study found that the MAO-B inhibitor L-deprenyl was superior to placebo (Tariot *et al.*, 1987). The anxiolytic action of beta-adrenergic blockers has not been tested in clinical trials. If increased activity at central dopaminergic synapses is contributing to anxiety, then agents that further increase synaptic dopamine should also, at least initially, increase anxiety, and dopamine receptor blockers should be anxiolytic. Although monoamine-oxidase inhibitors increase synaptic dopamine (in addition to other monoamine neurotransmitters), their anxiolytic efficacy in the cognitively intact elderly has not been demonstrated. Neuroleptics have not been formally tested either, but loxapine was found effective in anxiety occurring in dementia (Barnes *et al.*, 1982), offering some support for the idea that dopaminergic overactivity contributes to anxiety. Much recent work on the neurobiological basis of anxiety has focused on the role of serotonin (Kahn *et al.*, 1988; Petty *et al.*, 1996; Bell and Nutt, 1998). As with the other neurotransmitters, it is hypothesized that increased activity at serotonergic synapses is associated with anxiety (Nutt, 1990). Indeed, the selective serotonin reuptake inhibitors tend to initially be anxiogenic before later becoming anxiolytic, perhaps by a mechanism similar to that for noradrenaline uptake inhibition. The selective serotonin reuptake inhibitors have, however, not been proven as anxiolytics in the elderly. Indeed, in individuals with dementia, double-blind studies have been unable convincingly to show citalopram (Nyth and Gottfries, 1990) or fluvoxamine (Olafsson *et al.*, 1992) to be superior to placebo over periods of 16 and six weeks respectively. The azapirone buspirone, which is an agonist at 5-HT_{1A} presynaptic receptors that inhibit synaptic serotonin release (Nutt, 1990), should be anxiolytic. Four open studies (Napoliello, 1986; Singh and Beer, 1988; Robinson *et al.*, 1988; Levine *et al.*, 1989) and a double-blind randomized placebo-controlled trial (Bohm *et al.*, 1990), each of which lasted four weeks, suggest that the drug may have short-term anxiolytic properties that are superior to placebo in the elderly.

As GABA is the major inhibitory neurotransmitter, one would expect increased activity to diminish anxiety and decreased activity to exacerbate it. This is in fact what is found (Nutt, 1990). Benzodiazepine agonists act at the benzodiazepine-GABA receptor complex. One double-blind randomized controlled trial with 220 anxious elderly subjects found oxazepam to be superior to placebo over the four-week treatment period (Koepke *et al.*, 1982). Another with 63 subjects found ketazolam to be superior to placebo over 30 days (Bresolin, 1988). A further trial showed that alprazolam and buspirone had produced similar improvements in anxiety at the end of a 14-day period (Hart *et al.*, 1991). Therefore, benzodiazepines appear to also have short-term anxiolytic properties in the elderly. Some (Nutt, 1990) have gone so far as to argue that the most parsimonious explanation of generalized anxiety disorder is a dysfunction of central benzodiazepine function. However, as there appears to be multiple, perhaps global, involvement of neurotransmitter systems in anxiety, and blockade of any individual neurotransmitter system has only a limited anxiolytic effect in a limited proportion of individuals, perhaps a still more parsimonious explanation of chronic anxiety is that, like epilepsy, it is a diffuse neurophysiological abnormality involving thresholds and patterns of signalling between neurons with secondary neurochemical effects, rather than a primary neurochemical abnormality as such. The anticonvulsant phenytoin, whose major action at therapeutic concentrations is to block sodium channels and inhibit the generation of repetitive action potentials (Porter and Pitlick, 1989), was found in an open study to produce marked improvement in neurotic individuals unresponsive to treatment with antidepressants and anxiolytics (Haward, 1982).

Exorcizing the ghosts of anxiety past: 'unlearning the lessons' in phobic anxiety and compulsive disorder

Anxiety, whether of generalized, obsessional or panic form, may be associated with avoidance behaviour. If the anxiety is still diffusely (as opposed to specifically, as in phobic disorder) active, whether or not the precipitating stressor is, there may be *in vivo* avoidance of the originally feared and associated situations (phobia) with or without imaginal avoidance and ensuing harm-avoidant behaviour (compulsions). Anxiety may be compounded by secondary depression, which, by diminishing interest, energy and motivation, could perpetuate avoidant behaviours. As (transient) emotional events can lead to (lasting) learning effects, if and when diffuse anxiety is no longer active these behaviours may remain as specific 'fossil remnants' of the original fears. Consequently the anxiety–stress model predicts that interventions which reduce active diffuse anxiety should reduce avoidant behaviours to some degree. Additional benefit should result from any technique that re-educates the individual that the avoided situation or situations are in fact innocuous, and this approach should be the only one that works in individuals where there is no longer any diffuse anxiety.

Clinical recommendations for the treatment of phobias in the elderly embrace both pharmacological and psychotherapeutic approaches. Pharmacological intervention is advocated (Shader and Greenblatt, 1982; Schneider, 1993) for agoraphobia in particular and includes tricyclic antidepressants such as imipramine, monoamine-oxidase inhibitors, and benzodiazepines such as alprazolam (Turnbull and Turnbull, 1985). Recommended non-drug approaches (Shader and Greenblatt, 1982) include psychosocial interventions (Schneider, 1993) and behaviour therapy (Shader and Greenblatt, 1982). Flooding and desensitization are advocated for simple and social phobia (Turnbull and Turnbull, 1985) while progressive muscle relaxation with or without systematic desensitization is said to be the treatment of choice for all phobias in the elderly (Handen, 1991). In terms of the research findings, no pharmacological agents appear to have been evaluated for their efficacy in reducing the avoidant behaviour of elderly phobic individuals and thus the first prediction of the anxiety–stress model is supported only by clinical impression. However, a variety of case reports and case series suggest that enduring improvements in avoidant behaviour can be achieved using a behavioural approach. Specific phobia in the elderly will usually have started early in life and both diffuse and specific anxiety will usually be absent (Lindesay, 1991). One 70-year-old woman with dog phobia had complete resolution of avoidant behaviour with five sessions of *in vivo* exposure each lasting an hour and continued to be well at six-month follow-up (Thyer, 1981). Four elderly individuals with elevator (lift) phobia also had complete resolution of avoidant symptoms with systematic desensitization which was maintained at two-month follow-up (Hussian, 1981), as did a 64-year-old woman in a separate case report who additionally had agoraphobic avoidance (Woods and Britton, 1985). Long-standing agoraphobia in the elderly has been shown to respond to systematic desensitization, with at least partial resolution of avoidant behaviour maintained for up to 12 months (Garrison, 1978; Garfinkel, 1979). Perhaps the extent to which agoraphobic fear has generalized by association makes the creation of a comprehensive hierarchy of feared situations, and therefore full systematic desensitization, difficult. Nevertheless, these findings provide some support for the second prediction of the model.

Recommended treatment approaches for compulsive disorder in the elderly also include pharmacological and psychotherapeutic strategies. Tricyclic antidepressants, particularly imipramine (Turnbull and Turnbull, 1985) and clomipramine (Schneider, 1993; Jackson, 1995); buspirone

(Hocking and Koenig, 1995); beta-blockers (Hocking and Koenig, 1995); and selective serotonin reuptake inhibitors such as paroxetine, fluvoxamine, fluoxetine and sertraline (Jackson, 1995; Weiss, 1996) have been advocated. Psychotherapy (Turnbull and Turnbull, 1985; Hocking and Koenig, 1995) and in particular a behavioural approach (Schneider, 1993) involving the use of incompatible responses, *in vivo* exposure, modelling and response prevention (Handen, 1991) is also said to be effective. As in the case of phobia, there are no controlled trials of any treatments for compulsions in the elderly. There are isolated case reports reporting successful treatment of checking rituals with imipramine in a 65-year-old woman (Mavissakalian and Michelson, 1983) and cleaning, checking and hand-washing rituals with lithium in an 84-year-old woman (Casey and Davis, 1994). However, the available case reports and case series indicate that drug treatments such as tricyclic antidepressants (Casey and Davis, 1994), including imipramine (Junginger and Ditto, 1984; Bajulaiye and Addonizio, 1992) and clomipramine (Bajulaiye and Addonizio, 1992); phenelzine; fluoxetine (Bajulaiye and Addonizio, 1992; Casey and Davis, 1994); haloperidol (Casey and Davis, 1994); and alprazolam (Bajulaiye and Addonizio, 1992) are relatively ineffective when given alone for the compulsive component of obsessive-compulsive disorder in the elderly. On the other hand, *in vivo* desensitization of a 70-year-old woman with a 30-year history of compulsive hand-washing achieved complete resolution of compulsive behaviour which was maintained at 24-month follow-up (O'Brien, 1978). An 80-year-old man with a one-year exacerbation of lifelong checking and repeating rituals enjoyed substantial improvement after exposure and response prevention, which was maintained at eight-month follow up (Calamari, 1994). The beneficial effects of adding behavioural techniques to drug treatment which was not helping on its own have also been reported (Junginger and Ditto, 1984). Six treatments of ECT resulted in complete remission of cleaning, checking and hand-washing rituals in an 84-year-old woman, which was maintained for two months. However, further treatment was required and it was noted that there was a trend to briefer remissions with subsequent courses of treatment (Casey and Davis, 1994). Therefore, both predictions of the anxiety–stress model are upheld. Pharmacological intervention may have a general anxiolytic action and is usually partially effective at best, but behavioural re-education approaches seem to produce major and lasting improvement. One can only speculate about the effect of ECT on compulsive behaviour. Perhaps the neuronal pathways on which it is encoded, being particularly physiologically and therefore metabolically active at the time of treatment, are selectively 'stunned' by the ECT, take time to recover, and are in the process rendered more resistant to subsequent electrical insult.

CONCLUSION

The anxiety–stress model provides a framework for understanding the phenomenology of anxiety in relation to the neurophysiological and neurochemical processes that underlie it. By attempting to explain and generate predictions about how anxiety affects and is affected by other psychic and somatic phenomena, the model takes a holistic stance.

Research into the mechanisms and treatment of anxiety in elderly people is at a rudimentary stage. Future work will need to investigate how the stress response is switched on and off in the elderly and how chronicity of anxiety is established. The physiochemical processes giving rise to the putative

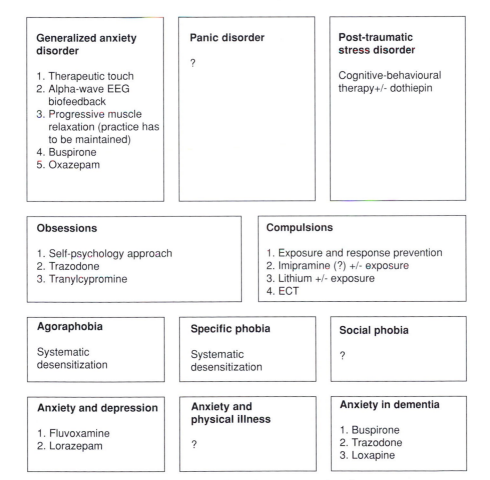

Figure 7. Evidence-based treatment of anxiety.

'engraving' and 'generalization by association' phenomena need to be established. Finally, the possibility of 'emergency' intervention at an early window of opportunity to prevent anxiety becoming chronic, and of course late intervention to reverse established chronic anxiety, are likely to be important areas of therapeutic research. Figure 7 summarizes the treatment recommendations one can make with the current evidence-base, listed in order of probable decreasing benefit:risk ratio. Clearly, there is much scope for the development and refinement of psychological treatments, and for clinical trials using the more modern psychotropics that are currently used for treating depression in the elderly.

REFERENCES

Ackerman, D.L., Greenland, S., Bystritsky, A. and Small, G.W. (1997) Characteristics of fluoxetine versus placebo responders in a randomized trial of geriatric depression. *Psychopharmacol Bull* **33**, 707–714.

American Psychiatric Association (1987). *Diagnostic criteria from DSM-III-R.* APA,Washington, DC.

American Psychiatric Association (1994). *Diagnostic and statistical manual of mental disorders,* fourth edition. APA, Washington, DC.

Appollonio, I., Carabellese, C., Frattola, L. and Trabucchi, M. (1996). Effects of sensory aids on the quality of life and mortality of elderly people: a multivariate analysis. *Age Ageing* **25**, 89–96.

Bajulaiye, R. and Addonizio, G. (1992). Obsessive compulsive disorder arising in a 75-year-old woman. *Int J Geriatr Psychiatry* **7**, 139–142.

Ballard, C.G., Mohan, R.N.C., Patel, A. and Graham, C. (1994). Anxiety disorder in dementia. *Ir J Psychol Med* **11**(3), 108–109.

Barbee, J.G. and McLaulin, J.B. (1990). Anxiety disorders: diagnosis and pharmacotherapy in the elderly. *Psychiatr Ann* **20**, 439–445.

Barbisoni, P., Bertozzi, B., Franzoni, S., Rozzini, R., Frisoni, G.B. and Trabucchi, M. (1996). Mood improvement in elderly women after in-hospital physical rehabilitation. *Arch Phys Med Rehabil* **77**, 346–349.

Barnes, R., Veith, R., Okimoto, J., Raskind, M. and Gumbrecht, G. (1982). Efficacy of antipsychotic medications in behaviourally distubed dementia patients. *Am J Psychiatry* **139**, 1170–1174.

Bell, C.J. and Nutt, D.J. (1998). Serotonin and panic. *Br J Psychiatry* **172**, 465–471.

Bergmann, K. (1971). The neuroses of old age. In: Kay, D.W.K. and Walker, A. (Eds), *Recent developments in psychogeriatrics.* Headley Bros, London, pp. 39–50.

Blazer, D., Hughes, D.C. and Fowler, N. (1989). Anxiety as an outcome symptom of depression in elderly and middle-aged adults. *Int J Geriatr Psychiatry* **4**, 273–278.

Bohm, C., Robinson, D.S., Gammans, R.E. *et al.* (1990). Buspirone therapy in anxious elderly patients: a controlled clinical trial. *J Clin Psychopharmacol* **10** (suppl), 48–51.

Brannon, L.J. (1976). The effects of biofeedback training of EEG alpha activity of the psychological functioning of the elderly [Thesis]. *Dissert Abstr Int* **37**, 5875B.

Bresolin, N., Monza, G., Scarpini, E. *et al.* (1988). Treatment of anxiety with ketazolam in elderly patients. *Clin Ther* **10**, 536–542.

Burchfield, S.R. (1979). The stress response: a new perspective. *Psychosom Med* **41**, 661–672.

Calamari, J.E. (1994). Treatment of obsessive compulsive disorder in the elderly: a review and case example. *J Behav Ther Exp Psychiatry* **25**, 95–104.

Cantillon, M., Molina, D. and Brunswick, R. (1994). Anxiety as a factor in agitation in the demented institutionalized elderly: randomized single blind treatment with azapirones versus neuroleptics. *Biol Psychiatry* **35**, 615–747.

Carstensen, L.L. (1988). The emerging field of behavioural gerontology. *Behav Ther* **19**, 259–281.

Casey, D.A. and Davis, M.H. (1994). Obsessive-compulsive disorder responsive to electroconvulsive therapy in an elderly woman. *South Med Journal* **87**, 862–864.

Cockburn, J. and Smith, P.T. (1994). Anxiety and errors of prospective memory among elderly people. *Br J Psychol* **85**, 273–282.

Cohen-Mansfield, J. (1986). Agitated behaviours in the elderly: II. Preliminary results in the cognitively deteriorated. *J Am Geriatr Soc* **34**, 722–727.

Cohen-Mansfield, J. and Billig, N. (1986). Agitated behaviours in the elderly: I. A conceptual review. *J Am Geriatr Soc* **34**, 711–721.

Crook, T. (1985). Diagnosis and treatment of mixed anxiety-depression in the elderly. *Int Med Special* **6**, 154–176.

Deahl, M.P., Gillham, A.B., Thomas, J. *et al.* (1994). Psychological sequelae following the Gulf War: factors associated with subsequent morbidity and the effectiveness of psychological debriefing. *Br J Psychiatry* **165**, 60–65.

Drozdek, B. (1997). Follow-up of concentration camp survivors from Bosnia-Herzegovina: three years later. *J Nerv Ment Dis* **185**, 690–694.

Engel, G.L. (1953). Homeostasis, behavioral adjustment and the concept of health and disease. In: Grinker, R. (Ed.), *Mid-century Psychiatry*. Charles C. Thomas, Springfield, IL.

Fernandez, F., Levy, J.K., Lachar, B.L. and Small, G.W. (1995). The management of depression and anxiety in the elderly. *J Clin Psychiatry* **56** (suppl 2), 20–29.

Flint, A.J., Cook, J.M. and Rabins, P.V. (1996). Why is panic disorder less frequent in late life? *Am J Geriatr Psychiatry* **4**, 96–109.

Fraser, R.M. and Glass, I.B. (1980). Unilateral and bilateral ECT in elderly patients: a comparative study. *Acta Psychiatr Scand* **62**, 13–31.

Garfinkel, R. (1979). Brief behaviour therapy with an elderly patient. *J Geriatr Psychiatry* **12**, 101–109.

Garrison, J.E. (1978). Stress management training for the elderly: a psychoeducational approach. *J Am Geriatr Soc* **9**, 397–403.

Gurian, B. and Goisman, R. (1993). Anxiety disorders in the elderly. *Generations* **17**, 39–42.

Haines, A.P., Imeson, J.D. and Meade, T.W. (1987). Phobic anxiety and ischaemic heart disease. *BMJ* **295**, 297–299.

Handen, B.L. (1991). Stress and stress management with the elderly. In: Wisocki, P.A. (Ed.), *Handbook of Clinical Behavior Therapy with the Elderly Client*. Plenum Press, New York.

Harp Scates, S.K., Randolph, D.L., Gutsch, K.U. and Knight, H.V. (1986). Effects of cognitive-behavioural, reminiscence, and activity treatments on life satisfaction and anxiety in the elderly. *Int J Aging Hum Dev* **22**, 141–146.

Hart, R.P., Colenda, C.C. and Hamer, R.M. (1991). Effects of buspirone and alprazolam on the cognitive performance of normal elderly subjects. *Am J Psychiatry* **148**, 73–77.

Haward, L.R.C. (1982). The use of phenytoin in neurotic disorders treated in general practice. *Curr Med Res Opin* **8**, 134–138.

Helzer, J.E., Robins, L.N. and McEvoy, L. (1987). Post-traumatic stress disorder in the general population. *N Engl J Med* **317**, 1630–1634.

Hershey, L.A. and Kim, K.Y. (1988). Diagnosis and treatment of anxiety in the elderly. *Ration Drug Ther* **22**(3), 1–6.

Himmelfarb, S. and Murrell, S.A. (1984). The prevalence and correlates of anxiety symptoms in older adults. *J Psychol* **116**, 159–167.

Hocking, L.B. and Koenig, H.G. (1995). Anxiety in medically ill older patients: a review and update. *Int J Psychiatry Med* **25**, 221–238.

Hussian, R.A. (1981). *Geriatric Psychology: A Behavioral Perspective*. Van Nostrand Reinhold, New York.

Jackson, C.W. (1995). Obsessive-compulsive disorder in elderly patients. *Drugs Aging* **7**, 438–448.

Jarvik, L.F. and Russell, D. (1979). Anxiety, aging and the third emergency reaction. *J Gerontol* **34**, 197–200.

Jenike, M.A. (1983). Treating anxiety in elderly patients. *Geriatrics* **38**, 115–119.

Jenike, M.A., Armentano, M.E. and Baer, L. (1987). Disabling obsessive thoughts responsive to antidepressants. *J Clin Psychopharmacol* **7**, 33–35.

Junginger, J. and Ditto, B. (1984). Multitreatment of obsessive-compulsive checking in a geriatric patient. *Behav Modif* **8**, 379–390.

Kahn, R.S., van Praag, H., Wetzler, S., Asnis, G.M. and Barr, G. (1988). Serotonin and anxiety revisited. *Biol Psychiatry* **23**, 189–208.

Karlsson, I. (1996a). Pharmacologic treatment of noncognitive symptoms of dementia. *Acta Neurol Scand* **165** (suppl), 101–104.

Karlsson, I. (1996b). Treatment of noncognitive symptoms in dementia. *Acta Neurol Scand* **168** (suppl), 93–95.

Koder, D. (1998). Treatment of anxiety in the cognitively impaired elderly: can cognitive-behaviour therapy help? *Int Psychogeriatr* **10**, 173–182.

Koepke, H.H., Gold, R.L., Linden, M.E., Lion, J.R. and Rickels, K. (1982). Multicentre controlled study of oxazepam in anxious elderly outpatients. *Psychosomatics* **23**, 641–645.

Krasucki, C., Bandyopadhay, D. and Hooper, E. (1995). Post World War II stress syndrome. *Lancet* **345**, 1240.

Krasucki, C., Howard, R. and Mann, A. (1998). The relationship between anxiety disorders and age. *Int J Geriatr Psychiatry* **13**, 79–99.

Larkin, B.A., Copeland, J.R.M., Dewey, M.E. *et al.* (1992). The natural history of neurotic disorder in an elderly urban population: findings from the Liverpool Longitudinal Study of Continuing Health in the Community. *Br J Psychiatry* **160**, 681–686.

Laws, D., Ashford, J.J. and Anstee, J.A. (1990). A multicentre double-blind trial of fluvoxamine versus lorazepam in mixed anxiety and depression treated in general practice. *Acta Psychiatr Scand* **81**, 185–189.

Lebert, F., Pasquier, F. and Petit, H. (1994). Behavioural effects of trazodone in Alzheimer's disease. *J Clin Psychiatry* **55**, 536–538.

Lemke, M.R. (1995). Effect of carbamazepine on agitation in Alzheimer's inpatients refractory to neuroleptics. *J Clin Psychiatry* **56**, 354-357.

Levine, S., Napoliello, M.J. and Domantay, A.G. (1989). An open study of buspirone in octagenarians with anxiety. *Hum Psychopharmacol* **4**, 51–53.

Lindesay, J. (1991). Phobic disorders in the elderly. *Br J Psychiatry* **159**, 531–541.

Lindesay, J. and Banerjee, S. (1994). Generalized anxiety and phobic disorders. In: Chiu, E. and Ames, D. (Eds), *Functional Disorders of the Elderly*. Cambridge University Press, Cambridge, New York, pp. 78–92.

Lindesay, J., Briggs, K. and Murphy, E. (1989). The Guy's/Age Concern Survey: prevalence rates of cognitive impairment, depression and anxiety in an urban elderly community. *Br J Psychiatry* **155**, 317–329.

McCarthy, P.R., Katz, I.R. and Foa, E.B. (1991). Cognitive-behavioural treatment of anxiety in the elderly: a proposed model. In: Salzman, C. and Lebowitz, B.D. (Eds), *Anxiety in the Elderly: Treatment and Research*. Springer, New York.

McCullough, P. K. (1992). Evaluation and management of anxiety in the older adult. *Geriatrics* **47**(4), 35–44.

McEwen, B.S., Gould, E.A. and Sakai, R.S. (1992). The vulnerability of the hippocampus to protective and destructive effects of glucocorticoids in relation to stress. *Br J Psychiatry* **160** (suppl 15), 18–24.

Martin, L.M., Fleming, K.C. and Evans, J.M. (1995). Recognition and management of anxiety and depression in elderly patients. *Mayo Clin Proc* **70**, 999–1006.

Mavissakalian, M. and Michelson, L. (1983). Tricyclic antidepressants in obsessive compulsive disorder: Antiobsessional or antidepressant agents? *J Nerv Ment Dis* **171**, 301–306.

Mynors-Wallis, L.M. and Gath, D.H. (1992). Brief psychological treatments. *Int Rev Psychiatry* **4**, 301–306.

Nakra, B.R.S. and Grossberg, G.T. (1986). Management of anxiety in the elderly. *Compr Ther* **12**(10), 53–60.

Napoliello, M.J. (1986). An interim multicentre report on 677 anxious geriatric out-patients treated with buspirone. *Br J Clin Pract* **40**, 71–73.

Nutt, D.J. (1990). The pharmacology of human anxiety. *Pharmacol Ther* **47**, 233–266.

Nutt, D. and Lawson, C. (1992). Panic attacks: a neurochemical overview of models and mechanisms. *Br J Psychiatry* **160**, 165–178.

Nyth, A.L. and Gottfries, C.G. (1990). The clinical efficacy of citalopram in treatment of emotional disturbances in dementia disorders: a Nordic multicentre study. *Br J Psychiatry* **157**, 894–901.

O'Brien, J.S. (1978). The behavioural treatment of a thirty year smallpox obsession and handwashing compulsion. *J Behav Ther Exp Psychiatry* **9**, 365–368.

O'Brien, M. and Nutt, D. (1998). Loss of consciousness and post-traumatic stress disorder: A clue to aetiology and treatment. *Br J Psychiatry* **173**, 102–104.

Olafsson, K., Jorgensen, S., Jensen, H.V., Bille, A., Arup, P. and Andersen, J. (1992). Fluvoxamine in the treatment of demented elderly patients: a double-blind, placebo-controlled study. *Acta Psychiatr Scand* **85**, 453–456.

Oxman, T.E., Barrett, J.E., Barrett, J. and Gerber, P. (1987). Psychiatric symptoms in the elderly in a primary care practice. *Gen Hosp Psychiatry* **9**, 167–173.

Pasnau, R.O. and Bystritsky, A. (1990). Importance of treating anxiety in the elderly ill patient. *Psychiatr Med* **8**, 163–173.

Petty, F., Davis, L.L., Kabel, D. and Kramer, G.L. (1996). Serotonin dysfunction disorders: a behavioural neurochemistry perspective. *J Clin Psychiatry* **57** (suppl 8), 11–16.

Pomara, N., Deptula, D., Singh, R. and Monroy, C.A. (1991). In: Salzman, C. and Lebowitz, B.D. (Eds), *Anxiety in the Elderly: Treatment and Research*. Springer, New York.

Porter, R.J. and Pitlick, W.H. (1989). Antiepileptic drugs. In: Katzung, B.G. (Ed.), *Basic and Clinical Pharmacology*. Prentice-Hall, London, pp. 287–303.

Post, R.M. (1992). Transduction of psychosocial stress into the neurobiology of recurrent affective disorder. *Am J Psychiatry* **149**, 999–1010.

Ramchandi, D. (1990). Trazodone for bowel obsession. *Am J Psychiatry* **147**, 124.

Rankin, E.J., Gilner, F.H., Gfeller, J.D. and Katz, B.M. (1993). Efficacy of progressive muscle relaxation for reducing state anxiety among elderly adults on memory tasks. *Percept Motor Skills* **77**, 1395–1402.

Reynolds, C.F., Frank, E., Perel, J.M. *et al.* (1996). High relapse rate after discontinuation of adjunctive medication for elderly patients with recurrent major depression. *Am J Psychiatry* **153**, 1418–1422.

Richardson, R.M. and Bell, J.A. (1989). Anxiety disorders in the elderly. *Postgrad Med* **85**(8), 67–80.

Rickard, H.C., Scogin, F. and Keith, S. (1994). A one-year follow-up of relaxation training for elders with subjective anxiety. *Gerontologist* **34**, 121–122.

Robinson, D., Napoliello, M.J. and Schenk, J. (1988). The safety and usefulness of buspirone as an anxiolytic drug in elderly versus young patients. *Clin Ther* **10**, 740–746.

Salzman, C. (1987). Treatment of the elderly agitated patient. *J Clin Psychiatry* **48** (suppl), 19–22.

Salzman, C. (1988). Treatment of agitation, anxiety and depression in dementia. *Psychopharmacol Bull* **24**, 39–42.

Salzman, C. (1990). Anxiety in the elderly: treatment strategies. *J Clin Psychiatry* **51**(10), 18–28.

Salzman, C. (1991). Conclusion. In: Salzman, C. and Lebowitz, B.D. (Eds), *Anxiety in the Elderly: Treatment and Research*. Springer, New York.

Schachter, S. and Singer, J.E. (1962). Cognitive, social, and physiological determinants of emotional state. *Psychol Rev* **69**, 379–399.

Schneider, L.S. (1993). Efficacy of treatment for geropsychiatric patients with severe mental illness. *Psychopharmacol Bull* **29**, 501–520.

Schneider, L.S. and Sobin, P.B. (1991). Non-neuroleptic medications in the management of agitation in Alzheimer's disease and other dementia: a selective review. *Int J Geriatr Psychiatry* **6**, 691–708.

Schreuder, J.N. (1996). Posttraumatic re-experiencing in older people: working through or covering up? *Am J Psychother* **50**, 231–242.

Scogin, F., Rickard, H.C., Keith, S., Wilson, J. and McElreath, L. (1992). Progressive and imaginal relaxation training for elderly persons with subjective anxiety. *Psychology and Aging* **7**, 419–424.

Seckl, J.R. and Olsson, T. (1995). Glucocorticoid hypersecretion and the age-impaired hippocampus: cause or effect? *J Endocrinol* **145**, 201–211.

Selye, H. (1956). *The Stress of Life*. McGraw-Hill, London.

Shader, R.J. and Greenblatt, D.J. (1982). Management of anxiety in the elderly: the balance between therapeutic and adverse effects. *J Clin Psychiatry* **43**(9), 8–16.

Simington, J.A. and Laing, G.P. (1993). Effects of therapeutic touch on anxiety in the institutionalized elderly. *Clin Nurs Res* **2**, 438–450.

Simpson, S., Morley, M. and Baldwin, B. (1996). Crime-related post-traumatic stress disorder in elderly psychiatric patients: a case series. *Int J Geriatr Psychiatry* **11**, 879–882.

Sinclair, J.M., Walsh, M.R., Valle-Jones, J.C. and Schiff, A.A. (1975). Treatment of anxiety/depressive conditions in the elderly: a double-blind comparative study of Motival and amitriptyline. *Age Ageing* **4**, 226–231.

Singh, A.N. and Beer, M. (1988). A dose range-finding study of buspirone in geriatric patients with symptoms of anxiety. *J Clin Psychopharmacol* **8**, 67–69.

Smith, S.L., Sherill, K.A. and Colenda, C.C. (1995). Assessing and treating anxiety in elderly persons. *Psychiatr Serv* **46**, 36–42.

Stein-Behrens, B., Mattson, M.P., Chang, I., Yeh, M. and Sapolsky, R. (1994). Stress exacerbates neuron loss and cytoskeletal pathology in the hippocampus. *J Neurosci* **14**, 5373–5380.

Stokes, P.E., Mourilhe, P.R., Barsdorf, A.I. and Ombid, H. (1996). Is post stress HPA response prolonged (disinhibited) in aged humans? *Biol Psychiatry* **39**, 554.

Stoudemire, A. (1996). Epidemiology and psychopharmacology of anxiety in medical patients. *J Clin Psychiatry* **57** (suppl 7), 64–72.

Tariot, P.N., Cohen, R.M., Sunderland, T. *et al.* (1987). L-deprenyl in Alzheimer's disease. *Arch Gen Psychiatry* **44**, 427–433.

Thyer, B.A. (1981). Prolonged *in vivo* exposure therapy with a 70-year-old woman. *J Behav Ther Exp Psychiatry* **12**, 69–71.

Turnbull, J.M. and Turnbull, S.K. (1985). Management of specific anxiety disorders in the elderly. *Geriatrics* **40**(8), 75–82.

Tyrer, P. (1986). Classification of anxiety disorders: a critique of DSM-III. *J Affect Disord* **11**, 99–104.

Tyrer, P. (1987). Outcome of neurotic disorders after outpatient and day hospital care. *Br J Psychiatry* **151**, 57–62.

Vetter, N.J. and Ford, D. (1989). Anxiety and depression in elderly fallers. *Int J Geriatr Psychiatry* **4**, 159–163.

Weiner, M.B. and White, M.T. (1985). The use of a self-psychology approach in treating a compulsive 84-year-old man. *Clin Gerontol* **3**, 64–67.

Weiss, K.J. (1996). Optimal management of anxiety in older patients. *Drugs Aging* **9**, 191–201.

West, H.L. (1978). The differential effects of biofeedback/relaxation training on elderly people. *Dissert Abstr Int* **39**, 1523B.

Whitbourne, S.K. (1976). Test anxiety in elderly and young adults. *Int J Aging Hum Dev* **7**, 201–210.

Woods, R.T. and Britton, P.G. (1985). *Clinical Psychology with the Elderly.* Aspen Systems, Rockville, MD.

World Health Organization (1992). *The ICD-10 Classification of Mental and Behavioural Disorders: Clinical Descriptions and Diagnostic Guidelines.* WHO, Geneva.

Yerkes, R.M. and Dodson, J.D. (1908). The relation of strength of stimuli to rapidity of habit-formation. *J Comp Physiol Psychol* **18**, 459–482.

17

Novel Antipsychotics in the Treatment of Late-Life Schizophrenia-Like Psychoses

ROBERT HOWARD

Section of Old Age Psychiatry, Institute of Psychiatry, London, UK

The major differences between standard antipsychotic drugs have always been in their potency and side-effect profile. Clozapine was the first antipsychotic to combine increased therapeutic efficacy and reduced levels of extrapyramidal side-effects and for this reason was termed 'atypical'. Three criteria have been proposed (Kinon and Lieberman, 1996) to define atypical antipsychotics. These are: (1) decrease or absence of the capacity to cause acute extrapyramidal side-effects and tardive dyskinesia; (2) increased therapeutic efficacy reflected by improvement in positive, negative or cognitive symptoms of schizophrenia; and (3) a decrease in or absence of the capacity to increase prolactin levels. As well as the newer drugs (clozapine, risperidone, olanzapine, sertindole, quetiapine and amisulpiride) which are discussed in this chapter, thioridazine and sulpiride are, strictly speaking, atypicals too. There are many new drugs but little information that is useful to the old age psychiatrist. Patients with late-onset schizophrenia-like psychosis have not yet been the subject of a systematic treatment trial with novel drugs. Much of what follows comes from trials which involved young schizophrenics or from open, often anecdotal, accounts of treatment of small numbers of elderly subjects. Most old age psychiatrists have had some experience with at least a couple of these drugs in their late-onset or 'graduate' schizophrenic patients and may even have used them in psychotic or behaviourally disturbed patients with dementia.

WHY WE NEED NEW DRUGS FOR LATE-ONSET PSYCHOSES

All elderly psychiatric patients are exquisitely sensitive to both the desired and undesired effects of antipsychotics. Those patients with onset of psychosis in old age, whether this be a functional or organic illness, are particularly sensitive. Although there is a paucity of controlled treatment trials, naturalistic treatment reports suggest that graduate schizophrenics are generally maintained on 50–75% of the young adult recommended antipsychotic dose, while late-onset (> 60 years) patients are successfully treated with 10–25% of young adult doses (Jeste et al., 1996; Howard and Levy, 1992). New drugs with better efficacy and fewer side-effects would be very welcome in old age psychiatry. Jeste has demonstrated that about one-third of elderly patients treated with conventional neuroleptics will have developed tardive dyskinesia after only a year of treatment (Jeste et al., 1993). Some of the symptoms which are a feature of late-onset psychosis, for example visual hallucinations, respond poorly to conventional antipsychotics. Finally, in terms of their appreciation of their own illness and the need for treatment, late-onset patients are a particularly insightless group. Unpleasant side-effects will at best make the patients reluctant to continue with treatment and at worst convince them that the psychiatric team are using debilitating poison as part of the general persecution that the patient believes he or she is experiencing.

Despite the apparently bewildering variety of receptor activities displayed by these new drugs, it is perhaps helpful to think of them as falling into three broad groups: the multireceptor antagonists (clozapine, olanzapine, quetiapine), the D_2-$5HT_2$-α_1 antagonists (risperidone, sertindole) and the D_2/D_3 antagonists (amisulpiride).

CLOZAPINE

The prototypical atypical antipsychotic, clozapine has affinity for the D_2 family, α_1 and α_2, $5HT_{1a}$ and $5HT_{1c}$, $5HT_2$, histaminic and both nicotinic and muscarinic receptors (Coward, 1992). Although its broad side-effect profile has caused problems, clozapine offered a clear 30–60% response advantage in treatment-resistant schizophrenia (Kane et al., 1988; Breier et al., 1993; Tamminga, 1997) and was useful in the treatment of patients with tardive dyskinesia. Although there have been some reports of successful use in elderly patients (Oberholzer et al., 1992; Chengappa et al., 1995), the drug is often poorly tolerated by patients, even at very low starting doses (as low as 6.25 mg) and long titration periods. Even with such low doses, side-effects in elderly patients (sedation, confusion, postural hypotension, excessive salivation) are common. The advent of clozapine analogues with more benign side-effect profiles means that there is no present justification for giving this drug to elderly patients.

RISPERIDONE

Generally far better tolerated by elderly patients than clozapine, risperidone has affinity for D_2, $5HT_2$ and α_1 receptors (Borison et al., 1992). The large multicentre trials of risperidone in young patients identified an optimum therapeutic dose of 6 mg/day which was superior to haloperidol 20 mg/day in terms of side-effects produced (Chouinard et al., 1993; Marder and Meibach, 1994). In younger patients, again, risperidone probably causes more extrapyramidal problems than clozapine (Daniel et al., 1996), and anecdotally this would seem to apply in the elderly. The notion of an optimum therapeutic dose, above which no increased therapeutic effect is seen, applies in elderly patients too. Graduate patients, and those with an onset of schizophrenia in middle age, respond optimally to doses of up to 4 mg/day (Berman et al., 1996; Jeste et al., 1996; Eastham and Jeste, 1997). The author's own experience with patients with onset after 60 years suggests that a dose of 2 mg/day should not be exceeded. Risperidone is the new atypical with which old age psychiatrists have most experience; it is also the antipsychotic for which there is most evidence of improvement in cognitive symptoms in elderly schizophrenics (reviewed below). Available in liquid as well as tablet form, a starting dose of 0.5 mg is generally well tolerated. Increases of 0.5 mg can be made every four to six days until symptoms disappear or a dose of 2 mg/day is reached. At these low doses, drowsiness, agitation or insomnia are the most common side-effects. Above 2 mg/day the drug appears to behave like a typical antipsychotic in these patients in that extrapyramidal side-effects become problematic. Activity at $5HT_2$ receptors (not unique to risperidone) appears to confer a useful action against visual hallucinations.

OLANZAPINE

Olanzapine is a clozapine analogue but without much of the original drug's nastiness. With particular regard to anticholinergic-induced confusion, although olanzapine blocks M_1, M_3 and M_5 muscarinic receptors, clinically significant anticholinergic effects were seen in the trials only at very high doses (Bymaster et al., 1996). This accords with the author's general experience of giving the drug to elderly patients, although some of these patients do experience sedation at low doses. Despite their marked chemical structural similarity, since the effective dose of olanzapine is only 5–20 mg, compared with 300 mg plus for clozapine, it may be that the much lower doses of olanzapine used are the main reason for the reduced side-effect potential observed. Data on olanzapine use in the elderly are sparse, but the drug is as effective as haloperidol in reducing positive symptoms in elderly schizophrenics (Reams et al., 1998); however, the extrapyramidal side-effect profile is not quite as good as that of clozapine. It has an important place in the treatment of dopaminomimetic psychosis in Parkinson's disease (Wolters et al., 1996), although there have been reports of significant worsening of motor symptoms in these patients at doses of 5 mg/day (Jimenez-Jimenez et al., 1998). The author's experience of treating psychosis in

Parkinson's disease with olanzapine has been that 2.5 or 5 mg/day is well tolerated, but increasing the dose above 5 mg causes a dramatic worsening of
extrapyramidal symptoms. In response to clinicians' requests, a 2.5 mg tablet is
now available which is an appropriate starting dose for late-onset patients.
Increasing doses of up to 10 mg/day appear to be well tolerated and the main
side-effects are drowsiness, weight gain and elevation of serum liver enzymes.

SERTINDOLE

Sertindole has high affinity for mesolimbic D_2 receptors, $5HT_2$ and α_1 receptors,
but little or no affinity for histaminic, muscarinic or α_2 receptors (Sanchez et al.,
1991) and is effective against positive and negative schizophrenic symptoms (van
Kammen et al., 1996; Zimbroft et al., 1997) and in treatment resistance (Geracioti
et al., 1998). Sertindole binds to mesolimbic D_2 receptors with 100 times the
avidity of striatal D_2 binding, and striatal D_2 binding is intermediate between
that seen with clozapine and conventional antipsychotics (Kasper et al., 1998).
This is reflected in low rates of extrapyramidal side-effects in young patients
treated with doses of up to 24 mg/day (van Kammen et al., 1996). Two adverse
events reported from the trials involving younger patients should be of particular concern to old age psychiatrists. First, through its α_1 activity, sertindole can
cause postural hypotension. Because of this a titration regimen is recommended.
Secondly, slight prelongation of the Q–T interval may be associated with use of
sertindole. The Q–T interval represents ventricular repolarization and shows
marked variability with age, sex and other factors. Prolongation of the Q–T
interval may be idiopathic or seen with quinidine-like drugs and the antihis-
tamine terfenadine. Q–T prolongation may cause cardiac arrhythmias, including
the potentially dangerous torsades de pointes. Such arrhythmias are more likely
to occur in the presence or bradycardia or hypokalaemia, so if a diuretic has to
be co-prescribed, the choice of a potassium-sparing drug is advisable. Sertindole
generally causes a mild tachycardia, and in order to evaluate the true impact of
Q–T changes, a correction factor for heart rate needs to be applied. The intrinsic α_1 antagonism of sertindole will also reduce the likelihood of arrhythmia, but
the data sheet cautions against the use of sertindole in patients with underlying
cardiac disease, bradycardia, hypokalaemia or hypomagnesaemia and in those
taking other drugs known to prolong the Q–T interval (Hale, 1998). As a general
precaution, all patients considered for the drug should have a baseline electrocardiogram (ECG) performed and this should be repeated at regular intervals.
It seems reasonable to exclude patients with a prolonged Q–T interval at
baseline. Many classical antipsychotics produce Q–T prolongation and this has
also been reported with risperidone. Hence good clinical practice guidelines
recommend a thorough cardiovascular evaluation of all psychotic patients before
antipsychotic treatment is initiated.

In a report of the tolerability of sertindole in 20 elderly patients with dementia (Buckley *et al.*, 1997), although we are not told why the patients were given the drug, they apparently tolerated a starting dose of 4 mg which was increased to 16 mg/day in 4 mg increments every four days.

Because of safety considerations, sertindole withdrawal is now advised, thus the information in this section may prove to be of purely historical interest.

QUETIAPINE

Quetiapine is a dibenzothiazepine with affinity for multiple receptors, rather similar to clozapine, and has a greater affinity for $5HT_2$ than D_2 receptors (Small *et al.*, 1997). The drug is well tolerated in younger patients in whom it is effective against positive and negative symptoms at high doses of at least 250 mg/day (Arvanitis *et al.*, 1997). The drug has also been used successfully to treat dopaminomimetic psychosis in Parkinson's disease without worsening extrapyramidal symptoms (Parsa and Bastani, 1998), and may turn out to be the agent of choice in this condition. There is little in the literature to suggest what dose range is appropriate for elderly patients. The British National Formulary recommends a starting dose in the elderly of 25 mg, increasing in steps of 25–50 mg/day, but does not give a maximum daily dose. It would seen prudent to limit the maximum dose to 50% of the usual dose range for young adults (300–450 mg/day),

AMISULPIRIDE

Amisulpiride is a mixed D_2/D_3 antagonist like sulpiride (Sokoloff *et al.*, 1990) and has only been recently introduced. There is very little published literature on its use, even in younger patients. It has activity against schizophrenic positive and negative symptoms, and is recommended at lower doses (50–300 mg/day) in the treatment of negative symptoms than in the management of an acute psychotic episode (400–800 mg/day). Side-effects include insomnia, agitation and anxiety, and gastrointestinal symptoms.

CAN THE ATYPICALS IMPROVE COGNITION IN ELDERLY PSYCHOTIC PATIENTS?

Cognitive improvement observed with a change in treatment to an atypical agent in a patient with schizophrenia could be attributable to several factors. Alleviation of positive symptoms of psychosis which might impair attention or co-operation, negative symptoms which themselves show overlap with features of dementia, and the effects of previously prescribed conventional neuroleptic drugs may be significant as well as a direct beneficial drug effect upon the cognitive symptoms of schizophrenia (Howard, 1998). Although no double-blind studies have been published in peer-reviewed journals, evidence from open trials of risperidone treatment of elderly schizophrenic patients suggests that the drug may improve their cognition. In an open-label study of 10 behaviourally disturbed chronic schizophrenics whose mean age was 71, Berman *et al.* (1996) carried out neuropsychological assessments before and during treatment with risperidone. Baseline assessments were made while patients received their conventional antipsychotic medication, which was then stopped, and a titrated (to a daily maximum of 6 mg) dose of risperidone was given. Patients were reassessed after at least one week on risperidone and showed significant improvements in Mini-Mental State Examination (MMSE) score (mean pre-treatment 22.4 and post-treatment 25.5), Digit Symbol Test, Word Recall and Constructional Praxis. Although the authors conceded that scores on the first assessment might have been deleteriously affected by conventional neuroleptics and that practice effects might have helped performance on risperidone, they were able to demonstrate that the increase in MMSE score did not correlate with improvement in psychotic symptoms. In a double-blind comparison of the cognitive effects of risperidone and haloperidol in 20 elderly schizophrenics (mean age 67.4 years) carried out by the same authors (Berman *et al.*, 1996 cited in Jeste *et al.*, 1996), those patients who received risperidone had significant improvement on MMSE score and the Boston Naming Test. Jeste and colleagues (1996) have themselves investigated the cognitive effects of risperidone treatment in middle-aged and elderly psychotic patients with an open uncontrolled study. Treatment was with low doses of risperidone, on average 2.1 mg/day, over a mean treatment period of 10.6 weeks. In a group of 19 patients (13 with schizophrenia), mean MMSE score increased from 24.2 to 28.2. The present quality of evidential data to support an improvement in cognitive function in elderly schizophrenic patients treated with atypicals is insufficient to be convincing, and controlled double-blind trials in both graduate and late-onset patients are needed before this effect can be ruled in or out. The results of such trials will have important implications for patients. Since cognitive impairment in schizophrenia appears to be chronic and stable, beneficial treatments are likely to be effective for years or even decades rather than the apparent short-term benefits of licensed cognition-improving drugs in Alzheimer's disease.

WEIGHT GAIN AND THE NEW ANTIPSYCHOTICS

Conventional antipsychotic drug use has always been associated with minor degrees of weight gain in patients, but with the atypicals this seems to be a more important problem. Both short-term and long-term weight gains are seen. In one trial involving olanzapine, within six to eight weeks patients had gained a mean of 2.8 kg and after 12 months 5.4 kg (Beasley *et al.*, 1996). There appears to be a dose–response relationship between dose of clozapine or olanzapine and degree of weight gain, so that young patients treated for 12 months with 5 mg/day olanzapine increased their weight by 2 kg, while the weight gain at 10 mg/day was 6 kg and at 15 mg/day 12 kg (Nemeroff, 1997). The gains appear to be progressive and with clozapine weight continues to increase after even 84 months of treatment (Umbricht *et al.*, 1994). Clozapine and olanzapine are probably the worst offenders, with risperidone and quetiapine intermediate between these drugs and those like haloperidol which have a low propensity to cause weight gain. Suggested mechanisms for the weight gain seen with the novel drugs have included drug-induced sedation, thirst or hormonal effects, but it is more likely that $5HT_2$ receptor antagonism impairs satiety directly. While weight gain may sound like a trivial or cosmetic side-effect, the risks of type 2 diabetes and hypertension associated with being overweight are important in elderly patients as are the effects on mobility of carrying around extra poundage. Sensible management of the problem involves discussion of this with the patient prior to drug commencement together with advice on diet. Weight can be monitored and exercise or dietary restriction introduced if appropriate.

THE FUTURE OF ATYPICALS IN ELDERLY PSYCHOTIC PATIENTS

Once old age psychiatrists have caught up with the explosion of information around newly available atypical antipsychotics, have tried them in practice and gained some experience and confidence in their use, these drugs will become as ubiquitous in our work as the selective serotonin reuptake inhibitors. At present there is a very serious dearth of trial data for these drugs from populations of older patients, although the makers of risperidone and olanzapine have already spotted the potential market within old age psychiatry and some trials are under way. If we can extrapolate from the data from young patients, the atypicals almost certainly offer better efficacy against positive, negative and cognitive symptoms.

Meanwhile, the atypical antipsychotics are most likely to be prescribed for elderly patients because of their benign motor side-effect profile rather than for any beneficial action on psychotic symptoms. Until depot preparations of the atypicals are available, it is difficult to see how they could replace conventional drugs in the treatment of isolated paranoid patients living in their own homes (Howard and Levy, 1992).

REFERENCES

Arvanitis, L.A., Miller, B.G. and the Seroquel Trial 13 Study Group (1997). Multiple fixed doses of 'Seroquel' (quetiapine) in patients with acute exacerbations or schizophrenia. A comparison with haloperidol and placebo. *Biol Psychiatry* **42**, 233–246.

Beasley, C.M., Tollefson, G., Tran, P., Satterlee, W., Sanger, T. and Hamilton, S. (1996). Olanzapine versus placebo and haloperidol: acute phase results of the North American double-blind olanzapine trial. *Neuropsychopharmacology* **14**, 111–123.

Berman, I., Merson, A., Rachov-Pavlov, J., Allen, E., Davidson, M. and Losonczy, M.F. (1996). Risperidone in elderly schizophrenic patients: an open-label trial. *Am J Geriatr Psychiatry* **4**, 173–179.

Borison, R.L., Pathiraja, A.P., Diamond and Meibach, R.C. (1992). Risperidone: clinical safety and efficacy in schizophrenia. *Psychopharmacol Bull* **28**, 213–272.

Breier, A., Buchanan, R.W., Irish, D. and Carpenter, W.T. (1993). Clozapine treatment of outpatients with schizophrenia: Outcome and longterm response patterns. *Hosp Commun Psychiatry* **44**, 1145–1149.

Buckley, P., Cutler, N., Silber, C., O'Neil, J. and Mack, P. (1997). The safety and tolerability of sertindole in elderly patients with dementia. *Schizophr Res* **24**, 201.

Bymaster F.P., Hemrick-Luecke, S.K., Perry, K.W. and Fuller, R.W. (1996). Neurochemical evidence for antagonism by olanzapine of dopamine, serotonin, α_1-adrenergic and muscarinic receptors *in vivo* in rats. *Psychopharmacology* **124**, 87–94.

Chengappa, K.N., Baker, R.W., Kreibrook, S.B. and Adair, D. (1995). Clozapine use in female geriatric patients with psychosis. *J Geriatr Psychiatry Neurol* **8**, 12–15.

Chouinard, G., Jones, B., Remington, G. *et al.* (1993). A Canadian multicenter placebo-controlled study of fixed doses of risperidone and haloperidol in the treatment of chronic schizophrenic patients. *J Clin Psychopharmacol* **13**, 25–40.

Coward, D.M. (1992). General pharmacology of clozapine. *Br J Psychiatry* **160** (suppl 17), 5–11.

Daniel, D.G., Goldberg, T.E., Weinberger, D.R. *et al.* (1996). Different side-effect profiles of risperidone and clozapine in 20 outpatients with schizophrenia or schizoaffective disorder: a pilot study. *Am J Psychiatry* **153**, 417–419.

Eastham, J.H. and Jeste, D.V. (1997). Treatment of schizophrenia and delusional disorder in the elderly. *Eur Arch Psychiatry Clin Neurosci* **247**, 209–218.

Geracioti, T.D., Parker, S., Lowther, N.B., Wortman, M. and Richtand, N.M. (1998). A case of treatment refractory psychosis responsive to sertindole. *Schizophr Res* **30**, 105–108.

Hale, A.S. (1998). A review of the safety and tolerability of sertindole. *Int Clin Psychopharmacol* **13** (suppl 3), S65–S70.

Howard, R. (1998). Cognitive impairment in late life schizophrenia: a suitable case for treatment? *Int J Geriatr Psychiatry* **13**, 400–404.

Howard, R. and Levy, R. (1992). What factors affect treatment response in late paraphrenia? *Int J Geriatr Psychiatry* **7**, 667–672.

Jeste, D.V., Lacro, J.P., Gilbert, P.L., Kline, J. and Kline, N. (1993). Treatment of late-life schizophrenia with neuroleptics. *Schizophr Bull* **19**, 817–830.

Jeste, D.V., Eastham, J.H., Lacro, J.P., Gierz, M., Field, M.G. and Harris, M.J. (1996). Management of late life psychosis. *J Clin Psychiatry* **57**, 39–45.

Jimenez-Jimenez, F.J., Tallon-Barranco, A., Orti-Pareja, M., Zurdo, M., Porta, J. and Molina, J.A. (1998). Olanzapine can worsen parkinsonism. *Neurology* **50**, 1183–1184.

Kane, J.M., Honigfield, G., Singer, J., Meltzer, H. and the Clozaril Collaborative Study Group (1988). Clozapine for the treatment-resistant schizophrenic: a double-blind comparison with chlorpromazine. *Arch Gen Psychiatry* **45**, 789–796.

Kasper, S., Tauscher, J., Kufferle, B. *et al.* (1998). Sertindole and dopamine D_2 receptor occupancy in comparison to risperidone, clozapine and haloperidol. A ^{123}I-IBZM SPECT study. *Psychopharmacology* **136**, 367–373.

Kinon, B.J. and Lieberman, J.A. (1996). Mechanisms of action of atypical antipsychotic drugs: a critical analysis. *Psychopharmacology* **124**, 2–34.

Marder, S.R. and Meibach, R.C. (1994). Risperidone in the treatment of schizophrenia. *Am J Psychiatry* **151**, 825–835.

Nemeroff, C.B. (1997). Dosing the antipsychotic medication olanzapine. *J Clin Psychiatry* **58** (suppl 10), 45–49.

Oberholzer, A.F., Hendriksen, C., Monsch, A.U., Heierli, B. and Stahelin, H.B. (1992). Safety and effectiveness of low-dose clozapine in psychogeriatric patients: a preliminary study. *Int Psychogeriatr* **4**, 187–195.

Parsa, M.A. and Bastani, B. (1998). Quetiapine (Seroquel) in the treatment of psychosis in patients with Parkinson's disease. *J Neuropsychiatry Clin Neurosci* **10**, 216–219.

Reams, S.G., Sanger, T.M. and Beasley, C.M. (1998). Olanzapine in the treatment of elderly patients with schizophrenia and related psychotic disorders. *Schizophr Res* **29**, 151–152.

Sanchez, C., Arnt, J., Dragsted, N. *et al.* (1991). Neurochemical and *in vivo* pharmacologic profile of sertindole, a limbic selective compound. *Drug Dev Res* **22**, 239–250.

Small, J.G., Hirsch, S.R., Arvanitis, L.A., Miller, B.G., Ling, C.G. and the Seroquel Study Group (1997). Quetiapine in patients with schizophrenia: a high- and low-dose double-blind comparison with placebo. *Arch Gen Psychiatry* **54**, 549–557.

Sokoloff, P., Giros, B., Martres, M.P., Bouthenet, M.L. and Schwartz, J.C. (1990). Molecular cloning and characterization of a novel dopamine receptor as a target for neuroleptics. *Nature* **347**, 146–151.

Tamminga, C.A. (1997). The promise of new drugs for schizophrenia treatment. *Can J Psychiatry* **42**, 265–273.

Umbricht, D.S., Pollack, S. and Kane, J.M. (1994). Clozapine and weight gain. *J Clin Psychiatry* **55** (suppl B), 157–160.

van Kammen, D.P., McEvoy, J.P., Targum, S.D., Kardatzke, D. and Sebree, T.D. (1996). A randomized, controlled, dose-ranging trial of sertindole in patients with schizophrenia. *Psychopharmacology* **124**, 168–175.

Wolters, E.C., Jansen, E.N., Tuynman-Qua, H.G. and Bermans, P.L. (1996). Olanzapine in the treatment of dopaminomimetic psychosis in patients with Parkinson's disease. *Neurology* **47**, 1085–1087.

Zimbroft, D., Kane, J., Tamminga, C. *et al.* (1997). Controlled, dose–response study of sertindole and haloperidol in the treatment of schizophrenia. *Am J Psychiatry* **154**, 782–791.

18

Psychodynamic Aspects of Old Age Psychiatry

MARK ARDERN

Department of Psychiatry of Old Age, St Charles' Hospital, London, UK

INTRODUCTION

How can psychodynamic theory and practice contribute to the work of the old age psychiatry team?

Two years ago the author wrote a chapter for a similarly compiled book on old age psychiatry. The title of the chapter was 'Psychotherapy and the elderly' (Ardern, 1997). Subsequently several colleagues commented that this placed too much emphasis on 'doing psychotherapy'. Since old age psychiatrists rarely have the opportunity to 'do psychotherapy' with their patients, what might be of greater relevance to our everyday work would be something which incorporated elements of psychodynamic thinking into the activity of the multidisciplinary team. Here, therefore, the author sets out to develop this broader theme. In doing so he provides material to answer the opening question above: one which was posed as an essay question in a recent MRCPsych Part II examination.

WHY 'PSYCHODYNAMIC'?

Our work in a psychiatric service for the elderly traditionally focuses on conscious phenomena. We hear what our patients, relatives and referrers report to us. We enquire about facts and memories of patients' earlier life experiences but not usually their role in the formation of character. Important external realities we have termed 'life events' are acknowledged as key triggers in illness. But these can seem disconnected: fragmented parts of an elusive whole. Social isolation, for example, is likely to be viewed as a

misfortune rather than an understandable expression of long-standing unconscious problems in relating. Psychodynamic understanding helps to shed light
on human behaviour. At its best it adds a three-dimensional quality to our
view of the patient's predicament: one which is unique to the individual.
From this we should be better placed to speculate on a particular patient's
response to whatever treatment regimen we choose.

WHAT ARE THE PRINCIPLES COMMON TO PSYCHODYNAMIC THEORISTS?

These can be summarized as follows:

1) The unconscious mind exists. It does so in all of us and can be responsible for apparently inexplicable thoughts, feelings and behaviour.
2) Early life experiences (along with genetic factors) are responsible for
   personality structure reflected in mental mechanisms used for ego defence.
3) Transference and countertransference, though universal phenomena
   between people, are of a particular quality and may be harnessed to
   beneficial effect in the clinical situation.
4) Interpretation is the psychodynamic therapist's tool. It aims to release
   unconscious phenomena and allow percolation into the conscious mind.
   With this, insight is deepened.

Strictly speaking, psychodynamic therapy can only be undertaken by qualified psychotherapists. There is a growing literature on the practice of
psychotherapy with elderly patients (Hildebrand, 1982; Porter, 1991;
Martindale, 1995) and the special problems pertaining to this age group. This
is outside the remit of this chapter.

Nevertheless, many of these theoretical principles could be made available
to the old age psychiatric team. Not surprisingly they require training,
practice and supervision. The technical skill of interpretation is akin to the
surgeon's knife. Many of our patients are not only unfit for surgery but
unable to withstand interpretation. And an unskilled therapist can severely
wound a vulnerable patient.

PSYCHODYNAMICS IN THE ASSESSMENT

As old age psychiatrists we can use psychodynamic skills in our assessments. A
preregistration surgical houseman may not be allowed much time in the operating theatre but spends a great deal of time taking histories, examining patients
and coming to diagnostic formulations. As he becomes more confident so the

houseman may be able to undertake some simple techniques. Similarly, incorporating psychodynamic assessment skills will increase knowledge of patients' difficulties. It does not imply that psychodynamic therapy will be applied to the patient who may be psychotic or have extensive organic brain disease.

Patient assessment begins even before the patient is seen. Letters of referral are mixtures of fact, opinion and request. Those which begin with 'This lovely old dear' may not just inform us about the referrer. It may reflect the effect that this patient has on people more generally. Will others have similar feelings when seeing the patient? Does this tell us something about the patient's way of relating? In a joint assessment by two professionals the countertransference produced in each can be sometimes usefully compared ('She reminded me of an ideal grandmother'; 'Me too, I wanted to give her a hug'). With this knowledge we begin to map out the patient's defensive structure.

It is generally agreed among old age psychiatrists that an initial home visit provides the most comprehensive information on patients. Clearly there is much sense in seeing the home environment especially for those patients who have dementia. Often patients' situations have a greater impact when first seen in this way. From a psychodynamic viewpoint fastidious order or chaotic turmoil provide valuable insights into the patient's inner mental world.

> A paranoid and inflexible lady was found living in a tumbledown house. There was no heating, no hot water, and the roof leaked. The reality of the disintegration of the house around her was denied by her. Life in the outside world could not penetrate the heavy curtains hung at the windows. Her mind appeared similarly sealed off and decaying. Access to both would prove a test of sensitivity and patience.

There are, however, disadvantages about invariably seeing patients at home. Boundaries can become blurred between the professional and social. Being a guest, perhaps an unwanted one in a patient's home, is entirely different from a first meeting in the outpatient clinic. In a patient's lounge the countertransference and transference can be difficult to unravel and provide more opportunities to 'act in'.

> A mildly depressed and lonely lady was seen at home by the author. The author made the mistake of accepting her tea and cake. He then found it difficult to ask essential personal questions about the lady's marital and sexual life. He supposed good nephews did not feel comfortable when asking such things of their aunties!

The division between assessment and management is somewhat artificial since all assessments involve elements of therapeutic (and sometimes countertherapeutic) activity. Psychotherapists, during their assessments, may offer up a 'trial interpretation'. This is done to gauge the receptiveness of the patient to making psychological connections: a test of psychological mindedness. It is not just a barometer of potential success or failure for future therapy but is also (if correct) simultaneously therapeutic.

Ideally the patient will feel relieved that a core anxiety has been unearthed and acknowledged by the therapist. With this the therapeutic alliance is strengthened. In old age psychiatry a concluding part of the assessment of patients who are reluctant to engage might include a comment to ease apprehensions.

> Mrs B, a middle-class religious lady, had suffered a series of bereavements. As a last straw she attributed the onset of her depression to her youngest son's marital break-up. On the wall of her living room all four of her children were proudly displayed in their wedding photographs. It appeared that her son's marriage failure not only reminded her of her own failed marriage and subsequent attempts to sublimate her life through her children's successes. She now had the double blow of failure as a wife and a mother. A simple explanation (barely an interpretation) of these connections allowed her to accept paroxetine. Until this moment she had declined, not having been a 'pill person'.

Psychotherapists (and occasionally candidates sitting the MRCPsych Part II exam) are expected to distil the essence of their initial analysis of the patient into a psychodynamic formulation. Later on we will see how it is possible to draw together the different threads into a useful working hypothesis. And, more important, show how this might point to improving the patient's outcome.

LISTENING AND LEARNING

> A Jewish lady, now 91, presented with anxiety and depression. She had lost all her family in Auschwitz apart from a daughter whom she brought up alone. The patient became a successful businesswoman of extrovert character. She remains determined to live at home, having a lively mind but increasingly severe osteoarthritis. Her daughter rarely visits. The patient manages briefly to attract students to live with her, who, in return for rent-free accommodation, are expected to be handmaidens serving her every need. Not surprisingly they do not stay long. She is seen as an outpatient complaining that she is all alone again. She berates the doctor for things about which he can do nothing. Soon he is aware of also feeling like a handmaiden who is nagged and wants to run away.

In fact the doctor did more than nothing. He observed the recurring pattern of people fleeing from the patient. Instead of repeating this experience he offered her regular but infrequent half-hours in which she was free to complain. This proved hard going until it became clear that the patient was not actually asking for anything more. An understanding had grown up that the patient's doctor would not disappear. In addition, the doctor was being nagged not only by the patient but also by a voice in his head which kept on saying 'You've got to do something to help'. Once he knew he was helping, his own self-nagging stopped. The doctor considered offering his interpretations but decided that the patient was not up to this and might be frightened away. One day she told him she appreciated seeing him and said she was less depressed.

Old age psychiatrists need to be task-orientated and probably enjoy managing to solve seemingly impossible situations. But listening is also work. In some ways psychodynamic listening in the clinical situation is similar to listening to classical music. The skill of the musicians playing, the balance of the orchestration, the juxtaposition of themes, developments, recapitulations and resolutions; these together with the affects and associations stimulated in the listener provide pleasure. This pleasure can be enhanced by training, so that we can learn to understand more about our patients' more unconscious communications.

Psychotherapists have learnt that a key therapeutic action is for the therapist to practise the art of silence. In the silence, observation is in the form of what Freud called 'evenly suspended attention'. Psychodynamic therapists would also rarely tell the patient how he should or should not feel or behave. This withholding of advice is an exceedingly difficult task, especially for the old age psychiatrist who is inclined to intervention and, dare it be said, 'super-egotism'.

Where the old age psychiatrist has the fortune not to be making decisions on behalf of the patient, he may be more able to concentrate on listening, watching and containing. One task can be to foster actively the patient's dependence, providing a reliable and safe setting in which the patient feels held. Theoretically this recreates the unconditional positive regard between mother and infant.

ATTACHMENT THEORY AND OLD AGE PSYCHIATRY

There is increasing evidence from research that elderly patients who have recovered from an episode of depression appear to be better protected from future relapse by extended contact between themselves and health professionals. Ong's study of patients in a weekly support group, which was not ostensibly psychoanalytic, demonstrated a reduction in both relapse and readmission rates over one year compared with controls who received traditional follow-up (Ong *et al.*, 1987). The Gospel Oak community study reported by Blanchard showed that depressed older people improved over a three-month period with simple and limited psychological intervention by a nurse (Blanchard, 1997). The author's own experience of running a weekly experimental psychodynamically orientated group supported these findings. The group was run jointly with a psychoanalyst over a period of five years. The patients were especially unpsychologically minded, all had long psychiatric histories, particularly depression, and came from a range of social classes. Most were socially isolated. The patients eventually told the therapists that what helped most was the fact that the group just went on meeting. One man said, 'We just want to be loved without having to love back'. This experience of 'going on being', or perhaps simply of the patient being borne in mind by his doctor, is frequently reported by patients. From a Kleinian perspective the consistency and reliability of the doctor can become introjected into the patient's unconscious as a good object. Most consultant psychiatrists have several long-term outpatients whom they see relatively infrequently. At some level they are aware of their patients' vulnerability, hence a reluctance to discharge. Here psychiatry may be being practised on a level of instinct and wisdom rather than more fashionable evidence-based logic.

There are no studies to quantify how often patients receiving long-term traditional outpatient 'support' require appointments. Indeed, until recently, application of psychodynamic theory to general psychiatric services has been lacking. Several psychotherapists have advocated a closer integration (Hobbs, 1990; Holmes, 1990; Holmes and Mitchison, 1995). Adshead's application of attachment theory to understanding management problems in psychiatric services could be especially relevant to old age psychiatry. The paper provides further theoretical underpinning of the sort of supportive work described above (Adshead, 1998).

PERSONALITY DISORDER AND ATTACHMENT

Elderly patients with personality disorders are notoriously exasperating for junior doctors. It is unlikely that trainees will, during their six-month posts in old age psychiatry, see significant benefits from their interventions. Strategic therapeutic input will require a much longer-term perspective.

> Miss C, a severely emotionally deprived and highly intelligent woman in her seventies, spent most of her life in contact with psychiatric services. In the early 1950s she received a leucotomy for depression. As the patient became blind and immobile, crises escalated. She complained bitterly about her carers at her sheltered accommodation, whom she constantly denigrated. She made several serious violent attempts at self-harm. It was

decided that in addition to attendance at the day hospital she might benefit from one-to-one sessions with the (female) clinical assistant, who saw the patient monthly for several years under the supervision of a consultant psychotherapist. The patient was envious of the young doctor's holidays and remembered any snippets of personal information in great detail. This she would recall, to the astonishment of the doctor. Despite the patient's attempts to undermine her, the doctor held her nerve and did not retaliate or allow herself to be bullied into more self-disclosure. Recently another crisis arose, the patient saying she could not stand living where she was and asking to come into hospital, having tried to hang herself with cord. Once in hospital she accused her doctor of holding her against her will. After about three weeks the patient stopped complaining. The doctor discussed with her supervisor a long-term goal of allowing her to have a continuing care bed, which might gratify the unconscious wish of the patient to be cared for.

There are several important matters here. First, the patient has never displayed clear evidence of mental illness. She does have an extremely paranoid personality and has almost no capacity to trust others. Her risk of suicide in the face of inaction is rising as her frailty increases. In times of crisis the panic generated among many different professionals had maintained the patient's uncertainty. A clinical assistant was chosen because of the relative permanency of her work. The patient appeared, albeit perversely, to be asking for help and over time her splitting and projections gradually lessened. She was helped to find a healthy part of herself (good object). The doctor had been severely tested but with the help of supervision had withstood the onslaught and survived. This survival was a revelation to the patient who still asks, 'Why do you [bother to] go on seeing me?'

Many of the patients we see do not want to change; they want to be looked after. But they want to make sure that the looking after is not a recreation of an earlier abusive experience. Without knowledge of Miss C's earlier abuse as a child and her later perception of the world in general as being abusive, no sense could be made of why she was nasty to those trying their best to help. Miss C's high intelligence enabled her envious attacks on staff to be especially sophisticated and wounding. If patient's attacks can be understood by staff then there is less chance of destructive retaliation.

THE INSTITUTION AS AN ATTACHMENT FIGURE

Clearly most patients will not be fortunate enough to receive one-to-one help from a single health professional. Previously the author has speculated that patients' transference projections appeared to be not only towards individuals but to the 'bricks and mortar' of the institution itself (Ardern, 1997). Adshead (1998) draws attention to the potentially negative as well as positive effects of the institution as an attachment figure, particularly the mixed messages conveyed to patients about their need to become more independent. In old age psychiatry, where patients are moving towards dependence, the institution needs to be especially self-aware. Martindale provides an analysis of the fears of staff provoked by patients' increasing dependence (Martindale, 1998).

In the day hospital where the author works, a psychodynamic under-standing helped instil confidence in changing the operational policy. Until this time there had been subtle but real pressures on the day hospital staff to provide statistics reflecting a rapid turnover of patients. It was neverthe-less observed that some patients were benefiting from the 'going on being' of the day hospital and that these needs would not be understood in a day centre. It was decided to designate a day (Thursdays) especially for long-term patients which was termed 'maintenance day'. Once a patient is metaphorically in receipt of a ticket for maintenance day then they only stop attending if they choose to leave – patients are given a kind of tenure, akin to a continuing care bed. Since throughput is hardly a measure of success on continuing care wards, so Thursday's statistics are gathered separately. The patients and purchasers are both happier. So too are the staff, who have a more clearly defined objective: the prevention of relapse. An initial survey of five years on by a trainee (Hepper, unpublished) suggests that mainte-nance day has enhanced such protection.

From these anecdotal accounts it seems that what we should be trying to establish are the specific psychodynamic factors responsible for maintaining mental health over the long term. These factors are likely to exist not just in the patients' psychological make-up but in the way the institution is run.

WHY STAFF NEED SUPPORT

A woman seen at home had a moderate degree of dementia. This was confined to severe problems with orientation and short-term memory. At the initial home visit the regularly involved district nurse was present. She was dressed in uniform. The author asked the patient who she (the nurse) was. The patient smiled, patted the author reassuringly and said, 'I've no idea, but she's very nice and that's the main thing'.

Such patients are unlikely to provide problems for professional carers. The severity of dementia in the lady above was of little relevance. Her inner calmness arising from a robust 'basic trust' was her biggest asset. One could not fail to be moved by the patient's acceptance of her predicament. Psychiatric services are more likely to be called upon where paranoid anxiety surrounds a similar degree of dementia. How often have we heard those desperate shrieks, 'Where's my handbag? Somebody's stolen my handbag!'. Here, the patient's mind is fragmented and split apart. The cognitive spaces become filled with malign intruders. Staff feel themselves to be persecuting rather than benevolent, which is painful for them too.

Previously, in the account of Miss C, we saw this pathological mistrust at work. Miss C and her doctor–therapist were, however, fortunate in having input from a qualified psychotherapist who was able to throw light on the reasons for her hostility. Once the doctor (if not the patient) had been able to understand her own discomfort, she was motivated to continue arduous but now more enjoyable work.

Organizations undertaking the task of caring for the elderly mentally ill therefore require support. The ability of staff to deal with troubled patients will depend on many factors: sensitivity, training, wisdom, empathy. But even the best staff will become demoralized in the contagious despair of a badly managed organization.

> A group analyst offered to run a staff support group for nursing staff on a ward caring for people with dementia. Staff were grateful and appreciative at first. However, the analyst rarely saw the same faces, as agency staff had been employed to fill gaps in the nursing establishment. New permanent staff had been forced to accept locally negotiated pay which meant loss of sick leave entitlement and no unsociable hours payments. The analyst felt impotent when hearing so many of these realities. She discussed the group with a new nurse manager who was sympathetic but powerless to change a policy which was being maintained by the Trust board.

What chance do patients have at the mercy of staff who are so demoralized? In the example above, management had consciously welcomed, and paid for, the services of the group analyst. Unconsciously, however, they seemed unable to change the sickness in the institution. With hindsight, input of an analyst had raised expectations which could not be made use of.

A situation commonly encountered in inpatient wards is the patient who 'ought to get better' but doesn't. The effect of this on staff can be dramatic. A psychodynamic insight with discussion of the care amongst all staff can help contain the frustrations and point a way forward. Holmes called this 'creating meaning out of confusion'. In the following example, staff took time out together to analyse a situation where they and the patient were stuck.

> Miss R was admitted with delusional depression. She had been an articulate, capable woman who had shunned intimacy. Now she was paranoid and believed staff were poisoning her. She refused an offer of

ECT and spat out her medication. She talked of feeling dead. Her behaviour oscillated between craving attention and yet rejecting help, accusing staff of incarcerating her (she remained informal). Discussion with her niece revealed that Miss R had been a likeable woman who by nature was independent and rather secretive. Her present situation was described as her worst nightmare come true. Staff discussed their frustration – they could not seem to do anything right. If they moved in too close the patient hit out; trials of ignoring unwanted behaviour seemed no better. What was striking was that all the staff had experienced similar feelings, of neither being able to get too close nor withdraw. They felt guilty every time they saw her. These were discovered to be similar to the patient's own experience. If the patient gave up fighting, staff might move in and give her treatment against her will. If the patient got too well she might be discharged. The patient and staff in their countertransference were trapped in a no man's land. Eventually the patient was helped by one-to-one sessions with an art therapist. The content of the patient's paintings revealed the dynamics of her despair, which was interpreted by the therapist to the patient and staff. Slowly there was an improvement all round. The patient was eventually discharged to a nursing home and staff were able to convey to her their genuine sadness at her leaving.

BRIEF ENCOUNTERS

Fortunately, psychodynamic understanding need not, however, require such time and effort.

A patient was seen at home with the referrer providing minimal information. Examining the mental state just didn't add up. The patient was jumping from subject to subject, possibly either thought-disordered or dysphasic. When the patient made no sense at all the doctor became panicky, not dissimilar to the patient's own experience. The doctor stopped the patient by saying, 'It all seems very confused', to which the patient replied with startling clarity, 'That's *exactly* me.' The patient turned out to be anxious, with a vascular dementia.

A universal apprehension among people as they grow old is about losing independence and having to accept help. For some patients who experienced inadequate parenting in their own lives the prospect of old age is approached not with trepidation but with terror. As a consequence it is not unusual for patients to be wary about engaging with professional services, which are seen as the thin edge of the wedge. None of these fears may be consciously considered by the patient or the old age psychiatry team. A simple comment made to patients during the initial assessment may help the patient to feel easier. 'I can see you are worried about losing your independence, maybe that we'll take over and you won't be able to have a say any more.' This comment does not exclude the possibility of the patient losing independence, or even being admitted compulsorily. It does though make it clear to the patient that their primary fear has been located and understood. The patient then is reassured that important decisions will not be made in ignorance.

ON FORMULATIONS

Not so many years ago, in the clinical part of the MRCPsych examination, candidates were routinely expected to produce formulations for their examiners. This practice has now been abandoned. Psychiatric trainees may nevertheless be asked to venture a psychodynamic formulation. Clearly it is unreasonable to be expected to produce more than a rudimentary attempt. Here are some basic ideas which might equally be of value to the old age psychiatry team.

A psychodynamic formulation is a working model of the patient's predicament. It draws together strands from the patient's past, his or her current relationships and how these may be generating symptoms. Consideration should be given to the patient's personality structure and mental mechanisms in operation. Where possible these are observed by way of transference and countertransference. A formulation is not fixed, but modified, as more insights into the patient's mental life are revealed.

The following demonstrates how an initial formulation may be determined from a first assessment of a patient seen on a medical ward for the elderly.

A 76-year-old lady presents with a second episode of an agitated depression. Her first was following the death of her husband four years ago and responded well to antidepressants. One month ago she fractured her femur and has failed to co-operate with postoperative physiotherapy. The geriatricians are asking for guidance on her refusal to eat or drink. In the history one learns that she came from a large family, her mother dying when she was 14. Subsequently she adopted the caring role for her younger siblings. She then trained as a nurse and married at 19. She was unable to have children and lived with a husband who drank heavily and was frequently violent towards her. She remained with him despite his having affairs throughout the marriage.

His death from a myocardial infarction followed a year's angina. The patient now ruminates on his loss. Financially she is hard-up, since his work's pension did not provide for a widow. She fell downstairs, fractured her femur and went into hospital. The social workers have talked to her about how she needs to think about an old people's home. The patient hears voices telling her she is no good and that she should kill herself.

SAMPLE PSYCHODYNAMIC FORMULATION

This 76-year-old widow shows evidence of dependent personality traits. She has overcompensated for these by spending her adult life providing for others, to her own detriment. These defences were probably mobilized at the time of her mother's death. She had an ambivalent relationship with her husband and believes, especially as a nurse, she should have taken more notice of his chest pains. Unconsciously she fears her aggressive fantasized attacks on him were responsible for his death, just as she experienced her mother's death as a reflection of her badness. Psychodynamically, depression is the result of a collapse of her defences and aggression directed inwards. The suggestion of being given ECT and being moved to an old people's home confirms her belief that she should be punished. Her current inertia may also have stimulated an overzealous enthusiasm for disposal by exasperated professionals. The patient's terror of dependency, having never experienced an unconditionally caring relationship, explains her preconceived assumption that an old people's home invariably involves abuse and neglect.

Here a formulation helps the professionals to prioritize clinical management. Since the patient is dangerously depressed, ECT is the appropriate first step towards rebuilding the patient's defences. The content of the depressive thinking reveals the long-standing battle with inadequacy. Once the patient has recovered the patient can be brought into longer-term decision-making about her future, perhaps using material revealed during the acute phase of her illness. It is unrealistic to try and change the patient's defences but helpful to acknowledge that future losses are likely to precipitate depression again. The patient may need lifelong follow-up and antidepressant medication. These could act as 'water wings' to help her stay afloat.

LEARNING ABOUT OURSELVES AT WORK

As old age psychiatrists we are usually busy people. But our work is very different from that of psychotherapists. Our contact with patients does not usually involve such privacy and we are more likely to work in teams, sharing information. Sometimes the 'hands off' approach and the sheer volume of work can lead to a feeling that our dealings with patients resemble marshalling trucks in a goods yard. A psychodynamic approach involves our having consciously to carve out time to reflect. At a conference a consultant colleague proudly informed the author that he never left work until after 7.00 p.m., saying that any old age psychiatrist 'worth their salt' should be doing the same. It seems unlikely that poor time management was the only explanation here. Another busy psychogeriatrician was asked at his retirement party if he would be continuing to do some private work. He replied that he intended to (clinically) avoid old people from that day on.

It may not be sufficient to benefit our patients by just working hard but to question *how* we work and examine feelings evoked by patients.

It is easy to understand the pleasure which comes from treating severely ill patients who get better and express grateful thanks. Unlike psychotherapists, old age psychiatrists do not choose their patients. We are called on to explain and manage difficult behaviour. In fact the more unpopular elderly people are those likely to be sent our way by frustrated and angry referrers.

The prospect of impending 'burn-out' is likely to arise, not just from being busy, but from being unable to control the workload. Manic defences, which may serve us well initially, do so unfortunately at the cost of avoiding insight. A philosophy of encouraging staff to question their own motives is unlikely to be welcomed in a department whose sole preoccupation is busyness. Doctors may fall into the trap of feeling obliged to respond to patients' unconscious wishes for fulfilment. The (younger) doctor is especially vulnerable when encountering patients who are elderly.

An intelligent widowed lady, previously addicted to diazepam, had moved from GP to GP looking for a doctor who 'understood' her. She looked much younger than her years, in contrast to 'the silly old people' at a day centre she reluctantly attended. The author offered her a series of appointments with him. At these she barely stopped talking. Mostly this was in the form of covert or explicit requests from him for help and advice. The author, feeling trapped, made the mistake of losing his temper, snapping at the patient. Later he reflected on his unusual irritation and his thoughts of how 'the patient shouldn't be so childish: she is a grown woman and should act her age'. He apologized to the patient at their next meeting, saying that he had the feeling of being drowned by her desperate floundering. This led to a useful disclosure by the patient as to the similar effects she had on other doctors who had thrown her off their lists. As a result she began to acknowledge how lonely she felt and how frightened she was of old age itself, and how she was a lost little girl inside an old woman's body. The author privately considered the fact that he was no longer a young man himself.

CONCLUSION

Old age psychiatry is by nature eclectic. Every week brings with it a new challenge, no matter how much theoretical knowledge we possess.

One aspect of our work involves the study of personality and behaviour. Psychodynamic theory can shed further light on our interaction with patients. Those patients unsuitable for formal psychotherapy are likely to remain the mainstay of our clinical work. Nevertheless, observation of the unconscious in action may help unpick knotty problems. Engagement, selection and support of patients may be helped by some practical skills such as careful use of interpretation. Staff, too, will need help in working with troubled older patients. The author believes that, ideally, every old age psychiatry department should consider input from a consultant psychotherapist. In this way, whatever we choose to do we will have a clearer idea of why we are doing it.

REFERENCES

Adshead, G. (1998). Psychiatric staff as attachment figures. Understanding management problems in psychiatric services in the light of attachment theory. *Br J Psychiatry* **172**, 64–69.

Ardern, M. (1997). Psychotherapy and the elderly. In: Holmes, C. and Howard, R. (Eds), *Advances in Old Age Psychiatry: Chromosomes to Community Care*. Wrightson Biomedical, Petersfield, pp. 265–276.

Blanchard, M. (1997). Non-drug treatment of depression in older people. In: Holmes, C. and Howard, R. (Eds), *Advances in Old Age Psychiatry: Chromosomes to Community Care*. Wrightson Biomedical, Petersfield, pp. 172–182.

Hildebrand, P. (1982). Psychotherapy with older patients. *Br J Med Psychol* **55**, 19–28.

Hobbs, M. (1990). The role of the psychotherapist as consultant to in-patient psychiatric units. *Psychiatr Bull* **14**, 8–12.

Holmes, J. (1990). What can psychotherapy contribute to community psychiatry and vice versa? The North Devon experience. *Psychiatr Bull* **14**, 213–216.

Holmes, J. and Mitchison, S. (1995). A model for an integrated psychotherapy service. *Psychiatr Bull* **19**, 209–213.

Martindale, B. (1995). Psychological treatment. II. Psychodynamic approaches. In: Lindesay, J. (Ed.), *Neurotic Disorders in the Elderly*. Oxford University Press, Oxford, pp. 114–137.

Martindale, B. (1998). On ageing, dying, death and eternal life. *Psychoanal Psychother* **12**, 259–270.

Ong, Y.-L., Martineau, F., Lloyd, C. and Robbins, I. (1987). A support group for the depressed elderly. *Int J Geriatr Psychiatry* **2**, 119–123.

Porter, R. (1991). Psychotherapy with the elderly. In: Holmes, J. (Ed.), *Textbook of Psychotherapy in Psychiatric Practice*. Churchill Livingstone, London, pp. 469–487.

19

Family Therapy with Older Adults

VASSILIS M. MOURATOGLOU

Old Age Directorate, The Bethlem Royal and Maudsley NHS Trust, London, UK

INTRODUCTION

Early philosophical and biblical writings refer to ageing as a process of change in sensory, cognitive, affective and personality terms (Pruchno and Lawton, 1991). Understanding those problems related to later life development and change enables individuals, families and professionals to deal with neuropsychological and affective difficulties associated with loss of physical health, cognitive abilities and identity. An older person's physical, emotional and social needs can be addressed through a combination of biological, intrapersonal and family therapies (Blazer, 1990).

  In this chapter the impact of ageing on family life and the way that family therapy is carried out with older adults will be described. Specific issues related to elderly people suffering from dementia, depression, substance misuse and physical disability will be explored. Interpersonal issues regarding caring, elder abuse and cultural issues are identified. Finally, considerations of the future for family therapy with this client group are discussed.

FAMILIES IN LATER LIFE

As the lifespan of the average person is increasing, the number of different generations still alive within families also increases. Three- and four-generation families are now common, with members' roles in transition. That is, it is not clear what could be great-grandparents' roles in relation to their children, who are grandparents themselves and whose role in turn towards their younger adult children may also change. Finally, the way children relate to or are influenced by two or three different adult generations may also be different and has not yet been researched.

Therefore each generation needs not only to deal with their own developmental difficulties, but also has to address cross-generational issues. Such an example is the effect on parents when their adult children divorce (Gray and Geron, 1995). The process of change in the relationship between grandparents and their adult children is interrupted during such divorce proceedings, frequently forcing the re-emergence of earlier parent–child relationships.

The stress–vulnerability model has been used in studies of mental health and illness during the later stages of the family life cycle (Shields and Wynne, 1997). According to this model, an individual's perceived level of strength, degree of vulnerability, health status and risk factors are influenced by life cycle issues (Erickson, 1959). Relationships between different generations can be influenced by the degree of conflict or congruence there exists in their developmental needs. The outcome of these interactions can produce stress (Qualls, 1997). Issues such as retirement, illness and loss can undermine the health- and strength-enhancing processes in individuals and families, and as a result older adults become more vulnerable to familial and mental health difficulties (Mouratoglou, 1991).

FAMILY THERAPY AND PSYCHOTHERAPY

A particular theme, which characterizes the ageing process, is the inherently limited amount of time that older people have available in order to come to terms with the death of their dreams (Oates, 1997). This particular type of grief can lead to embarrassment, isolation and dependency. Knight (1986) reports current therapeutic opinion, in that older adults are no longer considered to respond poorly to individual or family psychotherapy. Face-to-face contact with members of later-life-cycle families can enable functioning by giving advice, counselling and therapy (Mouratoglou, 1995; Tobin and Power, 1995). According to Sukosky (1994) marital and family life review can be a useful therapeutic tool, as it can provide insight into the past, offer clues concerning present behaviour and enable family members to face the future.

Erlanger (1997) has suggested that through normalizing the transitional changes expected within the later life cycle, and by reinforcing family strengths, competencies and resilience, these changes can be seen as opportunities rather than losses. Intergeneration of past and present experiences and the identification of new strengths to meet the future enable older adults and their families to overcome negative stereotyping of old age. By helping family members (Carter and McGoldrick (1980) referred to the entire family emotional system of at least three generations) cope with transitional points, they can be helped to move on to lead more fulfilling lives.

Family therapy clinics specializing in the care of older adults are very rare. Relatively recently they have started becoming integral parts of old age psychiatric services (Benbow *et al.*, 1990). The majority of family-focused interventions still cater for younger adults, despite the fact that understanding elderly clients' needs is crucial for their carers.

When to intervene

Later-life families who are in therapy present a unique example of group psychotherapy. Parental ageing, fragility, life-threatening illness and death influence surviving members' mental and social needs. These needs must be addressed if families are to cope with such crises (Doka, 1997). Virtanen (1993) suggests that a joint interview between the referred older person and his or her relatives should form a necessary part of the initial assessment.

Carpenter (1995) reported that of 54 referrals made over a period of three years from primary care for psychiatric illness, 30% identified marital or family problems. Despite the fact that only 9% had conjoint therapy as the primary means of intervention, in another 40% issues regarding family loss and conflict issues were addressed in therapy. What is remarkable regarding family work with elderly couples is the longevity of unresolved issues from the past (40 or 50 years before), especially those of infidelity. Forgiveness is a therapeutic construct resisted by clients as well as therapists (Sells and Hargrave, 1998). Marital and family environments constitute natural primary interpersonal contexts, and in addition to individual therapy there are advantages in treating the family as a whole.

The 10 most frequently met and generally agreed indications for family therapy with older adults (Mouratoglou, 1997) are as follows:

1) Inability to resolve conflicts, make decisions or solve problems.
2) Poor or rigid family organization which leads to a chaotic response or inability to deal with stress.
3) Over-closeness to the point that family members have lost sense of autonomy and individuality.
4) Open communication inhibited or blocked or so excessive that the speaker is either not heard, interrupted, or spoken for.
5) Such distance between family members that emotional and physical needs are not met.
6) Feelings responded to inappropriately.
7) Unresolved marital conflicts with repercussions on other family members.
8) Alliance across generations interfering with the smooth running of the family – for example overinvolved grandparent with child(ren) against parent(s).

9) Lack of congruence between verbal and nonverbal communication – for example an elderly person being severely told off by a smiling relative.
10) High expressed emotion among family members where a large number of critical comments are made.

When therapists join any elderly person's family for treatment they enter a complex intergenerational system where their role is to bring to the fore issues which hold families together or tear them apart. Family therapy is also called systemic therapy as the family is an example of a system; that is, it consists of a number of interacting individuals who have common aims and objectives (Neidhardt and Allen, 1993).

The participation of older adults in family therapy has long been established as presenting a particular challenge for systemic practitioners. Flori (1989) found a negative correlation between age and successful engagement in family therapy. The characteristics of elderly clients considered suitable for family therapy are as follows:

1) Elderly individuals who want to have a family consultation and/or therapy.
2) Individuals who can relate their personal difficulties to family functioning.
3) Older adults who have some insight into family relationships.
4) Those who consider the resolution of family difficulties (past or present) as necessary if they are to continue their family's normal development.
5) People who are not at an acute phase of their physical or mental health difficulties and have a stable medication regimen.

The primary difference between family and individual therapy is that, in the first case, the disorder is considered to lie primarily within family functioning, while, in the second it is primarily within an individual. As a result, in systemic terms the patient is always referred to as the IP, meaning the index person or identified patient. It is, therefore, assumed that it is the system that is in need of help, and not just a single family member. Atwood and Ruiz (1993) suggest that therapists should join the family system, learn that family's meaning system (the narrative about their problem), then challenge that meaning, in order to amplify and stabilize a new, more 'healthy' one.

What happens in session

A therapist sees families for approximately one hour. During that period the nature and history of the IP's presenting problem is considered (medical and/or psychiatric diagnosis) and a description of family environment (relationships and roles) is obtained. The sociocultural context and life cycle structure of the family (i.e. the function of the symptoms) is explored. More specifically, therapists are interested in and carefully observe:

- Family interactions – who talks to whom, where, when how?
- Affective structures – what happens when a family member becomes upset, angry or worried; who comforts whom, when, how?
- Control mechanisms – are family members allowed to express their own opinions; who, where, when and how can one control the expression of emotions, feelings and actions?
- Nurturance systems – whose physical, emotional and social needs are met, when, where, how and by whom?
- Communication patterns – who listens, disrupts, ignores or attacks other family members' communications, under what circumstances, in the presence of whom; what happens then?
- Secrets – how do they deal with family secrets, when did they come about, how do they influence the way family members relate to each other and to the outside world?
- Alliances – in disputes, who supports whom; when do alliances occur; who is the 'victim', 'victimizer' or 'rescuer'?
- Loyalties – to which part of the extended family do they belong; does a son/daughter belong to their family of origin – parental network – or do they belong to their family of choice – their own family?
- Boundaries – are relationships between people well defined but flexible enough to adjust to changing circumstances, such as dependency, loss and stress?

There will usually be an audiovisual recording made of the sessions. During the first meeting families are introduced to the special environment of the clinic, and their consent to have the session recorded is sought. Families can object to audio or visual recordings being made. Great efforts, however, are made to gain consent for the consultation team to observe the session.

The consultation team consists of two to three systemically informed clinicians, who observe the session via a television monitor or a one-way screen. If the family objects to the team observing, then a co-therapist may be identified and the rest of the team members are released. In most cases, however, consultation teams are accepted as an integral part of this treatment approach. The therapist meets with them three-quarters of the way through the session in order to discuss the issues raised and observations made, as well as to decide upon a home task.

The 'homework' is used to exemplify the points raised during the session, and promote change between sessions. Finally, the therapist shares these observations with the family before the session ends.

It is obviously important that the therapist and co-therapist or consultation team share the same systemic theoretical framework. Part of the aim of the early consultation of the therapist with the team is to decide which framework best addresses a specific family's needs and is most likely to bring about a successful outcome. The five main theoretical frameworks which are currently used for family therapy are as follows:

Family life cycle

Addresses: Transitional points in an elderly person's life, such as retirement, illness and bereavement

Focuses on: Chronic problems resulting from unmet needs of earlier life cycle stages

Enables: Family members to identify, adjust and evaluate their influence on their relative's transitional difficulties

This approach is most frequently used when elderly people have not found or were not allowed to find new roles within the family environment. Difficulties are viewed as life cycle issues. Elderly couples are helped to renegotiate their marital 'contract', while whole families renegotiate their relationships.

Interactional theory

Addresses: Communication styles

Focuses on: Misunderstandings, double messages, one-sided views, communication blocks

Enables: Each family member to listen to and be listened to by all participants

A major contribution of this approach in the care of older adult families is the use of reframing. As a result, an elderly person's problem is put into a different context (e.g. forgetfulness is seen as giving another family member an opportunity to care for them). This new perspective can result in a change in communication and behaviour patterns between family members.

Solution theory

Addresses: The solution process instead of the cause of a problem

Focuses on: Attempts made by family members to give solutions to their difficulties

Enables: Individuals make use of their family's strength-enhancing procedures by utilizing their skills and abilities

It makes use of older adults' previous experiences in dealing with difficulties in order to define goals that are attainable and identify first steps towards them. A small change in an elderly person's family environment may be sufficient to set the ball rolling. When past and current successes are defined as such, identified patients may start to see their world differently. When they start doing more of what is good for them, they may come to believe that they hold the key to the solution of their problems.

Structural theory
Addresses: Open communication and family organization
Focuses on: Boundaries among different generations expected to be well defined but flexible and permeable
Enables: Middle generation free of parental control and fully in charge of their younger children

This approach is relevant when an elderly person is 'triangulated' between different individuals or generations. A grandfather/mother may get involved in caring for a grandchild if they feel that their children are failing in their parental role. Similarly, if a younger couple want to avoid addressing their marital problems, focusing excessively on their parents' needs, this may handicap their parents' attempts to deal with their own difficulties.

Systems theory
Addresses: Interrelatedness and circularity of individuals and their difficulties
Focuses on: What happens between, rather than within, individuals
Enables: Family members to understand family relationships and what holds them together

It makes use of 'circular questioning' (ask a family member's opinion about another member's point of view on a certain topic; e.g. what do you think is your mother's opinion of going into a nursing home?) In this way, there is an enactment of the circularity of interaction notion. It challenges the contextual influences of cultural beliefs (such as ageism), and multigenerational family patterns.

Outcome is defined in terms of changes in symptomatology, familial patterns and relationships (Hargrave and Anderson, 1997). First-order change is defined as the reduction of an identified patient's (IP's) symptoms, while second-order changes refer to changes in the ways in which members of the system (e.g. a family) relate to each other. Typical expected outcomes are as follows:

First-order changes
1) Reduction of severity of IP's presenting problems
2) Reduction of frequency of IP's difficulties
3) IP experiences a fulfilling lifestyle

Second-order changes
1) Family members relate to each other in a mutually respectful manner with appropriate consideration for hierarchies and boundaries
2) New and more 'healthy' forms of communication have emerged
3) Interactions are characterized by reciprocity

4) Critical comments are kept to a minimum
5) Coalitions and alliances do not victimize any particular family members
6) Each family member acknowledges and observes their individual and other members' developmental needs

First-order changes are expected to be short-lived. When the elderly person comes up against another developmental difficulty (e.g. losing a partner, becoming ill or increasing dependency) they are likely to be in need of further family sessions. Following second-order changes are achieved when individuals learn to relate to each other in a different way and unite their personal and social resources in a joint effort to deal with such developmental problems; further formal sessions are then less likely to be needed.

Frequently, a 'booster' session is sufficient. Positive outcome of such interventions tends to be associated with the acceptance of one's own place within the family life cycle, rather than concrete changes in the future. This approach may serve as a possible preventative function in reducing future psychological distress in other family members.

The middle sessions of therapy, once the primary presenting problem is resolved, may lack aim, focus and intensity. This is the time that family members may blame their relative for 'not trying enough'. Erickson (1992) suggested the scheduling of two two-hour sessions, twenty-four hours apart, at this stage; as many members of the extended family as possible participate and are helped to deal with the crux of the matter as it affects the whole family, through the direct expression of feelings.

Resistance to therapeutic intervention can be anticipated in cases where there are distortions regarding the locus and degree of the problem, motivational issues and exclusive reliance on the medical model (Qualls, 1991). This resistance can be dealt with through increased collaboration between the therapist and the family and by providing additional information and facilitating problem-solving skills. Resistance is not always evident from participating family members. Therapists' failure to adapt their intervention to the capabilities of the families may be equally important.

SPECIFIC ISSUES

Dementia

According to Chaprazac (1996) families with a demented adult member tend to 'close in' on themselves and will only open to services when they can no longer contain the symptoms. Boundaries, either real or imaginary, between different subsystems of the family environment can be placed under threat by interventions made by health or social services professionals. There is a natural process of separation of offspring from their parents' ageing. Dementia can inhibit that process as continued involvement with the parental subsystem is required.

A typical case is that of Mrs T who suffered from a moderate degree of dementia. This 78-year-old woman was happy living independently, occasionally contacting her daughter (married with two children). Since diagnosis, however, there have been an inordinate number of 'crises' in which the daughter felt that she had to intervene. This made the daughter feel frustrated because she had difficulty attending to two households and felt resentful for becoming a carer, but at the same time would not allow services to be delivered to her mother (e.g. meals-on-wheels, home helps). She was not happy with the quality of those services, while her extended family network expected her to care for her mother. A family therapy meeting between the mother, daughter's family and involved service providers (as they were part of this identified patient's environment) addressed dysfunctional patterns of communication and ways of relating to each other.

Family therapy is a relevant psychological intervention needed to help carers cope with the burden of caring, thus helping to avoid pathological elder abuse (Huckle, 1994). For example, children may feel that they are 'entitled' to extra financial rewards from the parents, who may also collude with them, worried that they may lose contact with their offspring.

A good relationship and communication is possible within families of people suffering from dementia. Opinions differ regarding the participation of such patients in family meetings. Their presence, however, conveys a very important message to the whole family. That is, that in addressing such a patient's needs, it is necessary that the family acknowledge that:

- All family members work together.
- Individuals suffering from dementia are real people in their own right.
- They have valid needs.
- They occupy an important position in the family.

The presence of such patients in therapy makes it difficult for the family to scapegoat that person. The therapist is less likely to collude with the family's assumption of the patient's incompetence. As a result, overprotectiveness, invalidation of the patient and pressure to exclude him or her from the family is avoided.

Concerns about family members not expressing their true feelings or distorting facts in the presence of a demented family member are valid. Equally, when such a patient is confronted with the family, he or she can experience emotional pain and reduced self-esteem. Nevertheless, these worries should not be used to exclude the patient from family meetings. By drawing examples from the interview as it progresses and finding positive ways to talk about the patient's problems, the therapist can educate family members about what influences their relative's behaviour. Family members can thus be helped to 'survive' and tolerate such differences within the family (Cooklin, 1998).

Familial therapy permits family members to express their suffering, regulate conflicts, and decrease angst, which unchecked could deconstruct the patient's emotional system (Thomas *et al.*, 1997). It is important to acknowledge that different family members may be at different stages regarding their own adaptation to the diagnosis of dementia. Each family member will need to work on their own bereavement process, grieving for the 'intact' person who has been lost, as well as for future joint ventures which would have given them fulfilment and joy.

The family network needs to be helped to see themselves as a resource which can enhance the self-development of the older adult (either the caring spouse or the person with dementia). This is achieved through the provision of continuity, through maintenance of proximity over time, and through an enhanced quality and quantity of responsiveness for that individual, within their family network (Ungar and Levene, 1994). Family members need to stay in touch with older members who face challenges because of dementia and be prepared to offer time, tolerance and understanding.

Depression

In older adults, cognitive behaviour therapy and brief psychodynamic therapies appear to be equally effective in the treatment of depression (Woods, 1993). Family therapy is increasingly seen as another treatment modality for depression in older adults. Loss of spouse, sibling, physical integrity, vocational role and community contacts can be addressed through this therapeutic medium.

Mr C is a 68-year-old man with a history of moderate to severe depression for the last three years. He had a stroke two years before the referral was made. Around that time, his brother-in-law, who was very close to him and his wife, passed away. The couple were referred after a six-month history of deteriorating depressive symptomatology and increased, at times violent, arguments, especially after a disastrous holiday. In this case Mr and Mrs C had to deal with a number of losses and the implications for their everyday lives. The retirement process of this man was disrupted by his cerebrovascular accident, which limited his physical and cognitive abilities. Individual work with this patient had brought some improvement, but with limited effect. Mrs C was not made part of that change and, as a result, struggled to maintain the status quo (referred to as a homeostatic process). Addressing both partners' needs in a marital therapy session they were helped to understand each other's physical, emotional and social needs. Additionally, instead of working at cross-purposes, they were helped to unite their efforts in improving their life together, in the face of life cycle adversities. The significance of the disastrous holiday became apparent in session when it was realized that the couple had never had a holiday on their own; they had always been accompanied by the brother-in-law and his family. Their losses became more evident when his presence, help and support was missed. The conspiracy of silence, in avoiding talking about upsetting issues, was thus broken and the couple were ready to mourn their losses, before reconstructing their lives.

Leff (1998) conducted a clinical and economic evaluation of a random controlled trial of couple therapy versus antidepressants for people suffering from depression (older adults were also included, up to the age of 85). He concluded that for depressed people living with a partner, couple therapy was a much more acceptable mode of intervention than medication. Additionally, marital therapy was also found to be more efficacious, in both treatment and maintenance phases, and no more expensive.

Substance misuse

Segal *et al.* (1996) reported medication and drug misuse to be an important problem with the elderly. Many older people self-medicate with prescription and over-the-counter purchases. Frequently alcohol is also abused. The structure, dynamics and interactions among later-life family members may act to collude with substance misuse difficulties. Children abusing alcohol or drugs with their elderly parents are inadvertently reinforcing this type of behaviour. Even if an older adult is helped to detoxify, as he or she will return to a family or social environment which holds unchanged ideas and beliefs about substance misuse, it is, in most cases, a matter of time before relapse occurs.

Intergenerational family systems treatments have been used with success. In therapy, family members' relationships with substance misuse are examined in past and present generations. Help is thus provided through changing the identified patient's attitudes and belief system regarding misuse, as well as developing an appropriately supportive family environment. If an elderly drug user changes his or her value system regarding abstinence, and at the same time family members and friends are helped to encourage this change, they are more likely to sustain, at least, a moderate drug use.

Clinicians working with older problem drinkers need to be aware of over-identifying with the children of alcoholics and creating an alliance with them against the elderly drinker (Amodeo, 1990). The involvement of family members in the recovery process is very important, and as a result marital and/or family therapy can form an essential component of treatment. Families can encourage abstinence/moderation or, if that is not possible, help the elderly alcoholic to get drunk or face death with dignity.

Other conditions

Family work is not only beneficial in cases where psychiatric difficulties have been identified. Disability associated with physical illness or impairment can interact with institutional stresses to challenge the adaptive strength and integrity of the patient and their family environment (Remien and Christopher, 1996). For example, stroke patients and their families need time to adjust and utilize rehabilitation procedures offered in hospital and the community. Bed shortages and limited community resources create increasing pressure for early discharge. Slauenwhite and Simpson (1998) assessed 23 care recipients over the age of 60 years who had experienced a hip fracture, and their caregivers. They found that there was a high degree of mismatched care, especially in relation to care received from nursing staff, irrespective of whether they were in hospital or the community. They concluded that heightened communication involving clients, families and service providers, especially during the transition from hospital to home, can aid adaptation and successful discharge.

Pierce (1997) believes that family systems strive for stability, growth, control and spirituality. Nurses who practise within this framework can help individuals and their carers to adjust to the reality of chronic illness and disability. By facilitating a patient's familial system's maintenance and appropriate change, they can be helped to achieve coherence and individuation. The therapeutic utilization of narrative (that is, the 're-storying' of the negative aspects of carers' perceived reality) can help primarily elderly females caring for a disabled partner to transform their depression and burden into healthy acceptance (Clark and Standard, 1997).

INTERPERSONAL ASPECTS

Caring

In a caring society it is not necessarily the responsibility of any one person or group of people to ensure that the elderly receive care which is of high standard. For example, keeping an eye on an elderly person, supporting voluntary agencies, lobbying local and central government, working with the elderly, are all examples of caring. Some of the help is spontaneous, while some forms part of a care provision programme. Both aspects are important. Statutory and voluntary organizations increasingly rely on relatives' ability to care (Windmill, 1996).

The number of male caregivers of spouses is growing. It is widely assumed that women are best suited to provide care for ageing relatives. Such beliefs affect men negatively when they take up the carer's role, and place an unjust burden on women. Until society changes its beliefs about younger adult men and caring, it is important to prepare and support those male children who will later be asked or be expected to become involved. At the same time their female counterparts need to be helped in transferring their caregiving skills to male carers (Kriseman and Claes, 1997). As a result there is a need to develop interventions specifically designed for male caregivers and for carers of ethnic minorities if their stress and negative affect is to be addressed. According to Thompson and Gallagher (1996) family therapy can offer such an effective treatment schedule.

Placement of an elderly patient in a residential health care facility is very rarely perceived and appreciated as an act of caring by family members. According to Vassallo (1995) marital conflicts may emerge when a spouse is to be admitted to a nursing home's respite care services. A systemic intervention, which takes into consideration preadmission attitudes, choice in decision-making, and access to individual and family support, could facilitate a positive outcome in the process of adjustment to institutionalization.

Involvement of the extended family network in their relative's altered life situation is very important. Similarly, family members also need to adapt to this change (Saul, 1997). Information, education, emotional support, and opportunities for continuity or restoration of healthy relationships are required, as the means of addressing a resident's and their family members' needs. These processes need to take place during the admission period and often under exceptional circumstances, such as advanced dementia and terminal illness.

Elder abuse

The greater the number of dependent older persons, the higher the rate of financial, emotional and physical abuse they are likely to experience. Middle-aged and younger children struggle with problems of their own families and their finances may decline as a result of caring. Previous abusive relationships in a family increase the likelihood of elder abuse, and assistance of adult protection services may be urgently indicated (Pritchard, 1996).

It is not always the case that older adults are the victims of abuse, but they can be the perpetrators, too. Salomon (1998) reported a case of a woman in her late forties still living at home with her parents, who was being abused by her 82-year-old father. Family therapy is a useful context within which such destructive family dynamics can be addressed and change; particularly when carers feel that, in earlier years, they were taken advantage of or had their needs ignored by people who they now need to care for. Family therapy can help those people reconcile their differences, mourn for what has been lost (e.g. love, affection, abilities, opportunities), and facilitate their relating to each other in a mutually satisfying and respectful manner.

Cultural issues

Cultural and subcultural contexts influence the way inter- or intrapersonal difficulties are perceived by individual family members. Simon (1996) identified the significance of culture on expression of family beliefs, especially if they are in opposition to those that prevail in the 'host' community. More specifically, in Lebanese families family obligations supersede individuals' or marital needs. The role of the wife involves displays of submissiveness in public, but she may be much more influential within the home environment. By adhering to these rules, individuals can utilize the rich support system which is frequently used to care for older adults.

The impact of different cultural issues can also be seen in families of Chinese origin. Their family system is influenced by the Confucian philosophy, according to which the timing of tasks and rituals is very important in the life cycle. Gender and birth position are associated with responsibilities and privileges. Adult children are responsible for their elderly parents. Acculturation processes can adversely influence these filial roles and expectations (Hamilton, 1996).

Ben-David (1996) investigated the family therapist's perceptions of assessment and treatment as a function of immigrant families' cultural background (Russian and Ethiopian) and presenting problem. He found that neglect of an elderly family member was more likely to be attributed to the stresses of immigration in Ethiopian but not in Russian families. Most interestingly, the wider the cultural differences between therapists and families seen, the more sensitive and contextually appropriate were the therapist's assessment and treatment choices.

FUTURE CONSIDERATIONS

Despite advances on family interventions, empirical validation of systemic work with older adults is still very rare (Richardson, 1997). Further evaluation of systemic therapies is urgently needed. Mouratoglou (1998) conducted a comparative study of couples and families seen in traditional family therapy (adjoining rooms, recording facilities, therapy team) and outpatient (with a co-therapist only) clinics and found that:

- Family therapy and outpatient-based systemic interventions are not mutually exclusive, but necessary parts of the same service.
- The presenting difficulties (symptoms) of older adults can be reduced when they are addressed through systemic work, at either type of clinic.
- Family structures and relationships can become more functional and less troublesome when they are addressed within family therapy.

• The costs involved in the provision of family therapy are comparable to those of an outpatient clinic, provided that the number of therapists involved is kept to a minimum.

Another important aspect in dealing with older adults' familial difficulties is the health professionals' preoccupations with their own ageing. Therapists need to become aware and able to deal with their own preconceptions about old age. Gilleard *et al.* (1992), in a survey of professionals involved with family therapy with older adults, found that despite their positive attitude towards this type of treatment, scepticism regarding the potential for change may reflect latent ageist attitudes. It should be noted that it is not uncommon for systemic thinkers to share such beliefs.

Increasingly, systemic work with older adults is carried out less frequently in traditional family therapy settings; that is, in two adjoining rooms, with one-way mirror, video- and audio-recording equipment and the help of a consultation team. Community settings, such as identified patients' own homes and primary care practices, provide special challenges to family therapists. Systemic treatments may need to be adapted in order to take into consideration different environmental factors. The literature is very scanty with regard to the adaptation of family-based modes of intervention in caring for older adults and their families in the community. Research is urgently needed in this respect.

Graham *et al.* (1993) described the setting up of a specialist clinic run by general practitioners. It met with a high degree of acceptability for referrers and patients. Otherwise those identified patients and their families would have been referred to outside agencies, a process characterized by high nonattendance rates. Systemic work is not, and should not be, the exclusive privilege of relatively few people trained in its conceptualization and delivery. Leff (1998) concluded that primary care workers should be trained in couple therapy, as an efficient and effective way of addressing depressive symptomatology. Additionally, consultants in systemic intervention acting as members of multidisciplinary teams working with older adults in a variety of tertiary institutions can enhance the availability of therapeutic interventions, as well as advancing research and training opportunities.

REFERENCES

Amodeo, M. (1990). Treating the late life alcoholic: guidelines for working through denial integrating individual, family and group approaches. *J Geriatr Psychiatry* **23**, 91–105.

Atwood, J.D, and Ruiz, J. (1993). Social constructionist therapy with the elderly. *J Fam Psychother* **4**, 1–32.

Benbow, S., Egan, D., Marriott, A. and Tregay, K. (1990). Using the family life cycle with later life families. *J Fam Ther* **12**, 321–324.

Ben-David, A. (1996). Therapists' perceptions of multicultural assessment and therapy with immigrant families. *J Fam Ther* **18**, 23–41.

Blazer, D. (1990). *Emotional Problems in Later Life: Intervention Strategies for Professional Caregivers*. Springer Publishing Company, New York.

Carpenter, J. (1995). Older adults in primary health care in the United Kingdom: an exploration of the relevance of family therapy. *Fam Syst Med* **12**, 133–148.

Carter, E.A. and McGoldrick, M. (1980). The family life cycle and family therapy: an overview. In: Carter, E.A. and McGoldrick, M. (Eds), *The Family Life Cycle: A Framework for Family Therapy*. Gardner Press, New York, pp. 3–20.

Chaprazac, P. (1996). Economic and structural implications of the symptom in family therapy with demented elderly. *Psychol Med* **27**, 171–174.

Clark, M.C. and Standard, P.L. (1997). The caregiving story: how the narrative approach informs caregiving burden. *Issues Ment Health Nurs* **18**, 87–97.

Cooklin, A. (1998). Making connections through talking with children: from the 'return of the repressed' to 'dialectics'. *J Fam Ther* **20**, 153–164.

Doka, K.J. (1997). The effect of parental illness and loss on adult children. In: Deitch, I.E. and Candace, W. (Eds), *Counselling the Ageing and their Families. The Family Psychology and Counselling Series*. American Counselling Association, Alexandria, VA, pp. 147–155.

Erickson, B.M. (1992). The major surgery of psychotherapy: the extended family of origin session. *J Fam Psychother* **3**, 19–44.

Erickson, E. (1959). Identity and the life cycle. *Psychol Issues* Monograph 1, New York.

Erlanger, M.A. (1997). Changing roles and life-cycle transitions. In: Hargrave, T.D. and Hanna, S.M. (Eds), *The Ageing Family: New Visions in Theory and Reality*. Brunner/Mazel, New York, pp. 163–177.

Flori, D. (1989). The prevalence of later life concerns in marriage and family therapy journal literature (1976–1985): a content analysis. *J Marital Fam Ther* **15**, 289–297.

Gilleard, C., Lieberman, S. and Peeler, R. (1992). Family therapy for older adults: a survey of professionals' attitudes. *J Fam Ther* **14**, 413–422.

Graham, H., Senior, R., Dukes, S. and Lazarus, M. (1993). The introduction of family therapy to British general practice. *Fam Syst Med* **11**, 363–373.

Gray, C.A. and Geron, S.M. (1995). The other sorrow of divorce: the effects on grandparents when their adult children divorce. *J Gerontol Soc Work* **23**, 139–159.

Hamilton, B. (1996). Ethnicity and the family life cycle: the Chinese–American family. *Fam Ther* **23**, 199–212.

Hargrave, T.D. and Anderson, W.T. (1997). Finishing well: a contextual family therapy approach to the ageing family. In: Hargrave T.D. and Hanna, S.M. (Eds), *The Ageing Family: New Visions in Theory, Practice and Reality*. Brunner/Mazel, New York, pp. 61–80.

Huckle, P.L. (1994). Families and dementia. *Int J Geriatr Psychiatry* **9**, 735–741.

Kriseman, N.L. and Claes, J.A. (1997). Gender issues and elder care. In: Hargrave, T.D. and Hanna, S.M. (Eds), *The Ageing Family: New Vision in Theory, Practice and Reality*. Brunner/Mazel, New York, pp. 199–208.

Knight, B. (1986). *Psychotherapy with Older Adults*. Sage Publications, Newbury Park, CA.

Leff, J. (1998). The London Depression Intervention Trial: clinical and economic evaluation of an RCT of couple therapy versus antidepressants. *Family Research and Family Therapy Conference*, Institute of Psychiatry, London.

Mouratoglou, V.M. (1991). Older people and their families. *Context* **6**, 10–13.

Mouratoglou, V.M. (1995). Solution focused brief therapy: a workshop. *Psychologists' Special Interest Group in the Elderly Newsletter* **52**, 6–9.

Mouratoglou, V.M. (1997). Family therapy with older adults. *Psychologists' Special Interest Group in the Elderly Newsletter* **62**, 32–40.

Mouratoglou, V.M. (1998). The cost-effectiveness of family therapy and out-patient clinics for older adults. *Hellen Med J* **2**, 31–35.

Neidhardt, E.R. and Allen, J.A. (1993). *Family Therapy with the Elderly*. Sage Publications, Newbury Park, CA.

Oates, W.E. (1997). Reconciling with unfulfilled dreams at the end of life. In: Hargrave, T.D. and Hanna, S.M. (Eds), *The Ageing Family: New Visions in Theory, Practice and Reality*. Brunner/Mazel, New York, pp. 259–269.

Pierce, L.L. (1997). The framework of systemic organisation applied to older adults as family caregivers of persons with chronic disease and disability. *Gastroenterol Nurs* **20**, 168–175.

Pritchard, J. (1996). *Working with Elder Abuse: A Training Manual for Home Care, Residential and Day Care Staff*. Jessica Kingsley, London.

Pruchno, R. and Lawton, M. (1991). Gerontology. In: Walker, C. (Ed.), *Clinical Psychology: Historical Research and Foundations*. Plenum Press, New York, pp. 361–392.

Qualls, S.H. (1991). Resistance of older families to therapeutic interventions. *Clin Gerontol* **11**(1), 59–68.

Qualls, S.H. (1997). Ageing families: the personal, permanent group. *Group* **21** 175–190.

Remien, R.H. and Christopher, F. (1996). A family psychoeducational model for long term rehabilitation. *Phys Occup Ther Geriatr* **14**(2), 45–59.

Richardson, C. (1997). Family therapy. *Curr Opin Psychiatry* **10**, 333–336.

Salamon, M.J. (1998). Parents who continue to abuse. *Clin Gerontol* **18**(3), 60–63.

Saul, S. (1997). Placement of an elderly parent in a residential health care facility: impact on the family. In: Deitch, I. and Candace, W. (Eds), *Counselling the Ageing and their Families*. The Family Psychology and Counselling Series. American Counselling Association, Alexandria, VA, pp. 133–145.

Segal, D.L., Van-Hasselt, V.B., Hersen, M. and King, C. (1996). Treatment of substance abuse in older adults. In: Cautela, J.R. and Ishaq, W. (Eds), *Contemporary Issues in Behaviour Therapy: Improving the Human Condition*. Plenum Press, New York, pp. 69–85.

Sells, J.N. and Hargrave, T.D. (1998). Forgiveness: a review of theoretical and empirical literature. *J Fam Ther* **20**, 21–36.

Shields, C.G. and Wynne, L.C. (1997). The strength-vulnerability model of mental health and illness in the elderly. In: Hargrave, T.D. and Hanna, S.M. (Eds), *The Ageing Family: New Visions in Theory, Practice and Reality*. Brunner/Mazel, New York, pp. 131–160.

Simon, J.P. (1996). Lebanese families. In: McGordrick, M. and Giordano, J. (Eds), *Ethnicity and Family Therapy*, second edition. Guildford Press, New York, pp. 364–375.

Slauenwhite, C.A. and Simpson, P. (1998). Patient and family perspectives on early discharge and care of the older adult undergoing fractured hip rehabilitation. *Orthop Nurs* **17**, 30–36.

Sukosky, D.G. (1994). Life review in family psychotherapy. *J Fam Psychother* **5**(2), 21–39.

Thomas, P., Hasif, T.C. and Pradere, P. (1997). A systemic look at Alzheimer's disease: management of the demented elderly person's family using the systemic method. *Rev Psychiatry* **22**, 3–12.

Thompson, L.W. and Gallagher, T.D. (1996). Practical issues related to the maintenance of mental health and positive well being in family caregivers. In: Carstensen,

L.L. and Edelstein, B.A. (Eds), *The Practical Handbook of Clinical Gerontology.* Sage Publications, Thousand Oaks, CA, pp. 129–150.

Tobin, S.S. and Power, T.S. (1995). The diversity of direct practice. In: Smith, G.C. (Ed.), *Strengthening Ageing Families: Diversity in Practice and Policy.* Sage Publications, Newbury Park, CA, p. 290.

Ungar, M.T. and Levene, J.E. (1994). Selfobject functions of the family: implications for family therapy. *Clin Soc Work J* **22**, 303–316.

Vassallo, T. (1995). Systemic therapy and aged respite care: a neglected area. *Aust N Z J Fam Ther* **16**, 73–80.

Virtanen, H. (1993). Family therapy in old age. *Psychiatria Fennica* **24**, 87–95.

Windmill, V. (1996). *Caring for the Elderly.* Addison Wesley Longman Ltd, Harlow.

Woods, R.T. (1993). Psychosocial management of depression. *Int Rev Psychiatry* **5**, 427–436.

Index